EMG Pearls

D1452282

EMG Pearls

STEVEN A. GREENBERG, MD
Assistant Professor of Neurology
Harvard Medical School
Department of Neurology
Brigham and Women's Hospital
Boston, Massachusetts

ANTHONY A. AMATO, MD
Associate Professor of Neurology
Harvard Medical School
Chief, Neuromuscular Division
Director, Clinical Neurophysiology Laboratory
Vice-Chairman, Department of Neurology
Brigham and Women's Hospital
Boston, Massachusetts

Hanley & Belfus
An Imprint of Elsevier

HANLEY & BELFUS
An Imprint of Elsevier

The Curtis Center
170 S Independence W 300 E
Philadelphia, Pennsylvania 19106

EMG PEARLS   ISBN: 1-56053-613-6

Copyright © 2004 Elsevier Inc. All rights reserved.

No part of this publication may be reproduced or transmitted in any form or by any means, electronic or mechanical, including photocopy, recording, or any information storage and retrieval system, without permission in writing from the publisher.

Permissions may be sought directly from Elsevier Inc. Rights Department in Philadelphia, Pennsylvania, USA: telephone: (+1)215-238-7869, fax: (+1)215-238-2239, e-mail: *healthpermissions@elsevier.com*. You may also complete your request on-line via the Elsevier Science homepage *http://www.elsevier.com*, by selecting "Customer Support" and then "Obtaining Permissions."

Library of Congress Cataloging-in-Publication Data

Greenberg, Steven A. (Steven Alan), 1962-
    EMG pearls / Steven A. Greenberg, Anthony A. Amato.
        p. ; cm.
    Includes index.
    ISBN 1-56053-613-6
    1. Electromyography–Case studies. I. Title: Electromyography pearls. II. Amato,
Anthony A., 1960-III. Title.
    [DNLM: 1. Electromyography–methods–Case Reports. 2. Electromyography–methods–Problems and
Exercises. 3. Neuromuscular Diseases–diagnosis–Case Reports. 4. Neuromuscular
Diseases–diagnosis–Problems and Exercises. WE 18.2 G798e 2004]
    RC77.5.G745 2004
    616.7′407547–dc22   2004040545

Printed in the United States of America.

Last digit is the print number: 9 8 7 6 5 4 3 2 1

CONTENTS

Section VI.   EMG-Guided Botulinum Toxin Therapy of Focal Dystonias

PREFACE

This casebook of neuromuscular disorders focuses on electrodiagnostic studies. The reader is expected to have basic competence in the performance of nerve conduction and needle EMG studies. The case studies should be read carefully and not rushed through. We have aimed to convey how a neuromuscular specialist *thinks* about electrodiagnostic studies rather than focusing on technique.

All case descriptions are of actual patients and the studies performed on them; the case studies have not been altered or fictionalized to idealize the approach. Some of these studies are, therefore, not electrodiagnostically "ideal"; patient discomfort or limited studies done to answer specific questions are always practical considerations for the electromyographer.

The value of diagnostic procedures is usually dependent on normal values, and this is a surprisingly complex issue for nerve conduction studies. Limits of normality vary widely within the electrodiagnostic literature and reflect not only technical differences, but also differences in selection of "normal" subjects, design of the study, and statistical procedures. We like to think of electrodiagnostic results as ranges of clearly abnormal and normal values separated by a range of uncertainty and to interpret studies conservatively, erring on the side of normality. For the purposes of this book, we use the values listed below as the limits of normality:

Sensory			Motor		
Nerve	Amplitude μ(V)	Velocity (m/sec)	Nerve	Amplitude (mV)	DML (msec) or Velocity (m/sec)
Median	12	44	Median	4.8	4.5
Ulnar	10	44	Forearm		48
Sural	5	36	Upper arm		50
Superf. peroneal	3	36	Ulnar	4.5	3.9
F-waves			Forearm		48
			Across-elbow		48
Nerve	Min Latency	Persistence	Upper arm		50
Median	32 msec	50%	Peroneal	1.5	6.5
Ulnar	32 msec	50%	Leg		36
Peroneal	56 msec	0%	Across fib.		34
Tibial	56 msec	50%	Tibial	2.0	7.0
			Leg		36

Abbreviations used repeatedly in this book are standard and as follows:

- SNAP = sensory nerve action potential
- CMAP = compound muscle action potential
- CNAP = compound nerve action potential
- Median-APB = stimulating median nerve, recording abductor pollicis brevis
- Median-D2 = stimulating median nerve, recording digit 2
- Ulnar-ADM = stimulating ulnar nerve, recording abductor digiti minimi
- Radial-D1 = stimulating radial nerve, recording digit 1
- APB = abductor pollicis brevis
- ADM = abductor digiti minimi
- FDI = first dorsal interosseous
- EIP = extensor indicis proprius
- TA = tibialis anterior
- EDB = extensor digitorum brevis
- AH = abductor halluci

Steven A. Greenberg, MD
Anthony A. Amato, MD

ACKNOWLEDGMENTS

The authors gratefully acknowledge the contributions of the following electrodiagnostic technicians, residents, and fellows who have contributed to this book through their work in the Brigham and Women's Hospital Department of Neurology, Division of Neuromuscular Disease: Essa Kayd, Macharia Waruingi, Hannah Briemberg, Jayashri Srinivasan, Mary Beth Toran, Gisela Held, and Darlene Young.

SECTION I.   FOCAL NEUROPATHIES

Focal neuropathies are by definition disorders that affect a very limited portion of the peripheral nervous system, generally confined to a peripheral nerve at a single anatomical location. Nerve root disease (radiculopathies), plexus disease (plexopathy), and disorders of individual named nerves or their branches are all considered neuropathies.

The key principle for the electrodiagnosis of focal neuropathies is that of localization. The two methods of localization are

1. The "intersection" method
2. Demonstration of a focal nerve abnormality

The first method is the traditional one of localization for clinical neurology, adapted for electrodiagnosis. It consists of the demonstration of a nerve abnormality within two or more pathways and then consideration of where these pathways intersect. The point of intersection is in general the location of the focal neuropathy. For example, an absent median to second digit sensory nerve action potential implies a lesion anywhere between the C6 or C7 dorsal root ganglia and the median nerve sensory fibers in the digit, including the upper or middle trunk, lateral cord, or proximal or distal median nerve. When combined with needle electromyogram (EMG) abnormalities in deltoid and biceps (implying a lesion anywhere between the C5 or C6 cord anterior gray matter, nerve roots, or upper trunk), with appropriate other normal studies, the localization of an upper trunk lesion is made because of the common intersection of these two pathways. To use this method, detailed knowledge of the anatomy of the peripheral nervous system is crucial.

The second method is demonstration of a focal nerve abnormality—focal slowing, conduction block, or temporal dispersion—across a specific segment of a nerve. These are all usually aspects of focal demyelination, although on rare occasions other processes can produce these findings (i.e., early acute axonal injury). For example, a sufficiently prolonged median–abductor pollicis brevis (APB) distal motor latency localizes the lesion immediately to the across-wrist or palm segment of the median nerve. Note that this method can only be used when a technique exists to reliably stimulate supramaximally the nerve proximal to the affected segment.

It is also important to note that focal neuropathies do not always follow the rules of anatomy. In particular, partial focal nerve involvement occurs frequently. An L5 radiculopathy may result in needle EMG abnormalities in tibialis anterior and peroneus longus but not tibialis posterior or gluteus medius. An ulnar neuropathy at the elbow may result in focal slowing of the across-elbow motor fibers to the first dorsal interosseous (FDI) but not to the abductor digiti minimi (ADM). It is important in such cases to thoroughly examine all relevant parameters. In the first example above, the limited findings have a broad localization, including the anterior horn cells, plexus, and common peroneal nerve. One would want to perform needle EMG on L5 paraspinal muscles and the short and long heads of biceps femoris and pay attention to the amplitudes of the superficial peroneal sensory nerve action potentials (SNAPs) and peroneal–extensor digitorum brevis (EDB) compound muscle action potentials (CMAPs) on both sides, as well as the peroneal–EDB and peroneal–tibialis anterior (TA) across-fibular-head motor conduction velocities. The results may still be nonlocalizing.

Focal Neuropathies of the Upper Limb: Anatomy for the Electrodiagnostic Practitioner

Several anatomic points with regard to the upper limb are of great value in the interpretation of electrodiagnostic studies. The electromyographer should be fluent with the anatomy of the major portions of the brachial plexus and should be able to construct the plexus from memory (see Figure 1). In addition, the proximal course of the nerve fibers represented in various sensory and motor nerve conduction studies should be kept in mind, as shown in Table 1. Finally, knowledge of the innervation of the musculature of the arms, according to both nerve roots and plexus, is invaluable (see Table 2).

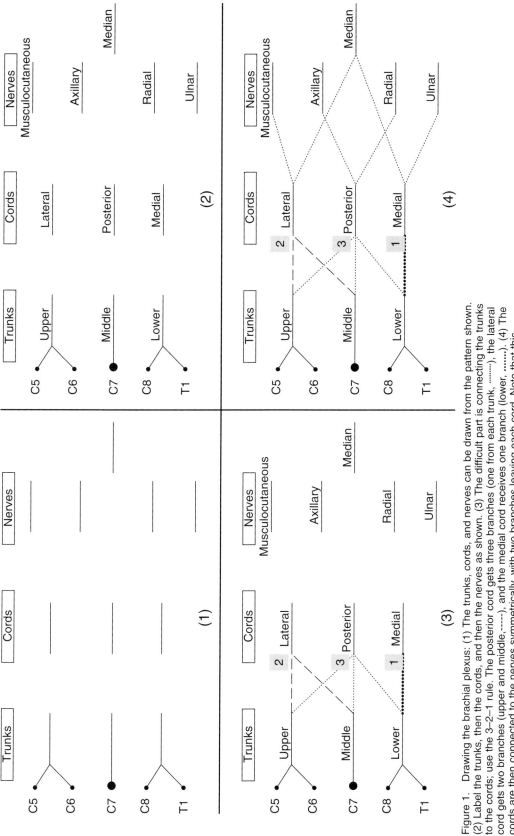

Figure 1. Drawing the brachial plexus: (1) The trunks, cords, and nerves can be drawn from the pattern shown. (2) Label the trunks, then the cords, and then the nerves as shown. (3) The difficult part is connecting the trunks to the cords; use the 3–2–1 rule. The posterior cord gets three branches (one from each trunk, ·······), the lateral cord gets two branches (upper and middle, ––––), and the medial cord receives one branch (lower, ······). (4) The cords are then connected to the nerves symmetrically, with two branches leaving each cord. Note that this common textbook representation of the plexus does not account for the C7, ulnar-innervated supply of several forearm muscles (flexor carpi ulnaris [FCU] and flexor digitorum profundus [FDP] digits 4 and 5). It is not clear how these fibers reach the ulnar nerve—whether it is directly from C7 to lower trunk or through middle trunk or posterior cord. Also note that the median nerve is the only nerve with supply from two different cords.

3

Table 1. Root, Trunk, Cord, and Nerve Innervation Relevant to Sensory and Motor Nerve Conduction Studies in the Upper Limb

Study	Root(s)	Trunk	Cord	Nerve
Sensory				
Lat anteb cutaneous	C6	Upper	Lateral	Musculocutaneous
Radial–webspace	C6	Upper	Posterior	Radial
Radial–D1	C6	Upper	Posterior	Radial
Median–D1	C6	Upper	Lateral	Median
Median–D2	C6, C7	Upper/middle	Lateral	Median
Median–D3	C7	Middle	Lateral	Median
Ulnar–D5	C8, T1	Lower	Medial	Ulnar
Dorsal ulnar cutaneous	C8, T1	Lower	Medial	Ulnar
Med anteb cutaneous	C8, T1	Lower	Medial	Med anteb cutaneous
Motor				
Radial–EIP	C7, C8	Middle	Posterior	Radial
Median–APB	T1 > C8	Lower	Medial	Median
Ulnar–FDI	T1 > C8	Lower	Medial	Ulnar
Ulnar–ADM	C8 > T1	Lower	Medial	Ulnar

Table 2. Root, Trunk, Cord, and Nerve Innervation Relevant to Needle EMG Studies in the Upper Limb

Muscle	Root(s)	Trunk	Cord	Nerve
Serratus anterior	C5, C6, C7	—	—	Long thoracic
Supraspinatus	C5, C6	Upper	—	Suprascapular
Infraspinatus	C5, C6	Upper	—	Suprascapular
Teres minor	C5, C6	Upper	Posterior	Axillary
Deltoid	C5, C6	Upper	Posterior	Axillary
Biceps	C5, C6	Upper	Lateral	Musculocutaneous
Brachioradialis	C5, C6	Upper	Posterior	Radial
Triceps	C6, C7, C8	All	Posterior	Radial
Supinator	C7, C8	Middle/lower	Posterior	Radial
Pronator teres	C6, C7	Upper/middle	Lateral	Median
Ext carpi radialis	C6, C7	Upper/middle	Posterior	Radial
Ext carpi ulnaris	C7, C8	Middle/lower	Posterior	Radial
Ext dig (EDC and EIP)	C7, C8	Middle/lower	Posterior	Radial
Flex carpi radialis	C6, C7	Upper/middle	Lateral	Median
Flex carpi ulnaris	C7, C8, T1	Middle/lower	Medial	Ulnar
Flex pollicis longus	C7, C8	Middle/lower	Medial	Median
Flex dig sup D2–5	C7, C8, T1	Middle/lower	Medial	Median
Flex dig prof D2–3	C7, C8	Middle/lower	Medial	Median
Flex dig prof D4–5	C7, C8	Middle/lower	Medial	Ulnar
Abd pollicis brevis	C8, T1	Lower	Medial	Median
Opponens pollicis	C8, T1	Lower	Medial	Median
Adductor pollicis	C8, T1	Lower	Medial	Ulnar
First dorsal interosseous	C8, T1	Lower	Medial	Ulnar
Abd digiti minimi	C8, T1	Lower	Medial	Ulnar

PATIENT 1

A 60-year-old man with numbness and tingling in his hands
for 1 year

This 60-year-old, left-handed man complained of nocturnal paresthesias in his left hand awakening him at night beginning 1 year ago. The intermittent tingling evolved into constant numbness in the left hand as well as intermittent paresthesias at night in both hands.

Electrodiagnostic Study:

Sensory NCS

Nerve	Sites	Recording Site	Onset (ms)	Peak (ms)	Amplitude (µV)	Distance (cm)	Velocity (m/s)
L. median–dig II	Wrist	Dig II	4.85	5.70	1.6	13	26.8
R. median–dig II	Wrist	Dig II	4.00	5.90	5.5	13	32.5
L. ulnar–dig V	Wrist	Dig V	2.45	3.30	13.1	11	44.9
R. ulnar–dig V	Wrist	Dig V	2.60	3.30	16.3	11	42.3
L. radial–sn box	Forearm	Sn box	1.85	2.50	24.0	10	54.1

Motor NCS

Nerve	Sites	Recording Site	Latency (ms)	Amplitude (mV)	Distance (cm)	Velocity (m/s)
L. median–APB	1. Wrist	APB	9.70	1.8	7	—
	2. Elbow	APB	15.20	1.4	27	49.1
R. median–APB	1. Wrist	APB	7.20	7.0	7	—
	2. Elbow	APB	12.10	6.5	25.5	52.0
L. ulnar–ADM	1. Wrist	ADM	3.05	13.1	7	—
	2. B. elbow	ADM	7.20	11.1	25	60.2
	3. A. elbow	ADM	9.40	10.0	13.5	61.4
R. ulnar–ADM	1. Wrist	ADM	3.10	11.0	7	—
	2. B. elbow	ADM	7.60	10.2	24.5	54.4
	3. A. elbow	ADM	9.35	10.2	12	68.6

EMG Summary Table

	IA	SA Fib	Fasc	Other	Amplitude (MUs)	Duration (MUs)	PolyP (MUs)	Activation	Recruitment Pattern
L. abd poll br	Nl	2+	0	0	Nl	Nl	Nl	Full	Mild red
R. abd poll br	Nl	0	0	0	Nl	Nl	Nl	Full	Nl

Question: What is the likely clinical diagnosis?

5

Answer: Bilateral carpal tunnel syndrome

Discussion: The electrodiagnostic abnormalities are:

- Reduced amplitudes, left worse than right, of bilateral median-D2 SNAPs
- Reduced conduction velocities, left slower than right, of bilateral median-D2 SNAPs
- Reduced amplitude of the left median-APB CMAP
- Prolongation, left more than right, of bilateral median–APB distal motor latencies
- Fibrillation potentials in left APB
- Mildly reduced recruitment of motor units in left APB.

The findings are those of bilateral median neuropathies at the wrists, left more severe than right. The electrodiagnostic approach to the patient with suspected carpal tunnel syndrome aims to:

- Demonstrate electrodiagnostic abnormalities of the median nerve.
- Localize abnormalities to the across-wrist segment of the median nerve.
- Demonstrate normal electrodiagnostic parameters of adjacent nerves, to exclude the presence of a more generalized nerve disorder.

In general, we focus on sensory studies before motor and amplitudes before velocities or latencies. Abnormalities in the median–D2 SNAP amplitude can be thought of as representative of the extent of sensory axon degeneration in the median fibers supplying the second digit. Abnormalities in the median–APB CMAP amplitude can similarly be thought of as representative of the extent of motor axon degeneration in the median motor fibers supplying APB. The caveat is that distal conduction block, of sensory or motor axons, may also produce low amplitudes. Reductions in median nerve conduction study amplitudes generally satisfy the first criterion above, although one should keep in mind that lesions of the lateral cord or upper trunk proximal to the median nerve may also cause SNAP amplitude loss, and lesions of the medial cord or lower trunk may cause CMAP amplitude reduction. Accordingly, a low median–D2 SNAP or median–APB CMAP suggests only a median neuropathy and never localizes the disorder to the wrist (*i.e.*, does not satisfy the second criterion).

To confidently localize any nerve lesion, it is usually necessary to demonstrate a focal electrodiagnostic abnormality: focal slowing, conduction block, or temporal dispersion across a specific nerve segment. For this purpose, either the median–D2 across-wrist sensory conduction velocity or the median–APB distal motor latency must be abnormal.

It can be very helpful to analyze the physiological implications of electrodiagnostic abnormalities one at a time to develop the skill of correlating electrophysiology with actual physiology and clinical findings. We proceed with this exercise for the above six electrodiagnostic abnormalities present in this case.

- *Median–D2 SNAP amplitude reduction.* Axonal degeneration of sensory axons in the median nerve at the wrist and supplying skin of digit 2. These axons come from dorsal root ganglion cells at the level of C6 and C7 principally, pass through the upper and middle trunk and lateral cord, and enter the median nerve in the axilla. Accordingly, a lesion anywhere along this pathway, including the C6 dorsal root ganglia (but not nerve root— why?), plexus, or proximal or distal median nerve could be the cause of this finding.
- *Median–D2 distal sensory conduction velocity reduction.* Focal demyelination of the median sensory fibers somewhere between the point of stimulation and the site of recording—that is, across the wrist (although conceivably a lesion in the palm could produce this finding as well). This provides definitive evidence for a median neuropathy at the wrist.
- *Left median–APB CMAP amplitude reduction.* Axonal degeneration of motor axons in the median nerve at the wrist and supplying APB. Again, as an isolated finding this would only imply a lesion anywhere along the course of the motor axons supplying this muscle and traveling within the median nerve at the wrist, including intramedullary lesions at the level of C8 or T1 myotomes (*i.e.*, syringomyelia or motor neuron diseases), lower trunk or medial cord lesions (*i.e.*, neurologic thoracic outlet syndrome), or proximal median neuropathies. In the context of the other abnormalities in this patient's study, the reduction in amplitude of the CMAP suggests a more severe involvement that might be affecting or threatening to affect the patient's strength. The caveat of distal conduction block as a cause of this reduction, without axonal degeneration, must still be kept in mind.
- *Median–APB distal motor latency prolongation.* Focal slowing of the median motor fibers across the wrist. This provides definitive evidence of a median neuropathy at the wrist. The left greater than right prolongation adds evidence of a more severe left median neuropathy than right.

6

- *Fibrillation potentials in left APB.* Acute denervation of this muscle. This provides support that the reduced CMAP amplitude (see third point above) is not entirely due to distal conduction block, and there is at least some element of axonal degeneration present.
- *Reduced recruitment of motor units in left APB.* Either chronic denervation or conduction block of motor axons can produce this finding. Physiologically, this reduced recruitment of motor units is the single electrodiagnostic parameter that most likely correlates with clinical weakness.
- Finally, it is important to note the normal studies of both ulnar nerves (motor and sensory) and the right radial nerve (sensory) to exclude a more generalized disorder, such as an acquired demyelinating neuropathy.

This study is characteristic of patients with moderate or moderate-severe median neuropathies. There are abnormalities of sensory and motor studies as well as needle EMG. Even though the slow median–D2 across-wrist sensory velocities are sufficient by themselves to establish the diagnosis of median neuropathies at the wrists, the other studies and parameters are essential for a fuller clinical understanding of the severity and extent of involvement.

Clinical Pearls

1. Confident localization of a median neuropathy to the wrist requires the presence of a focal abnormality: conduction block, focal slowing, or temporal dispersion.

2. Each individual electrodiagnostic abnormality has a physiological interpretation that you should train yourself to think of when performing and interpreting electrodiagnostic studies.

REFERENCES

1. Practice parameter: electrodiagnostic studies in carpal tunnel syndrome: report of the AAEM, AAN, and AAPMR, *Neurology* 2002; 58:1589–1592.
2. Jablecki, C.K., Andary, M.T., Floeter, M.K., Miller, R.G., Quartly, C.A., Vennix, M.J., Wilson, J.R., Second AAEM literature review of the usefulness of nerve conduction studies and electromyography for the evaluation of patients with carpal tunnel syndrome, *Muscle Nerve* 2002; 26.

PATIENT 2

A 48-year-old woman with numbness and tingling in her left hand

This 48-year-old woman complained of nocturnal paresthesias in her left hand for 3 months.
Electrodiagnostic Study:

Sensory NCS

Nerve	Sites	Recording Site	Onset (ms)	Peak (ms)	Amplitude (µV)	Distance (cm)	Velocity (m/s)
L. median–dig II	1. Wrist	Dig II	2.95	3.60	23.7	13	44.1
L. ulnar–dig V	1. Wrist	Dig V	2.10	2.60	22.2	11	52.4

Motor NCS

Nerve	Sites	Recording Site	Latency (ms)	Amplitude (mV)	Distance (cm)	Velocity (m/s)
L. median–APB	1. Wrist	APB	4.20	7.4	7	—
	2. Elbow	APB	8.15	7.1	22	55.7
L. ulnar–ADM	1. Wrist	ADM	2.65	9.7	7	—
	2. B. elbow	ADM	6.00	9.1	21	62.7
	3. A. elbow	ADM	7.40	8.8	8	57.1

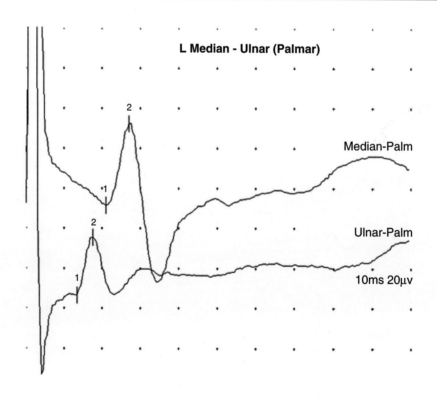

L Median - Ulnar (Palmar)

Median-Palm

Ulnar-Palm

10ms 20µv

Questions:

1. Do the above studies confidently diagnose or exclude carpal tunnel syndrome?
2. If not, what additional nerve conduction studies should be considered?
3. What study is illustrated in the figure and what does it show?

Answers:
1. No
2. A more sensitive study should be considered.
3. The median and ulnar palm-to-wrist mixed palmar study shows prolongation of the median response.

Discussion: The routine median and ulnar studies are within normal limits; however, the existence of more sensitive tests for carpal tunnel syndrome means this study is incomplete. An additional study was performed and is shown in the figure.

This study is abnormal for a prolonged median–ulnar mixed palmar interlatency difference (0.95 msec). The upper limit of normality for this technique has ranged from 0.2 to 0.5 in the medical literature. We prefer the conservative value of <0.5.

For detection of mild carpal tunnel syndrome, one often needs to use a more highly sensitive test than the standard wrist-digit recordings of SNAP latency. This need has stimulated a great deal of research. The main questions have been:

- Are sensory studies more sensitive than motor?
- Are comparison studies (*i.e.,* between median and ulnar or between median and radial) more sensitive than non-comparison studies?
- Are shorter segmental studies, such as median palm–wrist instead of digit–wrist, more sensitive?

The American Association of Electrodiagnostic Medicine (AAEM) second literature review answered "yes" to all of these questions. The AAEM concluded that sensory studies are more sensitive than motor studies, that comparison studies of median sensory or mixed nerve conduction through the carpal tunnel to radial or ulnar studies in the same hand are more sensitive than non-comparison studies, and that short segmental studies are more sensitive than wrist–digit studies. Accordingly, if median wrist–digit sensory conduction velocity is normal, one of these more sensitive tests should be used:

- Median–ulnar mixed palmar interlatency difference (the difference between median and ulnar palm–wrist mixed compound nerve action potential peak latencies)
- Median–ulnar D4 or median–radial D1 interlatency differences
- Median palm–wrist sensory latency compared to median wrist–digit or median elbow–wrist sensory latencies

In our experience, the first and second tests are used considerably more frequently than the third. Because a normal wrist–digit study should always be followed by a more sensitive test in patients with suspected carpal tunnel syndrome, one could argue that it would be more efficient to skip the wrist–digit study altogether and to routinely perform just the mixed palmar study or a comparison study to digit 4 or digit 1. We still prefer to perform the wrist–digit study because of the additional information obtained regarding the amplitude of the SNAP and its implication regarding axonal degeneration of sensory axons (see case 1 for further discussion).

Mixed Nerve CNAP Results from Figure

Nerve	Sites	Recording Site	Onset (ms)	Peak (ms)	Amplitude (μV)	Distance (cm)	Velocity (m/s)
L. median–ulnar (palmar)	1. Median–palmar	Wrist	2.10	2.70	41.0	8	38.1
	2. Ulnar–palmar	Wrist	1.35	1.75	28.9	8	59.3

Clinical Pearls

1. Sensory studies are more often abnormal in carpal tunnel syndrome than are motor studies.

2. If sensory median–digit studies are normal, one of several roughly equivalent sensory comparison studies should be done because of their increased sensitivity.

REFERENCES

1. Practice parameter: electrodiagnostic studies in carpal tunnel syndrome: report of the AAEM, AAN, and AAPMR, *Neurology* 2002; 58:1589–1592.
2. Chang, M.H., Wei, S.J., Chiang, H.L., Wang, H.M., Hsieh, P.F., Huang, S.Y., Comparison of motor conduction techniques in the diagnosis of carpal tunnel syndrome. *Neurology* 2002; 58(11):1603–1607.
3. Jablecki, C.K., Andary, M.T., Floeter, M.K., Miller, R.G., Quartly, C.A., Vennix, M.J., Wilson, J.R., Second AAEM literature review of the usefulness of nerve conduction studies and electromyography for the evaluation of patients with carpal tunnel syndrome, *Muscle Nerve* 2002; 26.
4. Kothari, M.J., Rutkove, S.B., Caress, J.B., Hinchey, J., Logigian, E.L., Preston, D.C., Comparison of digital sensory studies in patients with carpal tunnel syndrome. *Muscle Nerve* 1995; 18(11):1272–1276.
5. Preston, D.C., Logigian, E.L., Sensitivity of the three median-to-ulnar comparative tests in diagnosis of mild carpal tunnel syndrome. *Muscle Nerve* 1994; 17(8):955–956.

PATIENT 3

A 68-year-old woman with numbness and tingling in her hands

Electrodiagnostic Study:

Sensory NCS

Nerve	Sites	Recording Site	Onset (ms)	Peak (ms)	Amplitude (μV)	Distance (cm)	Velocity (m/s)
R. median–dig II	1. Wrist	Dig II	Absent	—	—	13	—
L. median–dig II	1. Wrist	Dig II	Absent	—	—	13	—
R. ulnar–dig V	1. Wrist	Dig V	1.90	2.50	41.2	11	57.9
L. ulnar–dig V	1. Wrist	Dig V	1.95	2.45	22.8	11	56.4
R. radial–sn box	1. Forearm	Sn box	1.55	2.05	23.3	10	64.5
L. radial–sn box	1. Forearm	Sn box	1.65	2.10	47.5	10	60.6

Motor NCS

Nerve	Sites	Recording Site	Latency (ms)	Amplitude (mV)	Distance (cm)	Velocity (m/s)
R. median–APB	1. Wrist	APB	Absent	—	—	—
L. median–APB	1. Wrist	APB	12.20	2.6	7	—
	2. Elbow	APB	17.25	2.7	22	43.6
R. ulnar–ADM	1. Wrist	ADM	2.85	7.3	7	—
	2. B. elbow	ADM	6.20	7.0	21	62.7
	3. A. elbow	ADM	8.30	6.7	13	61.9
L. ulnar–ADM	1. Wrist	ADM	2.60	9.6	7	—
	2. B. elbow	ADM	6.50	9.5	20	51.3
	3. A. elbow	ADM	9.00	9.1	13	52.0
R. ulnar–FDI	1. Wrist	FDI	3.70	9.8	—	—
	2. B. elbow	FDI	7.25	9.1	21	59.2
	3. A. elbow	FDI	9.30	9.3	13	63.4
L. median–vs. ulnar	1. Median	Lumb	9.90	0.5	10	—
	2. Ulnar	Inteross	3.05	6.4	10	—
R. median–vs. ulnar	1. Median	Lumb	11.65	0.5	10	—
	2. Ulnar	Inteross	3.15	6.2	10	—

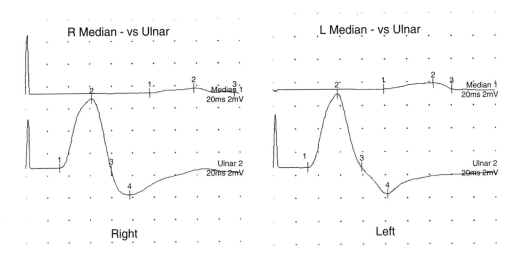

R Median - vs Ulnar

L Median - vs Ulnar

Median 1
20ms 2mV

Ulnar 2
20ms 2mV

Right

Left

Questions:

1. What finding is demonstrated in the figure?
2. How would the electrodiagnostic interpretation change if this particular study was not performed on the *right* side?
3. How would the electrodiagnostic interpretation change if this particular study was not performed on the *left* side?

Answers:
1. Abnormal bilateral median-lumbrical, ulnar interosseous interlatency differences
2. Unlocalized median neuropathy
3. No change

Discussion: The figure shows the result of the comparison of median-lumbrical vs. ulnar-second interosseous (2LIO) motor study. This comparison is made by stimulating at identical distances the median and ulnar nerves at the wrist and recording over a single surface location under which are both the second lumbrical (median innervated) and second palmar interosseous (ulnar innervated). As apparent in the figure and from the numerical values in the results table, there is a marked delay in both median responses. Without this study on the right, the absent median-D2 sensory and median-APB motor responses allow for a diagnosis of median neuropathy but not a more specific localization. A lesion anywhere along the course of the median nerve from the axilla to the palm could result in an absent median SNAP and CMAP. In this situation, the 2LIO study can be very helpful if a median-lumbrical CMAP is present, as it provides definitive localization of the median neuropathy at the wrist. Had the study not been performed on the left side, the interpretation would not have changed, as the recordable median–APB CMAP allows for determination of the distal motor latency, which is prolonged and provides a localization at the wrist, as well. As a general rule, carpal tunnel syndrome affects the SNAP amplitude before the median-APB CMAP amplitude, and this before the median–second lumbrical CMAP.

This special technique, first described in 1992 by Preston and Logigian,[4] generally does not provide insight beyond more standard electrodiagnostic techniques for patients with mild or moderate carpal tunnel syndrome but is invaluable in some patients with severe carpal tunnel syndrome. In many such patients, the absence of recordable median-digit SNAPs and median-APB CMAPs makes it otherwise impossible to localize the median neuropathy to the wrist. In the large study of Loscher *et al.*,[3] 36 patients had absent median-D2 and median-APB responses. Of these, 31 did have recordable median-lumbrical responses, abnormal in all cases. Preston and Logigian's technique has proven extremely valuable in this circumstance.

Clinical Pearl

Severe carpal tunnel syndrome, with absent median-digit sensory and median–APB motor responses, creates a diagnostic challenge in demonstrating a focal abnormality at the wrist. In this situation, the median-ulnar second lumbrical interosseous (2LIO) test is especially valuable.

REFERENCES

1. Boonyapisit, K., Katirji, B., Shapiro, B.E., Preston, D.C., Lumbrical and interossei recording in severe carpal tunnel syndrome, *Muscle Nerve* 2002; 25(1):102–105.
2. Chang, M.H., Wei, S.J., Chiang, H.L., Wang, H.M., Hsieh, P.F., Huang, S.Y., Comparison of motor conduction techniques in the diagnosis of carpal tunnel syndrome, *Neurology* 2002; 58(11):1603–1607.
3. Loscher, W.N., Auer-Grumbach, M., Trinka, E., Ladurner, G., Hartung, H.P., Comparison of second lumbrical and interosseous latencies with standard measures of median nerve function across the carpal tunnel: a prospective study of 450 hands, *J. Neurol.* 2000; 247(7):530–534.
4. Preston, D., Logigian, E.L., Lumbrical and interossei recording in carpal tunnel syndrome, *Muscle Nerve* 1992; 15:1253–1257.
5. Preston, D.C., Ross, M.H., Kothari, M.J., Plotkin, G.M., Venkatesh, S., Logigian, E.L., The median-ulnar latency difference studies are comparable in mild carpal tunnel syndrome. *Muscle Nerve* 1994; 17(12):1469–1471.

(See cases 1 and 2 for further references on carpal tunnel syndrome.)

PATIENT 4

A 53-year-old woman with right hand weakness and numbness after an axillary dissection

This 53-year-old woman underwent lumpectomy and axillary dissection of lymph nodes for breast cancer and immediately postoperatively noticed numbness of her right hand digits 1 to 3 and weakness. In particular, she had difficulty flexing her fingers, as noted in the figures.

Electrodiagnostic Study: Electrodiagnostic studies were performed 5 months later.

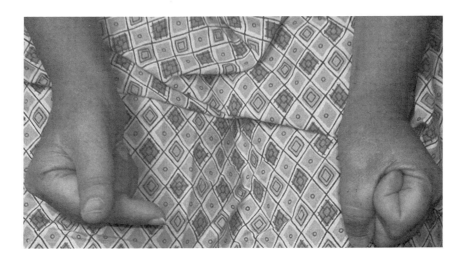

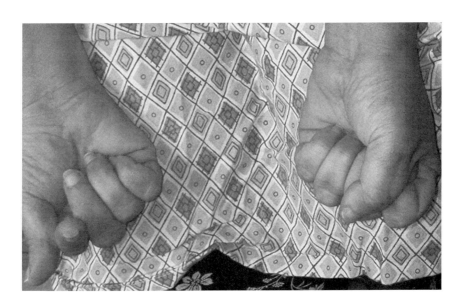

Sensory NCS

Nerve	Sites	Recording Site	Onset (ms)	Peak (ms)	BP Amplitude (µV)	Distance (cm)	Velocity (m/s)
R. median–dig II	1. Wrist	Dig II	2.95	3.70	2.8	13	44.1
L. median–dig II	1. Wrist	Dig II	2.30	3.00	108.3	13	56.5
R. ulnar–dig V	1. Wrist	Dig V	2.10	3.00	52.9	11	52.4
L. ulnar–dig V	1. Wrist	Dig V	1.95	2.75	85.7	11	56.4
R. radial–sn box	1. Forearm	Sn box	1.85	2.35	105.8	10	54.1
L. radial–sn box	1. Forearm	Sn box	1.75	2.30	79.5	10	57.1
R. lat AB cut	1. Elbow	Forearm	1.90	2.45	26.1	12	63.2
L. lat AB cut	1. Elbow	Forearm	1.30	1.75	23.5	12	92.3

Motor NCS

Nerve	Sites	Recording Site	Latency (ms)	Amplitude (mV)	Distance (cm)	Velocity (m/s)
R. median-APB	1. Wrist	ADM	—	Absent	7	—
R. ulnar–ADM	1. Wrist	ADM	3.85	7.8	7	—
	2. B. elbow	ADM	6.05	7.7	13	59.1
	3. A. elbow	ADM	8.05	7.4	10	50.0

F-Wave

Nerve	F_{min} (ms)	F_{max} (ms)	Max – Min (ms)	%F
R. median	Absent	—	—	—
R. ulnar	23.30	27.95	4.65	100

EMG Summary Table

Nerve	IA	SA Fib	SA Fasc	SA Other	Amplitude (MUs)	Duration (MUs)	PolyP (MUs)	Activation	Recruitment Pattern
R. pron teres	Nl	3+	0	0	Nl	Nl	Nl	Full	Single MU
R. flex poll ln	Nl	2+	0	0	Nl	Nl	Nl	Full	No activity
R. first dors int	Nl	0	0	0	Nl	Nl	Nl	Full	Nl
R. ext dig comm	Nl	0	0	0	Nl	Nl	Nl	Full	Nl
R. abd poll br	Nl	2+	0	0	Nl	Nl	Nl	Full	No activity

Questions:
1. What is the rationale for performing sensory nerve studies on the asymptomatic hand?
2. Do the nerve conduction studies alone localize the lesion? Could carpal tunnel syndrome produce these nerve conduction study abnormalities?
3. Could this patient have an anterior interosseous neuropathy?

Answers:
1. Side-to-side comparison of SNAP amplitudes provides greater sensitivity.
2. No; Yes
3. No. There is clinical sensory involvement.

Discussion: Because the range of normal for SNAP amplitudes is quite large, significant focal nerve lesions can produce amplitude reductions that remain within the normal range. Using the additional criterion of greater than 50% side-to-side reduction, subclinical abnormalities can sometimes be demonstrated. In evaluation of possible brachial plexus lesions, we often look at multiple sensory nerves bilaterally. In this case, no additional abnormalities outside of the median nerve territory were detected with this approach.

The nerve conduction studies are abnormal for reduced amplitude of the median sensory and absence of the median–APB motor responses, suggesting a median neuropathy, though without localization to the carpal tunnel. The first figure suggests weakness of thumb flexion (flexor pollicis longus) and digit 2 flexion at the distal interphalangeal (DIP) joint (flexor digitorum profundus [FDP], second digit) and proximal interphalangeal (PIP) joint (flexor digitorum superficialis [FDS], second digit). The second figure makes evident the weakness in the FDP and FDS for digit 3 and possibly for digit 4, though less so. These muscles are all supplied by the anterior interosseous nerve (AIN), a branch of the median nerve. Could this patient have an anterior interosseous neuropathy clinically? Not likely, as the patient noted numbness of digits 1 to 3; the AIN is purely motor. This would place the lesion more proximally, in the proximal median nerve. The electrodiagnostic studies confirm this, showing abnormalities in reduction in the median sensory potential amplitude and needle EMG abnormalities in pronator teres as well as the more distal median nerve territory.

This patient has a proximal median neuropathy as a perioperative complication. The cause is uncertain, and could relate to manipulation of the brachial plexus during the axillary dissection or compression of the median nerve in the upper arm during the procedure.

Clinical Pearls

1. The evaluation of brachial plexus abnormalities typically requires multiple bilateral sensory studies.

2. Consider proximal median neuropathy when routine studies demonstrate a median neuropathy that does not localize to the wrist.

REFERENCES

1. Gross, P.T., Jones, H.R., Jr., Proximal median neuropathies: electromyographic and clinical correlation, *Muscle Nerve* 1992; 15:390–395.
2. Gross, P.T., Tolomeo, E.A. Proximal median neuropathies, *Neurol. Clin.* 1999; 17:425–445.
3. Stewart, J.D., Proximal median neuropathies: electromyographic and clinical correlation, *Muscle Nerve* 1993; 16:321–322.
4. Veilleux, M., Richardson, P., Proximal median neuropathy secondary to humeral neck fracture, *Muscle Nerve* 2000; 23:426–429.

PATIENT 5

A 36-year-old man with 2 years of numbness in his left hand digits 4 and 5

This 36-year-old right-handed man noted progressive constant numbness and pins-and-needles paresthesias in his left hand digits 4 and 5 over 2 years. He worked as a laboratory researcher and spent many hours each day leaning on his fully flexed elbows. Neurological examination demonstrated a sensory disturbance in the left medial and dorsal hand up to the wrist crease and digits 5 and the medial half of digit 4.

Electrodiagnostic Study:

Sensory NCS

Nerve	Sites	Recording Site	Onset (ms)	Peak (ms)	Amplitude (µV)	Distance (cm)	Velocity (m/s)
L. median–dig II	1. Wrist	Dig II	2.35	2.90	36.6	13	55.3
R. median–dig II	1. Wrist	Dig II	2.30	2.75	51.9	13	56.5
L. ulnar–dig V	1. Wrist	Dig V	2.50	3.45	19.9	11	44.0
R. ulnar–dig V	1. Wrist	Dig V	2.15	2.75	44.4	11	51.2
L. ulnar dorsal	1. Wrist	Dors hand	—	Absent	—	10	—
R. ulnar dorsal	1. Wrist	Dors hand	1.80	2.35	12.4	10	55.6

Motor NCS

Nerve	Sites	Recording Site	Latency (ms)	Amplitude (mV)	Distance (cm)	Velocity (m/s)
L. median–APB	1. Wrist	APB	3.15	9.9	7	—
	2. Elbow	APB	7.05	9.3	22	56.4
L. ulnar–ADM	1. Wrist	ADM	2.40	7.4	7	—
	2. B. elbow	ADM	5.65	6.5	19	58.5
	3. A. elbow	ADM	8.55	7.0	14.5	50.0
R. median–APB	1. Wrist	APB	3.05	12.0	7	—
	2. Elbow	APB	6.80	12.2	23	61.3
R. ulnar–ADM	1. Wrist	ADM	2.15	9.6	7	—
	2. B. elbow	ADM	5.45	9.3	20	60.6
	3. A. elbow	ADM	8.10	8.5	14	52.8

Questions:
1. Would you consider any other nerve conduction studies at this point to clarify the diagnosis?
2. What is the likely diagnosis?
3. What electrodiagnostic studies would be helpful?
4. What abnormality is illustrated in the figure?

L Ulnar - ADM

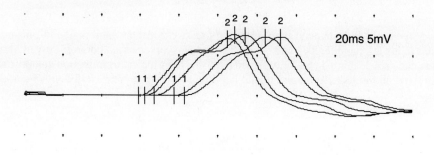

20ms 5mV

Answers:
1. Across elbow ulnar inching studies
2. Ulnar neuropathy at or near the elbow
3. Ulnar motor "inching" across the elbow
4. Prolongation of latencies between the third and fourth stimulation sites

Discussion: The electrodiagnostic study is notable for relative reduction in the amplitude of the left ulnar–D5 SNAP compared to the right ulnar–D5 SNAP. Greater than 50% reduction in side-to-side comparison of SNAP amplitudes is generally taken to be abnormal. In addition, the left dorsal ulnar cutaneous nerve response is absent on the left and robust ($12~\mu$V) on the right. These features, together with the other normal SNAPs, suggest a lesion of the lower trunk, medial cord, or ulnar nerve. The routine motor studies, including the ulnar-ADM across-elbow motor velocity of 50 m/sec are within normal limits, leaving the electromyographer unable to further localize the lesion.

The additional technique of "inching" across the elbow is quite helpful in further localizing the lesion. The results of this study are listed next.

The ulnar-ADM inching study demonstrates focal slowing of motor nerves in the elbow to the elbow + 2.5 cm proximally segment; this is the retroepicondylar segment that extends from the midpoint of a line drawn between the medial epicondyle and olecranon extending proximally. The figure shows a visible delay in onset latency between the third and fourth waveforms compared to the others, counting from the left. Although the overall motor conduction velocity across the 14.5-cm elbow segment in the routine ulnar study was 50 m/sec (normal), across this 2.5-cm segment there is a 1-msec delay (6.75 to 7.75 msec), translating to a velocity of 25 m/sec through this single short segment. This is an example of the value of short-segmental incremental studies in general, which also have value in the diagnosis of median neuropathies at the wrist.

In this case, the technique allows for precise localization of the ulnar neuropathy not just to the elbow but to the retroepicondylar segment. This provides excellent justification to discourage a cubital tunnel release as a surgical approach. Several technical caveats are noteworthy. One must be meticulous in inching study distance measurements, as shorter distance segments are prone to a greater percentage of error. Furthermore, rigorously defined normal values for inching are not available; 0.8 msec or greater across a single 2.5-cm elbow segment is generally taken as a conservative cutoff for abnormality. We also note a reduction in the amplitude of the dorsal ulnar cutaneous sensory study is generally taken as evidence of a lesion proximal to the wrist; however, 21% of normal individuals have a significant asymmetry, thus limiting the value of this technique.[5]

In general, one should note that the electrodiagnosis of ulnar neuropathy at the elbow is often not straightforward. Campbell[3] noted that Wilbourne referred to it as the "electromyographer's nightmare." The complexity of interpretation, particularly in relation to normal values that overlap substantially with abnormal values and that are highly dependent on technical factors, along with the very serious consequences of misdiagnosis leading to a failed operation, frequently lead to an ambiguous study.

Nerve	Sites	Recording Site	Latency (ms)	Amplitude (mV)
L. ulnar–ADM inching study	1. Elbow – 5.0	ADM	5.90	7.2
	2. Elbow – 2.5	ADM	6.25	7.6
	3. Elbow	ADM	6.75	7.5
	4. Elbow + 2.5	ADM	7.75	7.3
	5. Elbow + 5.0	ADM	8.30	7.3

Clinical Pearls

1. The localization of an ulnar neuropathy to the elbow is often difficult.

2. Short segmental studies ("inching") of the ulnar nerve across the elbow are a valuable technique when more routine studies are nonlocalizing.

3. The amplitude of the dorsal ulnar cutaneous SNAP may be significantly asymmetric in up to 21% of normal individuals, limiting its diagnostic utility.

REFERENCES

1. AAEM, Practice parameter for electrodiagnostic studies in ulnar neuropathy at the elbow: summary statement: American Association of Electrodiagnostic Medicine, American Academy of Neurology, American Academy of Physical Medicine and Rehabilitation, *Muscle Nerve* 1999; 22(suppl. 8):S171–S174.
2. AAEM. The electrodiagnostic evaluation of patients with ulnar neuropathy at the elbow: literature review of the usefulness of nerve conduction studies and needle electromyography, *Muscle Nerve* 1999; 22(suppl. 8):S175–S205.
3. Campbell, W.W., Ulnar neuropathy at the elbow, *Muscle Nerve* 2000; 23:450–452.
4. Campbell, W.W., Pridgeon, R.M., Sahni, K.S., Short segment incremental studies in the evaluation of ulnar neuropathy at the elbow, *Muscle Nerve* 1992; 15(9):1050–1054.
5. Dutra de Oliveira, A., Barreira, A.A., Marques, W., Limitations on the clinical utility of the ulnar dorsal cutaneous sensory nerve action potential, *Clin. Neurophysiol.* 2000; 111:1208–1210.

PATIENT 6

A 55-year-old man with numbness in hand digits 4 and 5

This 55-year-old man with diabetes and bilateral numbness, left more than right, in digits 4 and 5 of the hands was referred to "r/o cubital tunnel syndrome" by an orthopedic surgeon.

Electrodiagnostic Study:

Sensory NCS

Nerve	Sites	Recording Site	Onset (ms)	Peak (ms)	Amplitude (μV)	Distance (cm)	Velocity (m/s)
L. median–dig II	1. Wrist	Dig II	2.30	3.00	22.1	13	56.5
R. median–dig II	1. Wrist	Dig II	2.40	3.20	24.4	13	54.2
L. ulnar–dig V	1. Wrist	Dig V	3.65	4.70	10.3	11	30.1
R. ulnar–dig V	1. Wrist	Dig V	2.10	2.90	19.3	11	52.4
L. radial–sn box	1. Forearm	Sn box	1.50	2.10	21.3	10	66.7

Motor NCS

Nerve	Sites	Recording Site	Latency (ms)	Amplitude (mV)	Distance (cm)	Velocity (m/s)
L. median–APB	1. Wrist	APB	3.55	5.1	7	—
	2. Elbow	APB	8.45	4.8	25	51.0
L. ulnar–ADM	1. Wrist	ADM	3.00	6.9	7	—
	2. B. elbow	ADM	8.00	6.2	25	50.0
	3. A. elbow	ADM	12.35	1.4	12.5	28.7
R. ulnar–ADM	1. Wrist	ADM	2.75	7.7	7	—
	2. B. elbow	ADM	7.60	7.0	25	51.5
	3. A. elbow	ADM	9.50	6.5	10	52.6
L. ulnar–FDI	1. Wrist	FDI	4.35	11.8	—	—
	2. B. elbow	FDI	9.05	10.5	24	51.1
	3. A. elbow	FDI	13.10	4.1	11.5	28.4
R. ulnar–FDI	1. Wrist	FDI	3.95	10.1	—	—
	2. B. elbow	FDI	8.65	8.9	25	53.2
	3. A. elbow	FDI	10.90	8.6	11.5	51.1

EMG Summary Table

		SA							
	IA	Fib	Fasc	Other	Amplitude (MUs)	Duration (MUs)	PolyP (MUs)	Activation	Recruitment Pattern
L. first dors int	Inc	2+	0	0	Nl	Nl	Nl	Full	Mod red
L. abd poll br	Nl	0	0	0	Nl	Nl	Nl	Full	Nl
L. flex carp uln	Nl	0	0	0	Nl	Nl	Nl	Full	Nl

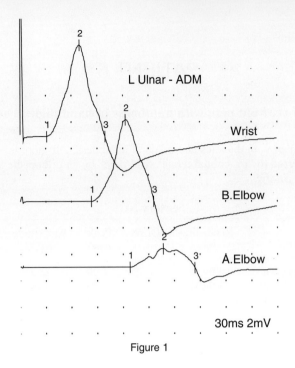

L Ulnar - ADM

Wrist

B.Elbow

A.Elbow

30ms 2mV

Figure 1

Questions:
1. What is the conclusion of the electrodiagnostic studies?
2. Do they confirm the presence of cubital tunnel syndrome and should the patient undergo ulnar nerve decompression at the cubital tunnel?
3. What finding is shown in the figure 1?

Answers:
1. A left ulnar neuropathy at or near the elbow is present.
2. No
3. Partial conduction block and focal slowing is shown.

Discussion: The electrodiagnostic studies are abnormal for borderline reduction in the amplitude of the left ulnar–D5 SNAP (nearly one-half the contralateral ulnar amplitude and at the lower limit of normal of 10 μV) and reveal slowing of both the ulnar-ADM and ulnar-FDI across-elbow motor segments and conduction block (>50% reduction in amplitude) in these same segments as well. These findings indicate a left ulnar neuropathy at or near the elbow. Also note the slowing of the left ulnar–D5 across-wrist sensory segment, which perhaps seems greater than one would expect as a consequence of the axonal loss alone.

Although the term *cubital tunnel syndrome* is often used synonymously with *ulnar neuropathy at or near the elbow*, doing so should be avoided. Ulnar neuropathies at or near the elbow (generally referred to as *ulnar neuropathy at the elbow*, or UNE) are grouped into several categories by localization, listed from proximal to distal: the medial intermuscular septum, the retroepicondylar groove, the humeroulnar arcade (HUA), and the point of exit from the flexor carpi ulnaris. The cubital tunnel is synonymous with HUA localization. Furthermore, even when localizing to the cubital tunnel, an ulnar neuropathy may be due to blunt trauma rather than ongoing compression. The use of the term *cubital tunnel syndrome* may lead to inappropriate surgical procedures for mistakes made in connection with either of these two points. Further electrodiagnostic studies including motor inching studies can clarify the localization. The results of inching studies are shown in the table below and in figure 2.

The inching studies demonstrate focal slowing and conduction block of the retroepicondylar (between the elbow and 2.5 cm proximally) and medial intermuscular septum (2.5 to 5.0 cm) segments. Although focal nerve conduction abnormalities do not always correlate with the precise site of compression, a cubital tunnel decompression was not recommended for this patient. If conservative treatment fails, ulnar nerve transposition could be considered, although it is of unproven value.

Ulnar Nerve Inching Study

Nerve	Sites	Recording Site	Latency (ms)	Amplitude (mV)	Distance (cm)	Velocity (m/s)
L. ulnar–ADM	1. 5.0 cm below elbow	ADM	8.20	6.0	2.5	—
	2. 2.5 cm below elbow	ADM	8.65	6.0	2.5	55.6
	3. At elbow	ADM	9.10	5.9	2.5	55.6
	4. 2.5 cm above elbow	ADM	10.70	2.2	2.5	15.6
	5. 5.0 cm above elbow	ADM	11.65	1.5	2.5	26.3

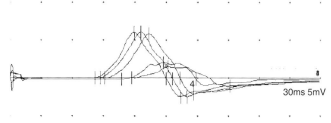

L Ulnar-ADM Across-Elbow Inching

30ms 5mV

Figure 2

Clinical Pearls

1. Ulnar neuropathy at or near the elbow is not synonymous with cubital tunnel syndrome; patients with ulnar neuropathies often have focal abnormalities at elbow sites proximal to the cubital tunnel.

2. Ulnar elbow inching studies, when abnormal, can demonstrate focal slowing, conduction block, or both.

REFERENCES

1. AAEM, Practice parameter for electrodiagnostic studies in ulnar neuropathy at the elbow: summary statement: American Association of Electrodiagnostic Medicine, American Academy of Neurology, American Academy of Physical Medicine and Rehabilitation, *Muscle Nerve* 1999; 22(suppl. 8):S171–S174.
2. AAEM. The electrodiagnostic evaluation of patients with ulnar neuropathy at the elbow: literature review of the usefulness of nerve conduction studies and needle electromyography, *Muscle Nerve* 1999; 22(suppl. 8):S175–S205.
3. Campbell, W.W., Ulnar neuropathy at the elbow, *Muscle Nerve* 2000; 23:450–452.
4. Campbell, W.W., Pridgeon, R.M., Sahni, K.S., Short segment incremental studies in the evaluation of ulnar neuropathy at the elbow, *Muscle Nerve* 1992; 15(9):1050–1054.
5. Dutra de Oliveira, A., Barreira, A.A., Marques, W., Limitations on the clinical utility of the ulnar dorsal cutaneous sensory nerve action potential, *Clin. Neurophysiol.* 2000; 111:1208–1210.

PATIENT 7

A 53-year-old woman with left hand weakness

This 53-year-old woman developed sudden weakness without sensory symptoms in her left hand. She was evaluated for electrodiagnostic studies 5 months later. Motor examination showed atrophy and weakness of left FDI with normal ADM, and no sensory loss was observed.

Electrodiagnostic Study:

Sensory NCS

Nerve	Sites	Recording Site	Onset (ms)	Peak (ms)	Amplitude (µV)	Distance (cm)	Velocity (m/s)
L. ulnar dorsal–hand	1. Wrist	Hand	1.55	1.95	25.0	10	64.5
L. median–dig II	1. Wrist	Dig II	2.10	2.85	43.9	13	61.9
L. ulnar dig V	1. Wrist	Dig V	1.95	2.75	35.8	11	56.4
R. ulnar–dig V	1. Wrist	Dig V	1.80	2.55	41.1	11	61.1

Motor NCS

Nerve	Sites	Recording Site	Latency (ms)	Amplitude (mV)	Distance (cm)	Velocity (m/s)
L. median–APB	1. Wrist	APB	3.45	11.9	7	—
	2. Elbow	APB	6.80	11.3	21	62.7
L. ulnar–ADM	1. Wrist	ADM	3.40	7.4	7	—
	2. B. elbow	ADM	6.65	7.5	21	64.6
	3. A. elbow	ADM	8.15	7.3	9	60.0
R. ulnar–ADM	1. Wrist	ADM	2.65	10.7	7	—
	2. B. elbow	ADM	6.10	10.2	21	60.9
	3. A. elbow	ADM	7.85	10.1	10	57.1
L. ulnar–FDI	1. Wrist	FDI	3.65	1.8	—	—
	2. B. elbow	FDI	7.10	1.6	21	60.9
	3. A. elbow	FDI	8.15	1.7	7	66.7
R. ulnar–FDI	1. Wrist	FDI	3.55	12.9	—	—
	2. B. elbow	FDI	6.80	12.0	21	64.6
	3. A. elbow	FDI	8.65	11.1	10	54.1
L. median–vs. ulnar	1. Median	Lumb	2.95	3.1	10	—
	2. Ulnar	Inteross	3.35	0.6	10	—
R. median–vs. ulnar	1. Median	Lumb	3.05	3.6	10	—
	2. Ulnar	Inteross	3.05	5.5	10	—

Needle EMG Summary Table

	SA				Amplitude (MUs)	Duration (MUs)	PolyP (MUs)	Activation	Recruitment Pattern
	IA	Fib	Fasc	Other					
L. abd poll br	Nl	0	0	0	Nl	Nl	Nl	Full	Nl
L. abd dig min	Nl	0	0	0	Nl	Nl	Nl	Full	Nl
L. ext indicis	Nl	0	0	0	Nl	Nl	Nl	Full	Nl
L. flex dig pr IV	Nl	0	0	0	Nl	Nl	Nl	Full	Nl
L. first dors int	Incr	3+	0	0	Nl	—	—	Full	Single MUP

Questions:
1. What are the electrodiagnostic abnormalities and conclusion?
2. What is the clinical localization of this lesion?

Answers:

1. Reduced amplitudes of the right ulnar-FDI, ulnar second palmar interosseous CMAPs, fibrillation potentials, and reduced motor unit recruitment in FDI suggest a lesion of the ulnar deep motor branch in the palm.
2. Ulnar neuropathy at the distal wrist or in the palm, affecting the deep motor branch only

Discussion: This patient has an ulnar neuropathy that spares the ulnar sensory and dorsal ulnar cutaneous nerve territories and the ADM. These features suggest a distal lesion. Distal ulnar neuropathies have four distinct patterns of presentation (figure 1):

- *At Guyon's canal:* the main trunk of the nerve is affected, so that deficits are apparent in both the superficial terminal branch (ulnar n. sensory loss, ventral medial palm, D5 and medial D4 sensory) and the proximal deep terminal branch (all ulnar-innervated intrinsic hand muscles).
- *Deep terminal branch proximal to hypothenar branches:* no sensory loss, with weakness of all ulnar innervated intrinsic hand muscles.
- *Deep terminal branch distal to hypothenar muscles:* no sensory loss, normal ADM, other ulnar intrinsic hand muscles weak.
- *Superficial terminal branch only:* ulnar territory sensory loss only.

This patient's deficits correspond electrodiagnostically to the third category.

Further evaluation included MRI of the wrist (see figure 2), which demonstrated a dumbell-shaped fluid collection adjacent to the hamate and Guyon's canal (arrow), displacing the ulnar nerve and artery (the neurovascular bundle, arrowhead). The appearance was typical of a ganglion cyst. Surgical exploration with removal of the mass and subsequent pathologic examination revealed a ganglionic cyst.

Ulnar neuropathy at the wrist is uncommon and may be due to a wide range of structural lesions, including hemorrhage, anomalous musculature, lipoma, or ganglionic cyst. External pressure, such as in bicycle riders and construction workers operating heavy drills, is another cause; note that the mechanism of external pressure is chronic compression but not entrapment (*i.e.,* compressive neuropathy ≠ entrapment neuropathy).

Electrodiagnostic techniques for specific use in the evaluation of ulnar neuropathies at the wrist include short segmental ("inching") studies recording from FDI, as well as the use of the median–ulnar second lumbrical–interosseous latency difference. The latter study, discussed in case 3, is generally of value in the diagnosis of severe carpal tunnel syndrome but may also be helpful for ulnar neuropathy at the wrist.

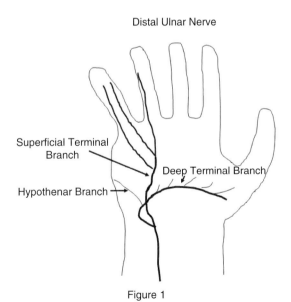

Distal Ulnar Nerve

Superficial Terminal Branch

Deep Terminal Branch

Hypothenar Branch

Figure 1

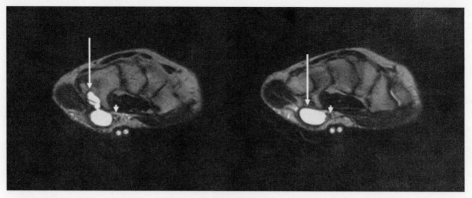

Figure 2

Clinical Pearls

1. Ulnar neuropathy at the wrist is uncommon; consideration of causes should always include masses.

2. Ulnar neuropathy at the wrist has a variety of patterns with varying sensory and motor involvement.

REFERENCES

1. Bui-Mansfield, L.T., Williamson, M., Wheeler, D.T., Johnstone, F., Guyon's canal lipoma causing ulnar neuropathy, *Am J Roentgenol.* 2002; 178:1458.
2. Elias, D.A., Lax, M.J., Anastakis, D.J., Musculoskeletal images: ganglion cyst of Guyon's canal causing ulnar nerve compression, *Can. J. Surg.* 2001; 44:331–332.
3. Kothari, M.J., Ulnar neuropathy at the wrist, *Neurol. Clin.* 1999; 17:463–476.
4. Kothari, M.J., Preston, D.C., Logigian, E.L., Lumbrical–interossei motor studies localize ulnar neuropathy at the wrist. *Muscle Nerve* 1996; 19:170–174.
5. McIntosh, K.A., Preston, D.C., Logigian, E.L., Short-segment incremental studies to localize ulnar nerve entrapment at the wrist, *Neurology* 1998; 50:303–306.
6. Olney, R.K., Hanson, M., AAEE case report #15: ulnar neuropathy at or distal to the wrist, *Muscle Nerve* 1988; 11:828–832.
7. Stewart, J.D., *Focal Peripheral Neuropathies*, 3rd ed., Lippincott Williams & Wilkins, Philadelphia, PA, 2000, pp. 267–268.

PATIENT 8

A 40-year-old woman referred for possible left carpal tunnel syndrome or ulnar neuropathy

Electrodiagnostic Study:

Sensory NCS

Nerve	Sites	Recording Site	Onset (ms)	Peak (ms)	Amplitude (µV)	Distance (cm)	Velocity (m/s)
L. median–dig II	1. Wrist	Dig II	2.50	3.30	51.4	13	52.0
L. ulnar–dig V	1. Wrist	Dig V	2.00	2.55	58.5	11	55.0
L. median–ulnar	1. Median–palm	Wrist	2.00	2.45	47.1	8	40.0
(palmar)	2. Ulnar–palm	Wrist	1.20	1.65	27.3	8	66.7
L. median–ulnar	1. Med wrist	Elbow	4.30	5.35	10.1	34	79.1
(elbow)	2. Uln wrist	Elbow	4.55	5.55	12.0	34	74.7

Motor NCS

Nerve	Sites	Recording Site	Latency (ms)	Amplitude (mV)	Distance (cm)	Velocity (m/s)
L. median–APB	1. Wrist	APB	3.85	7.3	7	—
	2. Elbow	APB	7.10	9.2	21	64.6
L. ulnar–ADM	1. Wrist	ADM	2.50	9.8	7	—
	2. B. elbow	ADM	5.70	7.1	21	65.6
	3. A. elbow	ADM	7.40	7.0	9	52.9
L. median–ADM	1. Med wrist	ADM	No response		—	—
	2. Med elbow	ADM	6.75	1.0	—	—
L. ulnar–FDI	1. Wrist	FDI	3.55	11.4	—	—
	2. B. elbow	FDI	6.85	7.3	—	—
	3. A. elbow	FDI	8.40	7.6	—	—
L. median–vs. ulnar	1. Median	Lumb	3.75	2.2	10	—
	2. Ulnar	Inteross	3.25	8.1	10	—

Questions:
1. What is the conclusion of the electrodiagnostic studies?
2. Do you think the drop in the amplitudes of the ulnar–ADM and ulnar–FDI CMAPs going from wrist to below-elbow stimulation are due to technical reasons? Look at the waveforms in the first two figures.
3. Note the increase in amplitude and change in morphology of the median–APB CMAP going from wrist to elbow stimulation. Does this clarify the situation? What additional nerve conduction study should be done?

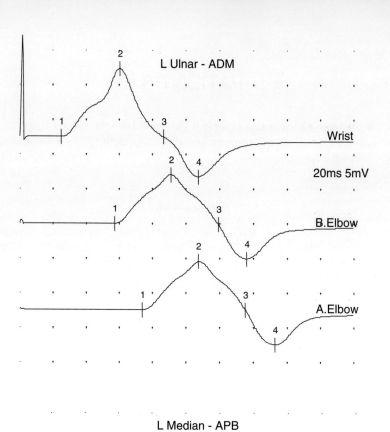

L Ulnar - ADM

Wrist

20ms 5mV

B.Elbow

A.Elbow

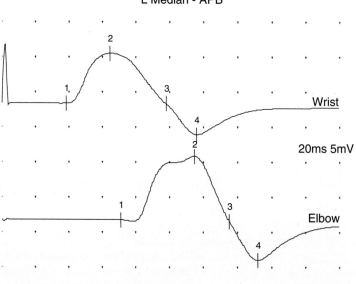

L Median - APB

Wrist

20ms 5mV

Elbow

L Median - ADM

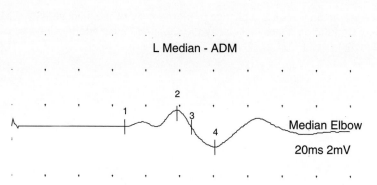

Median Elbow

20ms 2mV

Answers:
1. There is a Martin-Gruber anastomosis.
2. No.
3. Stimulate the median nerve at the elbow recording at ADM.

Discussion: The waveform from the additional study is shown in the third figure. The median nerve is stimulated at the elbow and a CMAP recorded from the ADM. An initial negative (upward) deflection indicates that axons innervating this muscle lie within the median nerve at the elbow. This anatomical variation is the Martin-Gruber anastomosis (MGA). The typical findings of an MGA are those of this case: (1) the median-APB CMAP *increases* with elbow stimulation, (2) the ulnar-ADM CMAP *decreases* with below-elbow stimulation, and (3) a CMAP is present in the ADM or FDI when stimulating the median nerve at the elbow. These findings are due, respectively, to (1) median nerve axons in the proximal forearm crossing over to the ulnar nerve distally and then innervating the flexor pollicis brevis (FPB) short head through the ulnar nerve at the wrist (because the FPB is adjacent to the APB, the thenar CMAP is summated by the FPB activation), and (2) the presence of axons innervating ADM in the ulnar nerve at the wrist but (3) in the median nerve in the proximal forearm. The changes in the proximal evoked median and ulnar CMAPs suggest the presence of an MGA. The only way to be sure of one is to stimulate the median nerve at the elbow and record over the ADM, as shown in the third figure. In rare circumstances, collision studies are required. Stimulating ulnar nerve (recording over thenar muscles) is not helpful, because the ulnar nerve normally innervates thenar muscles, including variably APB.

Clinical Pearls

1. Martin-Gruber anastomoses are common anatomical variants that should be considered when stimulation at the elbow results in a larger median and a smaller ulnar compound muscle action potential than distal stimulation.

2. Although several types of MGA exist, routine electrodiagnostic studies reliably detect only median-to-ulnar communications, through stimulation of the median nerve at the elbow and recording at ADM.

REFERENCES

1. Claussen, G.C., Ahmad, B.K., Sunwoo, I.N., Oh, S., Combined motor and sensory median-ulnar anastomosis: report of an electrophysiologically proven case, *Muscle Nerve* 1996; 19:231–233.
2. Crutchfield, C., Gutmann, L., Hereditary aspects of median–ulnar nerve communications, *J. Neurol. Neurosurg. Psychiatry* 1980; 43:53–55.
3. Oh, S.J., Claussen, G.C., Ahmad, B.K., Double anastomosis of median–ulnar and ulnar–median nerves: report of an electrophysiologically proven case, *Muscle Nerve* 1995; 18:1332–1334.
4. Streib, E.W., Sun, S.F., Martin–Gruber anastomosis: electromyographic studies, Part 1, *Electromyogr. Clin. Neurophysiol.* 1983; 23:261–270.
5. Sun, S.F., Streib, E.W., Martin–Gruber anastomosis: electromyographic studies, Part 2, *Electromyogr. Clin. Neurophysiol.* 1983; 23:271–285.

PATIENT 9

A 68-year-old-man with metastatic melanoma and progressive left wrist drop for several months

Electrodiagnostic Study:

Sensory NCS

Nerve	Sites	Recording Site	Onset (ms)	Peak (ms)	BP Amplitude (µV)	Distance (cm)	Velocity (m/s)
L. median–dig II	1. Wrist	Dig II	2.60	3.50	17.2	13	50.0
L. ulnar–dig V	1. Wrist	Dig V	2.60	3.25	10.8	11	42.3
L. radial–sn box	1. Forearm	Sn box	2.00	2.60	9.0	10	50.0
R. radial–sn box	1. Forearm	Sn box	2.10	2.75	19.7	10	47.6

Motor NCS

Nerve	Sites	Recording Site	Latency (ms)	Amplitude (µV)	Distance (cm)	Velocity (m/s)
L. median–APB	1. Wrist	APB	3.85	6.1	7	—
	2. Elbow	APB	9.25	6.4	26	48.1
L. radial–EIP	1. Forearm	EIP	3.25	0.5	7	—
	2. B. spiral gr	EIP	Not tolerated		—	—

F-Wave

Nerve	F_{min} (ms)	F_{max} (ms)	Max – Min (ms)	%F
L. median	33.50	36.95	3.45	—

Needle EMG Summary Table

		SA			Amplitude (MUs)	Duration (MUs)	PolyP (MUs)	Activation	Recruitment Pattern
	IA	Fib	Fasc	Other					
L. triceps	Incr	3+	0	0	Nl	Nl	Nl	Full	ModRed
L. brachiorad	Incr	4+	0	0	Nl	Nl	Nl	Full	SevRed
L. ext dig comm	Incr	3+	0	0	Nl	Long	Nl	Full	SevRed
L. deltoid	Nl	0	0	0	Nl	Nl	Nl	Full	Nl
L. biceps	Nl	0	0	0	Nl	Nl	Nl	Full	Nl
L. pron teres	Nl	0	0	0	Nl	Nl	Nl	Full	Nl
L. flex carp uln	Nl	0	0	0	Nl	Nl	Nl	Full	Nl

Questions:

1. What is the most likely localization suggested by the electrodiagnostic studies?
2. Are the nerve conduction studies alone, without the needle EMG findings, highly suggestive of this localization, or do they equally support other possible localizations? What single needle EMG muscle study would most distinguish among the remaining possibilities?

Answers:

1. Proximal radial neuropathy
2. There could be a posterior cord lesion as well. The deltoid also needs to be checked.

Discussion: The nerve conduction studies are abnormal for a greater than 50% reduction of the left radial–webspace SNAP compared to the right. The amplitude of the radial-extensor indicis proprius (EIP) distal evoked CMAP is also small, at 0.5 mV. These findings suggest a radial neuropathy or posterior cord plexopathy. Root disease does not generally reduce SNAP amplitudes, and the radial SNAP and CMAP have different trunk (upper vs. middle/lower) innervations; however, they both could be reduced from a posterior cord lesion. Accordingly, the needle EMG muscle study that would most readily distinguish between a radial neuropathy and posterior cord lesion is the deltoid muscle, supplied by the axillary nerve from the posterior cord. If normal, a radial neuropathy is more likely; if abnormal, a posterior cord lesion is more likely. This is a general rule: *Do not forget to study the deltoid in patients with suspected radial neuropathy to exclude a more proximal posterior cord lesion as the cause.*

This patient has a radial neuropathy. The reduction of the SNAP and the neurogenic abnormalities in the triceps and brachioradialis place the lesion proximal to the posterior interosseous nerve alone. Radial neuropathies typically produce wrist drop. A common cause is acute compression of the nerve, the so-called Saturday-night palsy. There is no accepted entrapment cause (the existence of an entrapment syndrome at the radial tunnel is dubious and extremely rare at best), and chronic compression is quite uncommon, but it does occur in patients using crutches. Confusing physical examination findings in patients with radial neuropathy may include mild arm flexion weakness (from brachioradialis weakness) and moderate to severe finger abductor weakness because of the flexed position of the fingers at the metacarpophalangeal (MCP) joints and the loss of mechanical advantage in this position.

Clinical Pearls

1. Radial neuropathy should always be distinguished from posterior cord lesions by needle examination of the deltoid.

2. Confusing clinical features of radial neuropathies are apparent ulnar hand weakness (from loss of mechanical advantage) and arm flexion weakness (from brachioradialis weakness).

REFERENCES

1. Carlson, N., Logigian, E.L., Radial neuropathy, *Neurol. Clin.* 1999; 17:499–523.
2. Stewart, J.D., *Focal Peripheral Neuropathies*, 3rd ed., Lippincott Williams & Wilkins, Philadelphia, PA, 2000.

PATIENT 10

A 43-year-old man with scapular winging after a cervical lymph node biopsy

This 43-year-old man with lymphoma developed recurrent lymphadenopathy in his left neck and underwent biopsy under local anesthesia. After returning home, he noticed difficulty raising his left arm over his head that persisted, and he was referred for electrodiagnostic studies 7 months later. General physical examination was notable for a well-healed scar in the posterior triangle of the left neck. Neurologic examination was notable for the appearance of enlargement of the suprascapular region when viewed anteriorly, as indicated by the arrowhead in figure 1B, and a slight drooping of the left shoulder (arrow). Arm abduction and flexion at the shoulder resulted in lateral and superior displacement of the scapula, as shown in the top portion of the figure, and mild posterior displacement off the back, as can be seen in the second figure. A dimpling in the area of the middle trapezius was noted with these maneuvers (arrow in figure 1A).

Electrodiagnostic Study: Sensory and motor nerve conduction studies are normal.

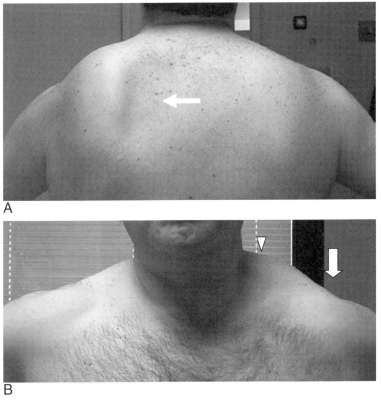

Figure 1

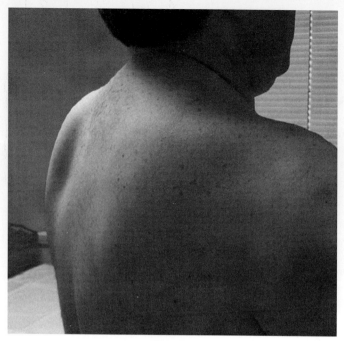

Figure 2

Needle EMG Summary Table

	IA	Fib	Fasc	Other	Amplitude (MUs)	Duration (MUs)	PolyP (MUs)	Activation	Recruitment Pattern
		SA							
L. deltoid	Nl	0	0	0	Nl	Nl	Nl	Full	Nl
L. serr ant	Nl	0	0	0	Nl	Nl	Nl	Full	Nl
L. infra-spinatus	Nl	0	0	0	Nl	Nl	Nl	Full	Nl
L. teres minor	Nl	0	0	0	Nl	Nl	Nl	Full	Nl
L. trapezius upper	Incr	1–2+	0	0	Nl	Nl	Few	Full	Nl
L. trapezius middle	Incr	2–3+	0	0					No units
L. trapezius lower	Nl	0	0	0	Nl	Nl	Few	Full	Nl
L. strenoclei domastoid	Nl	0	0	0	Nl	Nl	Few	Full	Nl

Questions:
1. What is the localization suggested by the electrodiagnostic studies?
2. What nerve lies in the posterior triangle of the neck?

Answers:
1. Spinal accessory nerve branch lesion
2. The spinal accessory nerve

Discussion: Scapula winging may be due to weakness of serratus anterior, trapezius, or rhomboid muscles. This patient has an iatrogenic injury to the accessory nerve, which is a recognized complication of cervical lymph node biopsy in the posterior triangle of the neck. Any surgeon performing such biopsies should be aware of this potential complication and must meticulously avoid this nerve. The lesion is distal to the branch to the sternocleidomastoid, which is not involved. Marked differential involvement of the three portions of the trapezius is present in this case; no motor units are recruited in the middle trapezius, and normal recruitment patterns are present in the upper and lower portions. Presumably, this is a lesion of the fascicle or branch of the nerve limited to supplying the middle trapezius.

Trapezius weakness results in drooping of the shoulder at rest. Figure 3 shows another patient with such drooping from a spinal accessory nerve palsy after radical neck dissection for oral cancer. Often there appears to be hypertrophy of the upper trapezius when the patient is viewed from the front (see arrowhead in figure 1B). In fact, upward displacement of the scapula because of middle and lower trapezius paralysis and the unopposed action of levator scapulae and rhomboids gives this appearance, which is evident from behind. With flexion or abduction, the scapula moves *laterally* and sometimes upward typically with only mild posterior displacement of the scapula (see figures 1 and 2). Atrophy of the trapezius may be evident (middle trapezius atrophy, as indicated by arrow in figure 1A).

Complete absence of recruitable motor units in the middle trapezius at 7 months suggests a very poor prognosis in this particular clinical setting, but not in all. The absence of demonstrable nerve continuity in the setting of a likely surgical lesion of the nerve makes recovery unlikely. In contrast, had this been a stretch or anesthetic injury to the accessory nerve, the absence of recruitable motor units at 7 months would warrant at least some optimism that recovery at 12 to 15 months was still possible.

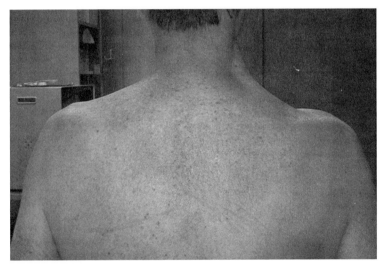

Figure 3

Clinical Pearls

1. The spinal accessory nerve lies in the posterior triangle of the neck and is susceptible to injury with lymph node biopsies.

2. Scapula winging may be due to weakness of serratus anterior, trapezius, or rhomboid muscles; the pattern of movement of the scapula with abduction and flexion of the arm is different among these different causes.

REFERENCES

1. Berry, H., MacDonald, E.A., Mrazel, A.C., Accessory nerve palsy: a review of 23 cases, *Can. J. Neurol. Sci.* 1991; 18:337–341.
2. Gordon, S.L., Graham, W.P., Black, J.T., Miller, S.H., Accessory nerve function after surgical procedures in the posterior triangle, *Arch. Surg.* 1977; 112:264–268.
3. Friedenberg, S.M., Zimprich, T., Harper, C.M., The natural history of long thoracic and spinal accessory neuropathies, *Muscle Nerve* 2002; 25(4):535–539.
4. Saeed, M.A., Gatens, P.F., Singh, S., Winging of the scapula, *Am. Fam. Physician* 1981; 42:139–143.
5. Stewart, J.D., *Focal Peripheral Neuropathies*, 3rd ed., Lippincott Williams & Wilkins, Philadelphia, PA, 2000.

PATIENT 11

A 51-year-old man with scapular winging after arthroscopic shoulder surgery

This 51-year-old man developed right shoulder pain while lifting the top on his convertible and could not use his arm for several days because of pain with movement. Weakness of external rotation was noted by an orthopedic specialist. Rotator cuff tear was suspected and confirmed with MRI arthrogram, which demonstrated a partial thickness tear of the supraspinatus and infraspinatus tendons. The patient underwent arthroscopic surgery performed with an interscalene brachial plexus block followed by general anesthesia. Postoperatively, he had difficulty with forward flexion of the arm and raising it above his head. Two weeks later, a physical therapist noted winging of his right scapula, and he was referred for electrodiagnostic consultation 6 months postoperatively. Neurologic examination was notable for a thin man with prominent scapula bilaterally. At rest, the right scapula was displaced superiorly compared to the left, and marked atrophy of infraspinatus was present (see figure 1). With arm abduction and forward flexion, marked winging of the right scapula was characterized by medial movement of the scapula as well as posterior displacement of the inferior angle of the scapula off the back (see figure 2).

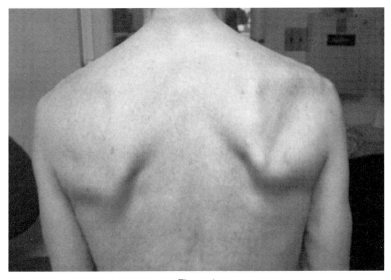

Figure 1

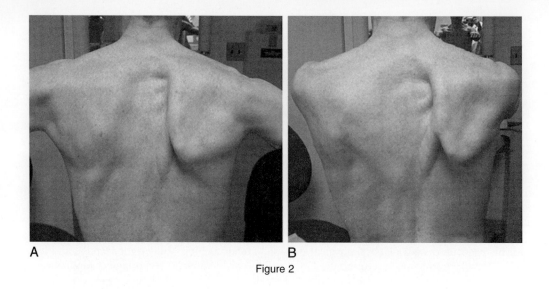

A   B

Figure 2

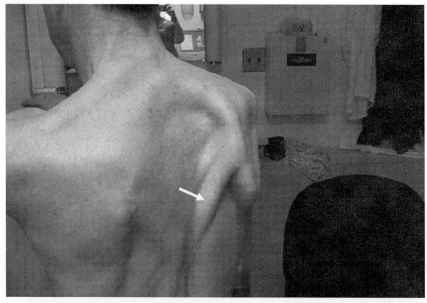

Figure 3

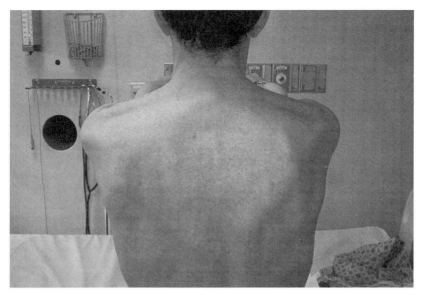

Figure 4

Stop and Consider: Scapular winging may be seen with weakness of any of three muscle groups. Name these groups and the distinct patterns of scapular winging seen with each. Plan the electrodiagnostic study.

Electrodiagnostic Study:

Sensory NCS

Nerve	Sites	Recording Site	Onset (ms)	Peak (ms)	Amplitude (µV)	Distance (cm)	Velocity (m/s)
R. median–dig II	1. Wrist	Dig II	2.55	3.40	46.9	13	51.0
R. ulnar–dig V	1. Wrist	Dig V	2.35	3.10	28.0	11	46.8
R. radial–sn box	1. Forearm	Sn box	1.75	2.35	47.8	10	57.1
R. med AB cut	1. Elbow	Forearm	2.00	2.50	23.5	—	—
R. lat AB cut	1. Elbow	Forearm	2.25	2.80	22.0	12	53.3

Motor NCS

Nerve	Sites	Recording Site	Latency (ms)	Amplitude (mV)	Distance (cm)	Velocity (m/s)
R. median–APB	1. Wrist	APB	3.95	13.8	7	—
	2. Elbow	APB	7.90	13.8	22	55.7
R. ulnar–ADM	1. Wrist	ADM	3.05	13.2	7	—
	2. B. elbow	ADM	6.60	13.1	21	59.2
	3. A. elbow	ADM	8.55	12.4	11	56.4

F-Wave

Nerve	F_{min} (ms)	F_{max} (ms)	Max − Min (ms)	%F
R. median	27.70	29.25	1.55	100

Needle EMG Summary Table

	IA	SA			Amplitude (MUs)	Duration (MUs)	PolyP (MUs)	Activation	Recruitment Pattern
		Fib	Fasc	Other					
R. serr ant	Incr	3+	0	0	Nl	Nl	Nl	Full	No activity
R. infraspinatus	Incr	3+	0	0	Nl	Nl	Nl	Full	No activity
R. deltoid	Nl	0	0	0	Nl	Nl	Nl	Full	Nl
R. supra spinatus	Nl	0	0	0	Nl	Nl	Nl	Full	Nl
R. levator scapulae	Nl	0	0	0	Nl	Nl	Nl	Full	Nl
R. rhomb maj	Nl	0	0	0	Nl	Nl	Nl	Full	Nl
R. trapezius (U)	Nl	0	0	0	Nl	Nl	Nl	Full	Nl
R. trapezius (L)	Nl	0	0	0	Nl	Nl	Nl	Full	Nl
R. lattisimus dorsi	Nl	0	0	0	Nl	Nl	Nl	Full	Nl
R. teres major	Nl	0	0	0	Nl	Nl	Nl	Full	Nl

Questions:
1. What muscle does the arrow in figure 3 point to?
2. What is the value of the sensory and motor studies in this case?
3. What is the conclusion of the electrodiagnostic studies?
4. Given this study 6 months postoperatively, what is the prognosis and what management do you recommend now?

Answers:

1. Lower trapezius
2. To exclude a more generalized brachial plexopathy
3. Long thoracic neuropathy and branch suprascapular neuropathy
4. Prognosis is uncertain; it is too early to assess. Conservative therapy is recommended.

Discussion: Scapula winging may be due to weakness of serratus anterior, trapezius, or rhomboid muscles (see patient 10 as well). Certainly more generalized shoulder girdle weakness—for example, from facioscapulohumeral muscular dystrophy or myasthenia gravis—can also result in scapula winging. When due to a focal neuropathy, the pattern of winging is distinctive among the three causes. This patient has a long thoracic neuropathy. Lesions of the long thoracic nerve result in serratus anterior weakness. Arm flexion and abduction result in *medial* movement of the scapula, particularly the inferior angle, as well as more marked posterior displacement off the back than that seen with trapezius or rhomboid weakness. The arrow in the third figure points to the contracting lower trapezius that is attempting to compensate for serratus anterior weakness and counteract the posterior displacement of the scapula.

Accessory nerve lesions result in trapezius weakness, which was shown in another patient in case 10 (see figures). Isolated dorsal scapular neuropathies resulting in rhomboid and possibly levator scapulae weakness are rare, and the resulting pattern of winging is not well described in the literature.

In this case, the electrodiagnostic studies demonstrate fibrillation potentials in the serratus anterior and infraspinatus, but not supraspinatus, suggesting lesions of the long thoracic nerve and a distal or fascicular lesion of the suprascapular nerve. The lack of sensory and motor abnormalities in the arm provides evidence against a more generalized brachial plexopathy, as might be seen in acute brachial neuritis. Additional EMG studies provide evidence against an accessory neuropathy, dorsal scapular neuropathy, or a lesion of the cervical plexus, from which the levator scapulae receives a predictable motor supply. The long thoracic neuropathy was likely a perioperative complication attributable to the interscalene plexus anesthetic block or surgical positioning or traction on the shoulder. The distal or fascicular lesion of the suprascapular nerve is not well understood in this case; the patient had weakness of external rotation prior to surgery. Complete absence of recruitable motor units in serratus anterior at 6 months suggested a poor prognosis, although it was considered too early to give this prognosis to the patient. Repeat clinical and electrodiagnostic assessment at 12 and 18 months was done. At 12 months, motor unit action potentials were present in the serratus and at 18 months movement of the scapula had nearly recovered (see figure 4 and compare to figure 2).

Clinical Pearls

1. In long thoracic nerve palsies, arm flexion and abduction result in *medial* movement of the scapula, particularly the inferior angle, as well as more marked posterior displacement off the back than that seen with trapezius or rhomboid weakness.

2. Unless surgical or traumatic laceration of the nerve is suspected, prognosis cannot be adequately predicted prior to 1 to 2 years.

REFERENCES

1. Friedenberg, S.M., Zimprich, T., Harper, C.M., The natural history of long thoracic and spinal accessory neuropathies, *Muscle Nerve* 2002; 25(4):535–539.
2. Frank, D.K., Wenk, E., Stern, J.C., Gottlieb, R.D., Moscatello, A.L., A cadaveric study of the motor nerves to the levator scapulae muscle, *Otolaryngol. Head Neck Surg.* 1997; 117(6):671–680.
3. Saeed, M.A., Gatens, P.F., Singh, S., Winging of the scapula, *Am. Fam. Physician* 1981; 42:139–143.
4. Stewart, J.D., *Focal Peripheral Neuropathies*, 3rd ed., Lippincott Williams & Wilkins, Philadelphia, PA, 2000.
5. Wiater, J.M., Flatow, E.L., Long thoracic nerve injury, *Clin. Orthop.* 1999; 368:17–27.

PATIENT 12

A 23-year-old woman with progressive weakness, atrophy, and numbness in one hand

This 23-year-old woman noted at age 13 intermittent right arm pain, numbness, and forearm finger flexor cramps. Progressive weakness and atrophy of the right hand and numbness in the medial forearm and medial palm developed at age 20. Examination showed moderate weakness without atrophy of ADM and severe atrophy and weakness of FDI and APB (see figure 1). Strength was normal for the pronator teres, flexor pollicis longus, all finger flexors, and flexor carpi ulnaris. A sensory disturbance was present in the right medial hand and forearm (see figure 2).

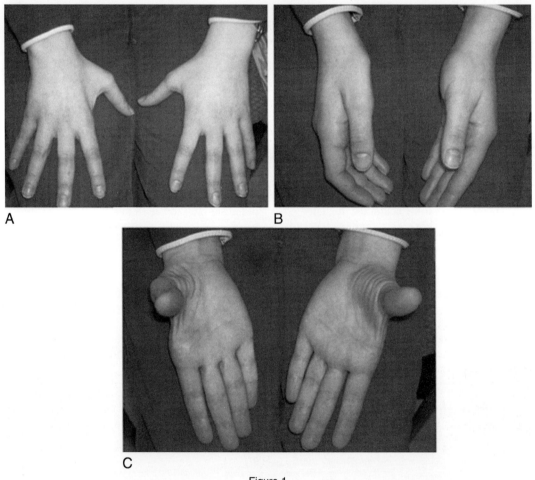

A

B

C

Figure 1

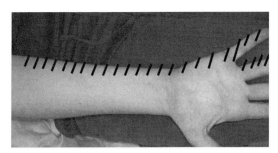

Figure 2

Electrodiagnostic Study:

Sensory NCS

Nerve	Amplitude (μV)	Velocity (m/s)
R. median–dig II	75	52.0
R. ulnar–dig V	Absent	—
R. ulnar dorsal	Absent	—
R. lat AB cut	19	61.5
R. med AB cut	Absent	—
L. median–dig II	64	52.0
L. ulnar–dig V	53	48.9
L. ulnar dorsal	19	62.5
L. med AB cut	12	63.2

Motor NCS

Nerve	Sites	Latency (ms)	Amplitude (mV)	Velocity (m/s)
R. median–APB	1. Wrist	—	Absent	—
R. ulnar–FDI	1. Wrist	4.55	4.7	—
	2. B. elbow	8.55	4.8	42.5
	3. A. elbow	9.95	4.7	71.4
	4. Axilla	12.10	4.3	46.5
R. ulnar–ADM	1. Wrist	3.85	5.3	—
	2. B. elbow	7.35	5.4	48.6
	3. A. elbow	8.75	5.3	71.4
	4. Axilla	10.70	5.2	51.3
L. ulnar–ADM	1. Wrist	2.55	9.8	—
	2. B. elbow	5.90	9.5	56.7
	3. A. elbow	7.45	9.8	64.5

F-Wave

Nerve	F_{min} (ms)	F_{max} (ms)	Max–min (ms)	Persistence
R. ulnar–ADM	34.65	37.00	2.35	6/10
L. ulnar–ADM	26.60	27.75	1.15	10/10

EMG Summary Table

	SA				Amplitude (MUs)	Duration (MUs)	PolyP (MUs)	Activation	Recruitment Pattern
	IA	Fib	Fasc	Other					
R. ext dig comm	Nl	0	0	0	Nl	Nl	Nl	Full	Nl
R. abd poll br	Nl	2+	0	0	Large	Nl	Nl	Full	Sev red
R. ext indicis	Nl	0	0	0	Nl	Nl	Nl	Full	Nl
R. abd dig min	Nl	1+	0	0	Nl	Nl	Nl	Full	Mild red

Questions:

1. Why is this not the combination of a median and ulnar neuropathy? Why is this not a T1 radiculopathy? What is the localization suggested by the electrodiagnostic studies?
2. Are there F-wave abnormalities and what are their significance?
3. What additional electrodiagnostic studies might be helpful?
4. Would the presence of a right Horner's syndrome be helpful for localization?

1. The median SNAP is normal; it is not T1 because the ulnar SNAP is abnormal. Electrodiagnostic studies suggest a medial cord lesion.
2. A prologed right ulnar F-wave minimum latency suggests focal demyelination.
3. Needle EMG of cervical paraspinals, pronator teres, and FDI
4. A Horner's syndrome would have suggested a T1 localization.

Discussion: This patient has the unusual combination of severe motor axonal loss to APB with a normal median SNAP, making a typical median neuropathy unlikely. The absence of the medial antebrachial cutaneous SNAP is not a feature of an ulnar neuropathy, as this nerve comes directly off the medial cord of the brachial plexus. Radiculopathy would also not account for the reduced amplitudes of SNAPs. The electrodiagnostic findings are those of a lesion of the medial cord of the brachial plexus. The lower trunk is also a reasonable localization to consider, although C8 motor axons in the posterior cord, such as those supplying the extensor digitorum communis (EDC) and extensor indicis proprius (EIP), are a part of the lower trunk, and needle EMG of the EDC and EIP was normal in this case. The right ulnar–ADM minimum F-wave latency is markedly prolonged compared to the other side and, in the setting of only mild reduction in the CMAP amplitude, provides evidence of focal demyelination of motor axons supplying the ADM. The localization of this study is defensible as is, although further EMG studies, including lower cervical paraspinal muscles, median nerve innervated lateral cord muscles (pronator teres and flexor carpi radialis), and additional ulnar-innervated medial cord muscles (FDI, flexor carpi ulnaris), would be of interest. Recall that the lateral cord does not contribute to the ulnar nerve.

In a young person with a longstanding progressive unilateral medial cord or lower trunk lesion, true neurologic thoracic outlet syndrome (n-TOS) is the most likely cause. The diagnosis of TOS is a wastebasket; many patients with strictly pain and no neurological abnormalities are given this diagnosis. Pain without neurologic symptoms is not usually due to a disease of the peripheral nervous system, and the diagnosis of n-TOS is reserved for patients with an actual neurologic deficit. Other processes that may affect the medial cord of the plexus in a young woman would include metastatic invasion and a schwannoma. Syringomyelia may produce hand wasting and a sensory deficit but does not produce this electrodiagnostic picture (*i.e.*, reduction in SNAP amplitudes).

This patient has n-TOS due to bilateral cervical ribs, which were seen on plain radiographs of the cervical spine (figure 3). MRI of the cervical spine and brachial plexus were interpreted as normal by experienced chest radiologists. Distinct angulations of the two cervical ribs probably accounts for the presence of a unilateral disorder. She underwent surgical decompression of the right plexus (figure 4), and at 6 months had moderate improvement, having regained the ability to snap her fingers and button on that side. n-TOS is rare and tends to present in young to middle-aged women. Greater involvement in thenar than hypothenar muscles is characteristic, as in this case. The disorder is often due to a rudimentary radiolucent band from the cervical rib or elongated C7 transverse process to the first thoracic rib. In this case, there was no band; the rib itself compressed and stretched the lower brachial plexus. It has also been stated that the sensory loss in n-TOS does not split the fourth finger but includes both medial and lateral portions; in this case, the sensory disturbance did split this digit.

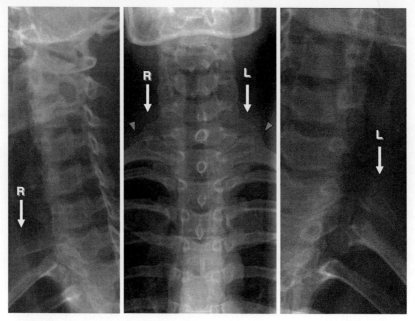

Figure 3

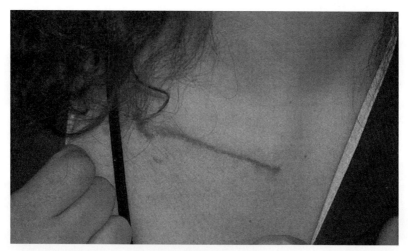

Figure 4

Clinical Pearls

1. The finding of thenar and FDI weakness with ulnar sensory loss is highly suggestive of true neurologic thoracic outlet syndrome.

2. Plain cervical spine films are more effective than MRI imaging for confirming this diagnosis.

REFERENCES

1. Le Forestier, N., Moulonguet, A., Maisonobe, T., Leger, J.M., Bouche, P., True neurogenic thoracic outlet syndrome: electrophysiological diagnosis in six cases, *Muscle Nerve* 1998; 21:1129–1134.
2. Wilbourn, A.J., Thoracic outlet syndromes, *Neurol Clin.* 1999; 17(3):477–497.

PATIENT 13

A 23-year-old man with right arm weakness after a motorcycle accident

This 23-year-old man suffered a severe right arm injury in a motorcycle crash. The patient, who was wearing a helmet, apparently lost control of his motorcycle and rolled the bike over on an exit ramp, leaving the highway at approximately 70 miles per hour. On physical examination, he was awake and alert. There was some soft tissue swelling of the cervical spine and of the right clavicular fossa. There was some thoracic spine tenderness and a laceration over the right scapula. There was a circumferential injury around the right upper extremity extending down to the biceps and triceps and deltoid muscles. His vascular examination was 2+ throughout. There was no motor function from the right elbow distally and no sensation in the right hand. Electrodiagnostic studies performed 18 and 22 months after the injury are presented below.

Electrodiagnostic Study:

Sensory NCS

Nerve	Sites	Recording Site	Onset (ms)	Peak (ms)	Amplitude (µV)	Distance (cm)	Velocity (m/s)
R. median–dig II	1. Wrist	Dig II	1.90	2.70	20.0	13	68.4
R. median–dig III	1. Wrist	Dig II	1.50	2.70	24.9	13	86.7
R. ulnar–dig V	1. Wrist	Dig V	1.75	2.65	27.7	11	62.9
R. radial–sn box	1. Forearm	Sn box	1.45	2.05	6.9	10	69.0
R. med AB cut	1. Elbow	Forearm	1.60	2.25	10.4	12	75.0
R. lat AB cut	1. Elbow	Forearm	1.40	2.05	16.3	—	—

Motor NCS

Nerve	Sites	Recording Site	Latency (ms)	Amplitude (mV)	Distance (cm)	Velocity (m/s)
R. median–APB	1. Wrist	APB	Absent	—	7	—
	2. Elbow	APB	Absent	—	—	—
R. ulnar–ADM	1. Wrist	ADM	Absent	—	7	—
	2. B. elbow	ADM	Absent	—	—	—
	3. A. elbow	ADM	Absent	—	—	—

Needle EMG Summary Table

		SA			Amplitude (MUs)	Duration (MUs)	PolyP (MUs)	Activation	Recruitment Pattern
	IA	Fib	Fasc	Other					
R. deltoid	Incr	3+	0	0	—	—	—	—	No activity
R. biceps	Incr	3+	0	0	—	—	—	—	No activity
R. triceps	Incr	3+	0	0	—	—	—	—	No activity
R. pron teres	Incr	3+	0	0	—	—	—	—	No activity
R. first dors int	Incr	3+	0	0	—	—	—	—	No activity

Continued

Needle EMG Summary Table—cont'd

		SA			Amplitude (MUs)	Duration (MUs)	PolyP (MUs)	Activation	Recruitment Pattern
	IA	Fib	Fasc	Other					
R. C5 paraspinal	Incr	3+	0	0	—	—	—	—	—
R. C6 paraspinal	Incr	3+	0	0	—	—	—	—	—
R. C7 paraspinal	Incr	3+	0	0	—	—	—	—	—
R. C8 paraspinal	Incr	3+	0	0	—	—	—	—	—

EMG Summary Table of Repeat EMG Studies Performed 5 Months Later

		SA			Amplitude (MUs)	Duration (MUs)	PolyP (MUs)	Activation	Recruitment Pattern
	IA	Fib	Fasc	Other					
R. deltoid	Incr	4+	0	0	—	—	—	—	No activity
R. biceps	Incr	4+	0	0	—	—	—	—	No activity
R. triceps	Incr	4+	0	0	—	—	—	—	No activity
R. pron teres	Incr	3+	0	0	—	—	—	—	No activity
R. first dors int	Incr	3+	0	0	—	—	—	—	No activity
R. ext dig comm	Incr	3+	0	0	—	—	—	—	No activity

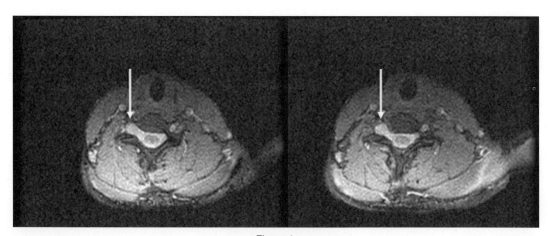

Figure 1

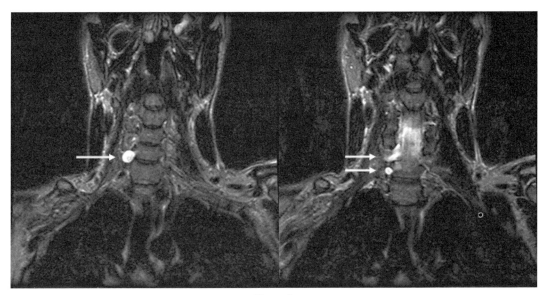

Figure 2

Questions:
1. What important prognostic question should be addressed in traumatic brachial plexopathy studies?
2. What abnormalities are demonstrated in the MRI images in the figures?

Answers:
1. Is there root avulsion?
2. The presence of pseudomeningoceles provides evidence of nerve root avulsion.

Discussion: The severe and diffuse motor involvement is evident from the absent CMAPs, widespread fibrillation potentials, and inability to recruit motor units. An important question in traumatic brachial plexopathy is whether the nerve roots remain intact or have been avulsed from their attachment to the spinal cord. Because the dorsal root ganglia contain the cell bodies of the primary sensory neurons, nerve root avulsion does not in general affect SNAP amplitudes. This allows for an important rule: a root distribution with severe motor axonal loss and normal SNAP amplitudes strongly suggests nerve root avulsion. Of course, root avulsion and more peripheral injury (with reduced SNAP amplitude) may coexist. Brachial plexus studies accordingly focus on the preservation of SNAPs from different root territories, as shown in the following table:

In this case, we note intact lateral antebrachial cutaneous (C6), median–D3 (C7), ulnar–D5 (C8), and medial antebrachial cutaneous (T1) SNAP amplitudes (although ideally they should have been compared to contralateral studies), but severe motor axonal loss in C6 (deltoid, biceps, pronator teres), C7 (triceps, pronator teres, EDC, paraspinals), C8 (EDC, FDI, paraspinals), and T1 (FDI) myotomes. This suggests nerve root avulsion of C6, C7, C8, and T1.

MRI imaging, shown in the figures, confirmed nerve root avulsion at least at C7 and C8 and showed the presence of pseudomeningoceles at these levels.

SNAP	Root
Radial–D1 or radial–webspace	C6
Lat antebrachial cutaneous	C6
Median–D3	C7
Ulnar–D5	C8
Med antebrachial cutaneous	C8/T1

Clinical Pearl

Root avulsion and more peripheral injury often coexist in severe brachial plexus trauma. Electrodiagnostic findings of normal SNAP amplitudes in root distributions with severe motor axonal loss are highly suggestive of root avulsion. Reduction in SNAP amplitudes indicates more peripheral injury, although root avulsion can be present as well.

REFERENCES
1. Aminoff, M.J., Olney, R.K., Parry, G.J., Raskin, N.H., Relative utility of different electrophysiologic techniques in the evaluation of brachial plexopathies, *Neurology* 1988; 38(4):546–550.
2. Di Benedetto, M., Markey, K., Electrodiagnostic localization of traumatic upper trunk brachial plexopathy, *Arch. Phys. Med. Rehabil.* 1984; 65(1):15–17.
3. Ferrante, M.A., Wilbourn, A.J., The utility of various sensory nerve conduction responses in assessing brachial plexopathies, *Muscle Nerve* 1995; 18(8):879–889.
4. Stewart, J.D., *Focal Peripheral Neuropathies*, 3rd ed., Lippincott Williams & Wilkins, Philadelphia, PA, 2000.
5. Wilbourn, A.J., Electrodiagnosis of plexopathies, *Neurol. Clin.* 1985; 3(3):511–529.

PATIENT 14

A 56-year-old woman 2 days after a left shoulder dislocation and closed reduction with diffuse left arm weakness

Neurological exam was notable for normal left shoulder shrug and slight arm abduction and otherwise complete paralysis of all other arm muscles.

Electrodiagnostic Study:

Sensory NCS

Nerve	Sites	Recording Site	Onset (ms)	Peak (ms)	Amplitude (µV)	Distance (cm)	Velocity (m/s)
L. median–dig II	1. Wrist	Dig II	3.05	3.95	17.3	13	42.6
L. ulnar–dig V	1. Wrist	Dig V	2.05	2.60	40.6	11	53.7
L. radial–sn box	1. Forearm	Sn box	1.65	2.15	26.4	10	60.6

Motor NCS

Nerve	Sites	Recording Site	Latency (ms)	Amplitude (mV)	Distance (cm)	Velocity (m/s)
L. median–APB	1. Wrist	APB	4.40	8.6	7	—
	2. Elbow	APB	8.10	7.6	20	54.1
	3. Axilla	APB	9.45	6.5	12	88.9
L. ulnar–ADM	1. Wrist	ADM	2.60	7.1	7	—

F-Wave

Nerve	F_{min} (ms)	F_{max} (ms)	Max – Min (ms)	%F
L. median	No response	—	—	—
L. ulnar	No response	—	—	—

EMG Summary Table

		SA			Amplitude (MUs)	Duration (MUs)	PolyP (MUs)	Activation	Recruitment Pattern
	IA	Fib	Fasc	Other					
L. deltoid	Nl	0	0	0	—	—	—	—	No activity
L. teres minor	Nl	0	0	0	—	—	—	—	No activity
L. biceps	Nl	0	0	0	—	—	—	—	No activity
L. triceps	Nl	0	0	0	—	—	—	—	No activity
L. pron teres	Nl	0	0	0	—	—	—	—	No activity
L. first dors int	Nl	0	0	0	—	—	—	—	No activity

Continued

EMG Summary Table—cont'd

	IA	Fib	Fasc	Other	Amplitude (MUs)	Duration (MUs)	PolyP (MUs)	Activation	Recruitment Pattern
		SA							
L. supra spinatus	Nl	0	0	0	Nl	Nl	Nl	Full	Nl
L. infra spinat	Nl	0	0	0	Nl	Nl	Nl	Full	Nl
L. lev scapuli	Nl	0	0	0	Nl	Nl	Nl	Full	Nl

A second follow-up electrodiagnostic study was performed 5 weeks later, and the results follow.

Sensory NCS

Nerve	Sites	Recording Site	Onset (ms)	Peak (ms)	Amplitude (µV)	Distance (cm)	Velocity (m/s)
L. median–dig II	1. Wrist	Dig II	Absent	—	—	—	—
L. ulnar–dig V	1. Wrist	Dig V	2.20	2.95	5.1	11	50.0
L. radial–sn box	1. Forearm	Sn box	1.40	1.95	23.8	10	71.4

Motor NCS

Nerve	Sites	Recording Site	Latency (ms)	Amplitude (mV)	Distance (cm)	Velocity (m/s)
L. median–APB	1. Wrist	APB	4.65	1.0	7	—
	2. Elbow	APB	10.65	0.7	21	35.0
L. ulnar–ADM	1. Wrist	ADM	2.95	3.7	7	—
	2. B. elbow	ADM	6.55	3.1	18	50.0
	3. A. elbow	ADM	8.55	3.1	10	50.0

F-Wave

Nerve	F_{min} (ms)	F_{max} (ms)	Max − Min (ms)	%F
L. ulnar	Absent	—	—	—
L. median	Absent	—	—	—

EMG Summary Table

	IA	Fib	Fasc	Other	Amplitude (MUs)	Duration (MUs)	PolyP (MUs)	Activation	Recruitment Pattern
		SA							
L. deltoid	Nl	3+	0	0	Nl	Nl	Nl	—	No activity
L. biceps	Nl	4+	0	0	Nl	Nl	Nl	—	No activity
L. first dors int	Nl	4+	0	0	Nl	Nl	Nl	—	No activity
L. abd dig min	Nl	4+	0	0	Nl	Nl	Nl	—	No activit

		SA			Amplitude (MUs)	Duration (MUs)	PolyP (MUs)	Activation	Recruitment Pattern
	IA	Fib	Fasc	Other					
L. flex dig pr II	Nl	4+	0	0	Nl	Nl	Nl	Full	Single MU
L. flex dif pr III	Nl	4+	0	0	Nl	Nl	Nl	Full	Single MU
L. ext dig comm	Nl	3+	0	0	Nl	Nl	Nl	Full	Single MU

Questions:

1. What electrodiagnostic studies are most likely to be abnormal immediately after an acute motor nerve lesion?
2. An experienced clinician's assessment of the patient was conversion disorder or hysterical paralysis. What features of the neurological exam and the electrodiagnostic study refute or support this opinion?
3. What abnormalities did you expect to see in this follow-up study?
4. After reviewing the follow-up study, how would you account for the combination of findings related to the radial sensory study and the needle EMG study of the deltoid and biceps? What additional studies not performed would have been of value in this regard?

Answers:

1. Needle EMG interference pattens and possibly F-waves
2. Hysterical paralysis of an arm usually includes shoulder shrug.
3. Correlates of axonal degeneration
4. Stretch lesions are often not discrete; paraspinal needle EMG should have been performed.

Discussion: This case illustrates the value and limitations of electrodiagnostic studies in the period of time immediately after a nerve lesion. Even complete nerve transection is followed by normal distal evoked amplitudes, distal latency and velocities, and no fibrillation potentials in the hyperacute period, typically for several days. F-wave abnormalities are then quite valuable in demonstrating the proximal nature of the lesion. If the lesion is incomplete, than needle EMG will generally show a reduced (neurogenic) interference pattern in weak muscles. If the lesion is complete, the complete absence of recruited motor units makes it impossible to say whether the weakness is suprasegmental (*i.e.*, reduced effort, unconscious hysterical paralysis, or upper motor neuron weakness) or truly due to lower motor neuron weakness.

In this case, the abnormalities are the absence of F-wave responses (despite normal distal CMAPs) and the complete lack of motor unit recruitment in multiple arm muscles. In hyperacute nerve lesions, the F-wave studies and needle EMG interference patterns are generally the only studies likely to be abnormal. Occasionally, median and ulnar somatosensory evoked potentials may be useful as well.

In addition to the absent F-wave responses noted above, two additional features serve to argue strongly against an hysterical cause of this patient's weakness. Hysterical paralysis of an arm usually includes the upper trapezius; patients generally are not aware that the spinal accessory nerve accounting for shoulder shrug has an anatomic pathway distinct from the other nerves supplying arm function. In addition, both the infraspinatus (suprascapular nerve) and teres minor (axillary nerve) contribute to external rotation of the arm at the shoulder. In this case, the former has a full interference pattern, and the latter shows no recruitable motor units. It is doubtful that such a discrepancy can be attributed to a conscious or unconscious psychogenic mechanism.

The second electrodiagnostic studies demonstrate the correlates of axonal degeneration not yet present in the first study. To summarize the implications:

- Absent median–D2 SNAP suggests an upper trunk or lateral cord lesion; the normal radial SNAP favors the lateral cord localization.
- Reduced ulnar–D5 SNAP, median–APB CMAP, and ulnar–ADM CMAP suggest a lower trunk or medial cord lesion.
- Moderately reduced ulnar–ADM CMAP but inability to recruit motor units voluntarily suggests at least partial focal demyelination of motor nerves in addition to the axonal loss evidenced by the abundant fibrillation potentials present.
- Normal radial SNAP with complete inability to recruit motor units in deltoid is suggestive of C6 nerve root avulsion. An alternative possibility would be combined lesions of the axillary nerve and musculocutaneous nerves.

The last finding is surprising in light of the clinical history. Neglected in this study was examination of the paraspinal muscles, which can be invaluable in determining nerve root avulsion. This possibility was not considered by the electromyographer during the study. Finally, it can be noted that stretch injuries of the plexus are not discrete lesions, and it is possible to differentially affect fibers within the same nerve bundle; this may be the explanation for findings that do not precisely localize.

Evolution of electrodiagnostic abnormalities after acute axonal injury is generally occurs as follows:

- Abnormalities in F-wave, H-reflexes, and needle EMG interference patterns
- Reduction in CMAP amplitude without fibrillation potentials due to neuromuscular transmission failure
- Reduction in SNAP amplitude after Wallerian degeneration has proceeded distally to the point of nerve stimulation
- Continued reduction in CMAP amplitude with development of fibrillation potentials as Wallerian degeneration reaches distally

Clinical Pearl

Although fibrillation potentials may take several weeks to develop after an acute axonal injury, other abnormalities (F-waves, motor unit recruitment patterns) are present immediately, and electrodiagnostic studies can be helpful even early after an injury.

PATIENT 15

A 56-year-old man with painful left hand weakness

This 56-year-old man developed aching pain in his left upper arm that lasted several days and was followed by an inability to bend his thumb, index, and middle fingers. Pain resolved, but weakness persisted, and he underwent electrodiagnostic studies at 8 months. There was no numbness in his hand or arm. Neurological exam was notable for normal sensation and weakness of forearm pronation and supination; the findings are shown in the figure.

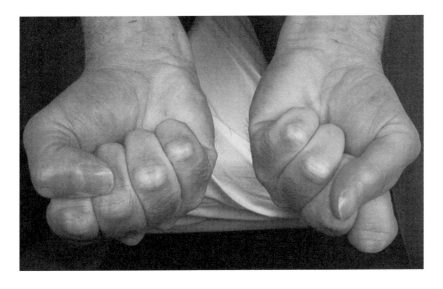

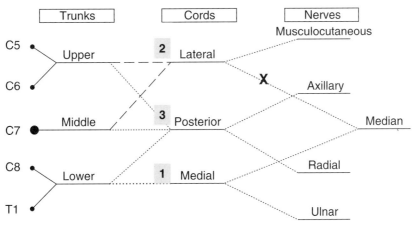

Electrodiagnostic Study:

Sensory NCS

Nerve	Sites	Recording Site	Onset (ms)	Peak (ms)	BP Amplitude (μV)	Distance (cm)	Velocity (m/s)
L. median–dig II	1. Wrist	Dig II	2.30	3.05	26.0	13	56.5
R. median–dig II	1. Wrist	Dig II	2.80	3.45	22.4	13	46.4
L. ulnar–dig V	1. Wrist	Dig V	2.25	2.85	21.2	11	48.9
L. radial–sn box	1. Forearm	Sn box	1.60	2.35	19.8	10	62.5
L. med AB cut	1. Elbow	Forearm	1.90	2.40	7.4	12	63.2
R. med AB cut	1. Elbow	Forearm	2.10	2.55	6.0	12	57.1
L. lat AB cut	1. Elbow	Forearm	2.65	3.15	5.9	12	45.3
R. lat AB cut	1. Elbow	Forearm	2.45	2.95	7.5	12	49.0

Motor NCS

Nerve	Sites	Recording Site	Latency (ms)	Amplitude (mV)	Distance (cm)	Velocity (m/s)
L. median–APB	1. Wrist	APB	3.35	7.0	7	—
	2. Elbow	APB	7.80	6.2	22.5	50.6
L. ulnar–ADM	1. Wrist	ADM	3.05	8.5	7	—
	2. B. elbow	ADM	6.25	8.5	21	65.6
	3. A. elbow	ADM	7.75	8.3	10	66.7

F-Wave

Nerve	F_{min} (ms)	F_{max} (ms)	Max – Min (ms)	%F
L. median	29.70	32.30	2.60	70
L. ulnar	29.70	31.05	1.35	90

Needle EMG Summary Table

		SA			Amplitude (MUs)	Duration (MUs)	PolyP (MUs)	Activation	Recruitment Pattern
	IA	Fib	Fasc	Other					
L. deltoid	Nl	0	0	0	Nl	Nl	Few	Full	Nl
L. biceps	Nl	0	0	0	Nl	Nl	Nl	Full	Nl
L. triceps	Nl	0	0	0	Nl	Nl	Nl	Full	Nl
L. pron teres	Nl	3+	0	0	Nl	Nl	Nl	Sub max	Nl
L. flex carp rad	Nl	2+	0	0	Nl	Nl	Nl	Full	Nl
L. flex poll ln	Nl	2+	0	0	Nl	Nl	Nl	Full	No activity
L. supinator	Nl	1+	0	0	Nl	Nl	Nl	Full	Nl
L. ext dig comm	Nl	0	0	0	Nl	Nl	Nl	Full	Nl
L. brachio-rad	Nl	0	0	0	Nl	Nl	Nl	Full	Nl
L. APB	Nl	0	0	0	Nl	Nl	Nl	Full	Nl

1. How do you best explain the pronator teres and flexor carpi radialis involvement without the APB involvement in this case? Putting aside the supinator involvement for a moment, are the remaining findings best explained by a proximal median neuropathy? Give three electrophysiological reasons why "no" is the answer to this question.
2. The patient was asked to make a fist with both hands (see figure). What are the findings present?

Answers:

1. The median-D2 SNAP is of normal amplitude, the median-APB CMAP is of normal amplitude, and the needle EMG study of APB is normal.
2. Weakness of left FPL and flexion of digits 2 and 3

Discussion: The figure shows severe weakness of flexion of the left thumb distal phalanx and less ability to fully flex the left second and third digits (note that the proximal interphalangeal joints of the index and ring fingers are not as fully tucked in on the left as on the right). The thumb weakness is that of flexor pollicis longus (FPL), and one cannot tell from the picture if the difficulty with digits 2 and 3 is due to weakness of flexion at the distal interphalangeal joints (flexor digitorum profundus, FDP) or at the proximal interphalangeal joints (flexor digitorum superficialis, FDS). Clinical exam demonstrated weakness of FDP digits 2 and 3 with normal strength for FDS 2 and 3. Strength was normal for FDP digits 4 and 5.

The electrodiagnostic study showed symmetric amplitudes of all sensory nerve action potentials. The needle EMG study was notable for the complete absence of recruitable motor units in the FPL, as well as fibrillation potentials in the pronator teres, flexor carpi radialis, and supinator. Clinically, the patient appears to have at least an anterior interosseous neuropathy, with weakness of flexion of the distal tips of digits 1 to 3, a deficit he reported in the initial history. Given the involvement of the pronator teres and flexor carpi radialis as well, one is tempted to suggest a proximal median neuropathy rather than an anterior interosseous neuropathy. There are three arguments against this: (1) the median–D2 SNAP has normal amplitude, (2) the median–APB CMAP has normal amplitude, and (3) the needle EMG study of APB was normal. Recall also that the patient did not have any sensory symptoms or findings.

The involvement of the pronator teres (PT) and flexor carpi radialis (FCR) is probably best explained by a lesion of the median nerve portion of the lateral cord. Recall the median nerve receives a branch from the lateral cord and from the medial cord; PT and FCR are the two lateral cord median-innervated muscles, while all other median-innervated muscles are medial cord. In this case, the patient appears to have a lesion of the anterior interosseous nerve and of the unnamed branch from the lateral cord to the median nerve (marked with an X in the figure). A more proximal lateral cord lesion is probably not present given the normal lateral antebrachial cutaneous SNAP and the normal needle EMG study of the biceps. In addition, the patient seems to have isolated supinator involvement, without other features of a radial neuropathy (normal radial SNAP and EMG of brachioradialis), posterior cord lesion (normal radial SNAP, deltoid, triceps, brachioradialis, and EDC), or C7 or C8 root lesion (normal triceps and EDC). Such isolated and unusual focal neuropathies are characteristic of the diagnosis of acute brachial neuritis.

Acute brachial neuritis, also referred to as neuralgic amyotrophy or the Parsonnage–Turner syndrome, is a disorder of unknown cause, with typical features of acute and severe pain in the shoulder, shoulder blade, or arm for several days or a week or so, followed by multifocal weakness of the arm with variable and usually relatively minor sensory symptoms and findings. The diversity of this disease is impressive and includes remarkable focality such as involvement of the nerve branch to a single muscle. Involvement of certain nerves, such as the anterior interosseous or posterior interosseous, occurs so regularly in this disorder, and not in the much more common compression syndromes, that their involvement always raises acute brachial neuritis as a consideration.

Clinical Pearls

1. Acute brachial neuritis may present with more distal appearing lesions.
2. Two median nerve muscles are lateral cord innervated—pronator teres and flexor carpi radialis.

REFERENCES

1. England, J.D., Sumner, A.J., Neuralgic amyotrophy: an increasingly diverse entity, *Muscle Nerve* 1987; 10:60–68.
2. Lahrmann, H., Grisold, W., Authier, F.J., Zifko, U.A., Neuralgic amyotrophy with phrenic nerve involvement, *Muscle Nerve* 1999; 22:437–442.
3. Malamut, R.I., Marques, W., England, J.D., Sumner, A.J., Postsurgical idiopathic brachial neuritis, *Muscle Nerve* 1994; 17:320–324.

4. Parsonage, M.J., Turner, J.W.A., Neuralgic amyotrophy: the shoulder girdle syndrome, *Lancet* 1948; i:973–978.
5. Pierre, P.A., Laterre, C.E., Van Den Bergh, P.Y., Neuralgic amyotrophy with involvement of cranial nerves IX, X, XI, and XII, *Muscle Nerve* 1990; 13:704–707.
6. Turner, J.W.A., Parsonage, M.J., Neuralgic amyotrophy (paralytic brachial neuritis), *Lancet* 1957; ii:209–212.

PATIENT 16

A 71-year-old man with left arm weakness for 1 week

This 71-year-old man had brief loss of consciousness and fell in the shower 1 week prior to this study and awoke with painless weakness of his left arm, with no sensory disturbance.

Electrodiagnostic Study:

Sensory NCS

Nerve	Sites	Recording Site	Onset (ms)	Peak (ms)	BP Amplitude (μV)	Distance (cm)	Velocity (m/s)
L. median–dig II	1. Wrist	Dig II	3.10	4.15	19.2	13	41.9
L. ulnar–dig V	1. Wrist	Dig V	2.45	3.30	13.2	11	44.9
L. radial–sn box	1. Forearm	Sn box	1.95	2.50	24.6	10	51.3

Motor NCS

Nerve	Sites	Recording Site	Latency (ms)	Amplitude (mV)	Distance (cm)	Velocity (m/s)
L. median–APB	1. Wrist	APB	4.50	7.2	7	—
	2. Elbow	APB	8.90	7.2	24	54.5
L. ulnar–ADM	1. Wrist	ADM	3.00	6.0	7	—
	2. B. elbow	ADM	7.30	6.2	23	53.5
	3. A. elbow	ADM	10.00	5.9	13	48.1

EMG Summary Table

		SA			Amplitude (MUs)	Duration (MUs)	PolyP (MUs)	Activation	Recruitment Pattern
	IA	Fib	Fasc	Other					
L. deltoid	Nl	0	0	0	Nl	Nl	Nl	Full	SevRed
L. biceps	Nl	0	0	0	Nl	Nl	Nl	Full	SevRed
L. triceps	Nl	0	0	0	Nl	Nl	Nl	Full	ModRed
L. pron teres	Nl	0	0	0	Nl	Nl	Nl	Full	ModRed
L. first dors int	Nl	0	0	0	Nl	Nl	Nl	Full	Nl
L. ext dig comm	Nl	0	0	0	Nl	Nl	Nl	Full	Nl
L. supra spinatus	Nl	1–2+	0	0	Nl	Nl	Nl	Full	MildRed
L. infra spinat	Nl	1–2+	0	0	Nl	Nl	Nl	Full	MildRed
L. C4 paraspinal	Nl	0	0	0	—	—	—	—	—
L. C5 paraspinal	Nl	3–4+	0	0	—	—	—	—	—
L. C6 paraspinal	Nl	3–4+	0	0	—	—	—	—	—

Question: How do you explain the presence of fibrillation potentials in some but not all muscles supplied by a common nerve root?

Answers: Ongoing wallerian degeneration of motor axons creates a "proximal-to-distal" gradient of fibrillation potentials.

Discussion: The results of nerve conduction studies are normal. The results of EMG studies are abnormal for: (1) fibrillation potentials with a proximal-to-distal gradient in left C5 and C6 cervical paraspinal muscles and supraspinatus and infraspinatus, and (2) reduced recruitment of motor unit action potentials that is severe for the left deltoid and biceps, moderate for the pronator teres and triceps, and mild for the supraspinatus and infraspinatus.

The presence of marked reduction in interference patterns in the deltoid, biceps, and pronator teres with the absence of fibrillation potentials could be due to a purely demyelinating lesion or to acute axonal injury prior to the development of Wallerian degeneration. In this case, the latter is more likely given the fibrillation potentials present in more proximal C6 muscles including paraspinals. The most proximal muscles, the paraspinals, had 3 to 4+ fibrillation potentials; the next distal muscles, supraspinatus and infraspinatus, had 1 to 2+ fibrillation potentials; and more distal muscles did not show fibrillation potentials. The presence of this "proximal-to-distal gradient"

of fibrillation potentials is a typical sign of acute axonal injury, as Wallerian degeneration proceeds from proximal to distal muscles. Follow-up needle EMG study in 2 weeks would likely show abundant fibrillation potentials in the distal muscles as well.

In general, the electrodiagnostic examination of suspected radiculopathy targets muscles that both sample and overlap the C5–T1 roots. For example, the muscles shown in the first table below serve this purpose. This set of muscles samples all these roots, with at least two muscles for each root, as well as the five major nerves of the arm. The specific pattern of needle EMG abnormalities in cervical radiculopathies is generally distinct for each root, although one should be cautious because published myotome tables are quite variable and individual variation clearly exists. An excellent discussion of these patterns is noted by Levin et al.,[1] whose findings are summarized in the second table below. In this case, the abnormalities are most suggestive of a C6 localization and do not fit neatly into the scheme suggested by Levin et al.

Five Muscles Useful for Needle EMG Screening of the Arm, Sampling All Roots with at Least Two Muscles per Root and All Five Major Nerves of the Arm

Muscle	Root	Trunk	Cord	Nerve
Deltoid	C5–C6	Upper	Posterior	Axillary
Biceps	C5–C6	Upper	Lateral	Musculocut
Pronator teres	C6–C7	Upper	Lateral	Median
Extens dig comm	C7–C8	Middle	Posterior	Radial
First dorsal inteross	C8, T1	Lower	Medial	Ulnar

Pattern of Needle EMG Abnormalities in Single Root Lesions as Determined by Levin et al.[2]

Root	Muscles Involved
C5	Rhomboids, spinati, deltoid, biceps, brachialis, and brachioradialis
C6	Either the above-C5 or below-C7 pattern
C7	Triceps, anconeus, pronator teres, and flexor carpi radialis
C8	All ulnar innervated + finger extensors + flex pollicis longus

Clinical Pearl

Needle EMG screening for radiculopathy should include muscles with overlapping root segments and cover all trunks, cords, and the five major nerves to the arm. The first table above suggests one possible combination that achieves this.

REFERENCES

1. Levin, K.H., Maggiano, H.J., Wilbourn, A.J., Cervical radiculopathies: comparison of surgical and EMG localization of single-root lesions, *Neurology* 1996; 46:1022–1025.
2. Wilbourne, A.J., Aminoff, M.J., AAEM minimonograph 32: the electrodiagnosis examination in patients with radiculopathies, *Muscle Nerve* 1998; 21:1612–1631.

PATIENT 17

A 61-year-old woman with breast cancer, right neck and shoulder pain, and hand weakness and numbness 3 months prior to evaluation

Electrodiagnostic Study:

Sensory NCS

Nerve	Sites	Recording Site	Onset (ms)	Peak (ms)	BP Amplitude (µV)	Distance (cm)	Velocity (m/s)
R. median–dig II	1. Wrist	Dig II	2.35	3.00	27.1	13	55.3
L. median–dig II	1. Wrist	Dig II	1.95	2.70	35.8	13	66.7
R. ulnar–dig V	1. Wrist	Dig V	2.05	2.70	27.5	11	53.7
L. ulnar–dig V	1. Wrist	Dig V	1.70	2.45	25.3	11	64.7
R. ulnar dorsal	1. Wrist	Dors hand	Absent	—	—	—	—
L. ulnar dorsal	1. Wrist	Dors hand	Absent	—	—	—	—
R. radial–sn box	1. Forearm	Sn box	1.50	2.00	34.5	10	66.7
L. radial–sn box	1. Forearm	Sn box	1.45	1.90	34.6	10	69.0
R. med AB cut	1. Elbow	Forearm	1.65	2.10	10.1	12	72.7
L. med AB cut	1. Elbow	Forearm	1.65	2.25	10.0	12	72.7
R. lat AB cut	1. Elbow	Forearm	1.85	2.25	11.0	12	66.0
L. lat AB cut	1. Elbow	Forearm	2.00	2.40	14.0	12	60.0

Motor NCS

Nerve	Sites	Recording Site	Latency (ms)	Amplitude (mV)	Distance (cm)	Velocity (m/s)
R. median–APB	1. Wrist	APB	3.35	10.5	7	—
	2. Elbow	APB	6.90	10.3	20.5	57.7
L. median–APB	1. Wrist	APB	3.15	8.8	7	—
	2. Elbow	APB	6.80	8.4	21.5	58.9
R. ulnar–ADM	1. Wrist	ADM	2.70	5.5	7	—
	2. B. elbow	ADM	5.65	5.3	19	64.4
	3. A. elbow	ADM	7.40	5.1	12	68.6
L. ulnar–ADM	1. Wrist	ADM	2.20	10.0	7	—
	2. B. elbow	ADM	5.15	9.3	19.5	66.1
	3. A. elbow	ADM	6.70	8.6	10	64.5
R. ulnar–FDI	1. Wrist	FDI	3.55	4.7	—	—
	2. B. elbow	FDI	6.75	4.6	19	59.4
	3. A. elbow	FDI	8.25	4.6	10	66.7
L. ulnar–FDI	1. Wrist	FDI	3.25	11.7	—	—
	2. B. elbow	FDI	6.25	10.7	20	66.7
	3. A. elbow	FDI	7.80	9.8	10	64.5

F-Wave

Nerve	F_{min} (ms)	F_{max} (ms)	Max – Min (ms)	%F
R. median	25.95	27.35	1.40	—
R. ulnar	27.05	29.75	2.70	—

Needle EMG Summary Table

		SA			Amplitude (MUs)	—	Duration (MUs)	—	PolyP (MUs)	Activation	Recruitment Pattern
	IA	Fib	Fasc	Other							
R. first dors int	Incr	1+	0	0	Many	Large	Many	Long	Many	Full	Discrete
R. abd poll br	Nl	0	0	0	Many	Large	Many	Long	Few	Full	Mod red
R. abd dig min	Incr	Rare	0	0	Many	Large	Many	Long	Nl	Full	Mild red
R. flex poll ln	Nl	0	0	0	Most	Large	Most	Long	Nl	Full	Discrete
R. ext poll ln	Incr	2+	0	0	Many	Large	Many	Long	Many	Full	Mod red
R. deltoid	Nl	0	0	0	Nl	—	Nl	—	Nl	Full	Nl
R. triceps	Nl	0	0	0	Nl	—	Nl	—	Nl	Full	Nl
R. pron teres	Nl	0	0	0	Nl	—	Nl	—	Nl	Full	Nl
R. C7 para-spinal	Nl	0	0	0	Nl	—	Nl	—	Nl	Full	Nl
R. C8 para-spinal	Incr	2+	0	0	Nl	—	Nl	—	Nl	Full	Nl
R. T1 para-spinals	Incr	2+	0	0	Nl	—	Nl	—	Nl	Full	Nl
R. thoracic PSP upper	Nl	0	0	0	Nl	—	Nl	—	Nl	Full	Nl
L. first dors int	Nl	0	0	0	Nl	—	Nl	—	Nl	Full	Nl
L. C8 para-spinal	Nl	0	0	0	Nl	—	Nl	—	Nl	Full	Nl

Questions:
1. Are the nerve conduction studies more suggestive of a radiculopathy or a plexopathy?
2. What is the electrodiagnostic diagnosis?

Answers:

1. Radiculopathy
2. C8 radiculopathy

Discussion: The nerve conduction studies show symmetric and normal sensory studies. Given the patient's sensory complaints, this immediately favors a root more likely than plexus localization. The bilateral absence of the dorsal ulnar cutaneous SNAPs is a normal finding in some individuals. The motor studies show relatively reduced amplitudes (approximately or less than 50% those of contralateral studies) of the right ulnar–ADM and ulnar–FDI CMAPs, suggesting motor axonal loss in these muscles. As their innervation is in the C8 and T1 roots, lower trunk, or medial cord and the ulnar nerve, a normal ulnar–D5 SNAP suggests the proximal root localization. The needle EMG study abnormalities in the ulnar-innervated FDI and ADM muscles, as well as in the radial finger extensor EPL and median muscle FPL and APB, is the pattern of a C8 lesion (see discussion and tables for patient 16).

Clinical Pearl

Sensory nerve action potential amplitudes are normal in cervical radiculopathy despite sensory symptoms and signs—this is because a lesion proximal to the dorsal root ganglion does not result in degeneration of the peripheral sensory axons.

REFERENCES

1. Levin, K.H., Maggiano, H.J., Wilbourn, A.J., Cervical radiculopathies: comparison of surgical and EMG localization of single-root lesions, *Neurology* 1996; 46:1022–1025.
2. Wilbourne, A.J., Aminoff, M.J., AAEM minimonograph 32: the electrodiagnosis examination in patients with radiculopathies, *Muscle Nerve* 1998; 21:1612–1631.

Focal Neuropathies of the Lower Limb: Anatomy for the Electrodiagnostic Practitioner

As with the arm, the electromyographer needs to think about the anatomy of the leg from the perspective of nerve conduction studies and needle EMG. The five lumbar roots L1 to L5 and first three sacral roots S1 to S3 supply the leg. The lumbosacral plexus (figure I.2) is formed from a combination of the lumbar plexus and the sacral plexus. The lumbar plexus is formed from the ventral rami of L1–L4; the sacral plexus is formed from the ventral rami of S1–S4 together with a communication between the two, the lumbosacral trunk, which distally gives rise to the lateral portion of the sciatic nerve and eventually the common peroneal nerve. The electrodiagnostic tools available for examination of the leg are more restricted than those for the arm. Table 1 shows the nerve conduction studies available and the portions of the peripheral nervous system from which they are derived. As can be seen, nerve conduction studies reliably assess axons derived from the L5, S1, and S2 roots, the lumbosacral trunk, and the sacral plexus, but they do not reliably assess the lumbar plexus. The saphenous SNAP, which could possibly be of value in assessing the lumbar plexus, unfortunately has not been obtainable in some healthy controls in several studies.[1,4,6] The absence of sensory nerve studies of the lumbar plexus limits the diagnostic power to separate root from plexus disease, particularly as the presence of lumbar paraspinal muscle abnormalities (the only other electrodiagnostic technique available) can be seen in healthy individuals.[2]

It is also noteworthy that, unlike the arm, the dorsal root ganglia for lumbosacral dorsal roots sometimes lie within the spine canal; thus, intraspinal processes may result in amplitude reductions for the superficial peroneal SNAP[2] and, in theory, the sural SNAP.

Table 1.   Root, Plexus, and Nerve Innervation Relevant to Sensory and Motor Nerve Conduction Studies in the Lower Limb

Study	Root(s)	Plexus	Nerve
Sensory			
Sural	S1	Sacral	Tibial
Superficial peroneal	L5	Lumbosacral trunk	Superficial peroneal
Saphenous	L4	Lumbar	Femoral
Lateral femoral cut	L2,3	Lumbar	Lateral femoral cutaneous
Lateral plantar	S1	Sacral	Tibial
Medial plantar	?L5, S1	Sacral	Tibial
Motor			
Peroneal-EDB	L5, S1	Lumbosacral trunk	Deep peroneal
Tibial-AH	S1, 2	Sacral	Tibial
Peroneal-TA	L4, 5	Lumbosacral trunk	Deep peroneal

Table 2.   Root and Nerve Innervation Relevant to Needle EMG Studies in the Lower Limb

Muscle	Root(s)	Nerve
Iliopsoas	L2, L3	Lumbar plexus
Adductor magnus	L2, L3, L4	Obturator + Sciatic
Adductor longus	L2, L3, L4	Obturator

Continued

Table 2. Root and Nerve Innervation Relevant to Needle EMG Studies in the Lower Limb

Muscle	Root(s)	Nerve
Quadriceps	L2, L3, L4	Femoral
Tibialis anterior	L4,5	Peroneal
Peroneus longus	L5, S1	Peroneal
Tibialis posterior	L5, S1	Tibial
Biceps femoris, short head	L5, S1	Sciatic, lateral
Biceps femoris, long head	L5, S1	Sciatic, medial
Extensor hallucis longus	L5, S1	Peroneal
Flexor hallucis longus	L5, S1	Tibial
Gastrocnemius	S1, S2	Tibial
Gluteus medius	L4, L5, S1	Superior gluteal
Tensor fascia lata	L4, L5, S1	Superior gluteal
Gluteus maximus	L5, S1, S2	Inferior gluteal

The Lumbosacral Plexus

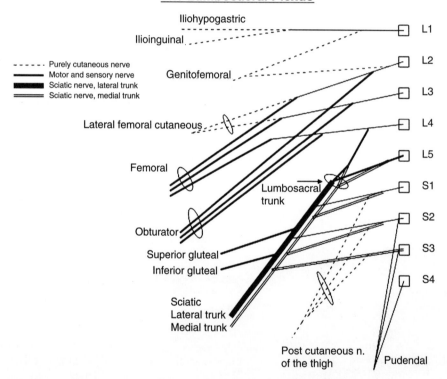

REFERENCES

1. Izzo, K.L., Sridhara, C.R., Rosenholtz, H., Sensory conduction studies of branches of superficial peroneal nerve, *Arch. Phys. Med. Rehabil.* 1981; 62:24–27.
2. Levin, K.H., L5 radiculopathy with reduced superficial peroneal sensory responses: intraspinal and extraspinal causes, *Muscle Nerve* 1998; 21:3–7.
3. Nardin, R.A., Raynor, E.M., Rutkove, S.B., Fibrillations in lumbosacral paraspinal muscles of normal subjects, *Muscle Nerve* 1998; 21(10):1347–1349.
4. Senden, R., Van Mulders, J., Ghys, R., Rosselle, N., Conduction velocity of the distal segment of the saphenous nerve in normal adult subjects, *Electromyogr. Clin. Neurophysiol.* 1981; 21:3–10.
5. Subramony, S.H., Wilbourn, A.J., Radicular derivation of sensory action potentials in lower extremity, *Arch. Phys. Med. Rehabil.* 1981; 62(11):590–592.
6. Tranier, S., Durey, A., Chevallier, B., Liot, F., Value of somatosensory evoked potentials in saphenous entrapment neuropathy, *J. Neurol. Neurosurg. Psychiatry* 1992; 55(6):461–465.

PATIENT 18

A 64-year-old man with right foot drop 6 weeks prior

This man could not recall the precise onset of his right foot weakness but believed it had not changed since first noticed. There was no numbness or pain that he was aware of. His wife noted his tendency to fall asleep with his right leg crossed over his left. Examination showed grade 2/5 strength in the right tibialis anterior, eversion, and toe extensors, with all other muscles 5/5. There was a sensory disturbance to light touch over the dorsum of his foot and lateral leg to the mid lower leg.

Electrodiagnostic Study:

Sensory NCS

Nerve	Sites	Recording Site	Onset (ms)	Amplitude (μV)	Distance (cm)	Velocity (m/s)
L. sural–lat mall	1. Mid calf	Ankle	4.2	16.2	14	33.3
R. sural–lat mall	1. Mid calf	Ankle	4.5	19.9	14	31.1
R. sup peroneal	1. Lat leg	Ankle	3.8	9.2	14	36.8
L. sup peroneal	1. Lat leg	Ankle	3.9	6.3	14	36.0

Motor NCS

Nerve	Sites	Recording Site	Latency (ms)	Amplitude (mV)	Distance (cm)	Velocity (m/s)
R. peroneal–EDB	1. Ankle	EDB	7.8	0.8	8	—
	2. Fib head	EDB	14.7	0.8	24	34.7
	3. Pop fossa	EDB	Absent	—	—	—
R. peroneal–tib ant	1. Fib head	Tib ant	4.2	0.8	8	—
	2. Pop fossa	Tib ant	9.4	0.3	9	17.3
R. tibial–AH	1. Ankle	AH	5.3	2.2	8	—
	2. Pop fossa	AH	14.5	1.5	35	38.0

EMG Summary Table

		SA						
	IA	Fib	Fasc	Other	Amplitude (MUs)	Duration (MUs)	PolyP (MUs)	Activation	Recruitment Pattern
R. tib ant	Nl	2+	0	0	None			Full	Sev dec
R. per long	Nl	2+	0	0	Nl	Nl	Nl	Full	Sev dec
R. tib post	Nl	0	0	0	Nl	Nl	Nl	Full	Nl
R. bic fem SH	Nl	0	0	0	Nl	Nl	Nl	Full	Nl

Questions:
1. What is the clinical differential diagnosis?
2. What specific nerve conduction and EMG studies should be performed to address this differential diagnosis?
3. If the nerve conduction velocities had all been normal, what additional nerve conduction and needle EMG studies might have been helpful?

Answers:

1. Common peroneal neuropathy vs. L5 radiculopathy
2. SNAP amplitudes, across fibular head conduction velocity, and tibialis posterior needle EMG
3. Contralateral nerve conduction studies and ipsilateral more proximal needle EMG studies

Discussion: The clinical localization of a unilateral foot drop is typically either a common peroneal neuropathy or L5 radiculopathy. A sciatic neuropathy, although uncommon, may show differential involvement of the lateral portion, which is the common peroneal nerve. Other localizations may occur, including central. The clinical features that may distinguish an L5 radiculopathy from a common peroneal neuropathy at the fibular head include the presence of low back and posterior leg pain, weakness of foot inversion and hip internal rotation (L5 but not common peroneal nerve), and a pattern of sensory disturbance. In an L5 lesion, this may include a portion of the distal sole and ventral surfaces of the toes, as well as the lateral calf above the mid-leg to the knee. In a peroneal neuropathy at the fibular head, the sensory loss does not usually go onto the ventral foot or above the mid-lower leg (lateral cutaneous nerve of the calf territory, a branch of the lateral cord of the sciatic nerve and essentially common peroneal nerve, but above the popliteal fossa). In addition, signs of mechanical irritability of the peroneal nerve at the fibular head (*i.e.*, tingling paresthesias in its distribution provoked by tapping or rubbing the nerve over the fibular head) may also be helpful in localization.

The electrodiagnostic parameters that may be of help include:

- The amplitude of the superficial peroneal SNAP—SNAPs may be helpful in distinguishing root from more peripheral lesions, although not always;[3] however, common peroneal nerve lesions at the fibular head due to compression are often predominantly demyelinating, which will not affect the distal evoked superficial peroneal SNAP amplitude unless there has been secondary Wallerian degeneration.
- The amplitude of the peroneal-EDB CMAP—The peroneal-EDB CMAP amplitude is often not affected by an L5 lesion but may be by a common peroneal neuropathy at the fibular head (although, again, pure demyelinating lesions will not affect it).
- The presence of focal slowing or conduction block across the fibular head of peroneal–

EDB or peroneal-TA motor segments—As we have emphasized before, a focal abnormality such as these are definitive in localization.

- Peroneal–EDB F-wave minimum latency and persistence, compared to the other side—Particularly when the distal evoked CMAP is normal, the absence of F-waves on one side with good persistence on the other provides good evidence of a proximal demyelinating (or too recent) lesion but will not distinguish peroneal nerve from L5 lesions.
- Needle EMG abnormalities in common peroneal innervated muscles (tibialis anterior, peroneus longus) but not L5 non-peroneal nerve-innervated muscles (tibialis posterior, gluteus medius, L5 paraspinal muscles)—Additionally, the short head of biceps femoris is supplied by the common peroneal division of the sciatic nerve, while the long head is supplied by the tibial division. Demonstrating normality of these helps to exclude L5 and sciatic neuropathies as the cause of the foot drop.

In this particular case, the clinical features suggested a peroneal neuropathy, particularly the full strength for ankle inversion and the sensory deficit sparing the territory of the lateral cutaneous nerve of the calf (L5, but off of peroneal division of sciatic nerve at or just above the popliteal fossa). The electrodiagnostic abnormalities include reduced amplitude of the peroneal–EDB CMAP (uncommon but does occur with L5 lesions) and a definitive focal abnormality—an across-fibular-head velocity of 17 m/s for the peroneal–TA motor segment—localizing the lesion to a peroneal neuropathy at the fibular head. The needle EMG studies provide more support of this. Additional nerve conduction studies that would have been helpful if focal slowing was not present would have included contralateral peroneal–EDB and peroneal–TA CMAP and superficial peroneal SNAP amplitudes to compare to the symptomatic side. Additional needle EMG studies would have included both heads of biceps femoris, gluteus medius, and paraspinal muscles.

Clinical Pearls

1. The differential diagnosis of a foot drop includes upper motor neuron lesions, L4 or L5 anterior horn or root lesions, lumbosacral trunk, sciatic or peroneal neuropathies, and disorders of the neuromuscular junction and muscle.

2. When the tibialis anterior has needle EMG abnormalities in patients with foot drop, other muscles that should be examined include peroneus longus (distinguishes common peroneal from deep peroneal neuropathies), tibialis posterior (abnormal in L5 but not peroneal neuropathies), and gluteus medius or lumbar paraspinal muscles (both abnormal in L5 but not sciatic neuropathies).

REFERENCES

1. Bendszus, M., Koltzenburg, M., Visualization of denervated muscle by gadolinium-enhanced MRI, *Neurology* 2001; 57:1709–1711.
2. Katirji, B., Peroneal neuropathy, *Neurol. Clin.* 1999; 17:567–591.
3. Levin, K.H., L5 radiculopathy with reduced superficial peroneal sensory responses: intraspinal and extraspinal causes, *Muscle Nerve* 1998; 21:3–7.

PATIENT 19

A 70-year-old woman with right foot drop after hip replacement

This woman was referred for right foot drop immediately after right hip replacement several months prior. Examination was notable for severe weakness of tibialis anterior and ankle eversion with probable normal ankle inversion and plantarflexion. The sensory disturbance included the dorsal and lateral aspects of the foot and the lateral leg up to the knee.

Electrodiagnostic Study:

Sensory NCS

Nerve	Sites	Recording Site	Onset (ms)	Peak (ms)	Amplitude (μV)	Distance (cm)	Velocity (m/s)
R. sural–lat mall	1. Mid calf	Ankle	Absent	—	—	—	—
R. sup peroneal	1. Lat leg	Ankle	Absent	—	—	—	—
L. sural–lat mall	1. Mid calf	Ankle	3.10	3.60	4.3	14	45.2
L. sup peroneal	1. Lat leg	Ankle	2.10	2.90	10.6	12	57.1

Motor NCS

Nerve	Sites	Recording Site	Latency (ms)	Amplitude (mV)	Distance (cm)	Velocity (m/s)
R. peroneal–EDB	1. Ankle	EDB	Absent	—	8	—
L. peroneal–EDB	1. Ankle	EDB	3.60	3.1	8	—
	2. Fib head	EDB	9.55	2.9	27	45.4
	3. Pop fossa	EDB	10.55	2.8	6	60.0
R. peroneal–tib ant	1. Fib head	Tib ant	Absent	—	—	—
L. peroneal–tib ant	1. Fib head	Tib ant	2.70	4.6	7	—
	2. Pop fossa	Tib ant	3.90	3.6	—	—
R. tibial–AH	1. Ankle	AH	3.60	6.0	8	—
	2. Pop fossa	AH	11.25	3.7	36	47.1
L. tibial–AH	1. Ankle	AH	3.35	10.8	8	—
	2. Pop fossa	AH	10.70	7.4	33	44.9

EMG Summary Table

		SA			Amplitude (MUs)	Duration (MUs)	PolyP (MUs)	Activation	Recruitment Pattern
	IA	Fib	Fasc	Other					
R. tib ant	Inc	3+	0	0	None		—	None	None
R. tib post	Nl	0	0	0	Nl	Nl	Nl	Full	Nl
R. gastroc med	Nl	0	0	0	Nl	Nl	Nl	Full	Nl
R. vast med	Nl	0	0	0	Nl	Nl	Nl	Full	Nl
R. bic fem SH	Inc	2+	0	0	Nl	Nl	Many	Full	Mild red
R. glut Nl med	Nl	0	0		Nl	Nl	Nl	Full	Nl
R. L5 paraspinals	Nl	0	0	0	—	—	—	—	—

Questions:
1. What are the main clinical considerations?
2. What is the localization, based on the electrodiagnostic studies?

Answers:
1. Peroneal neuropathy, sciatic neuropathy, or L4 or L5 rdiculopathy
2. Sciatic neuropathy

Discussion: As discussed in case 18, the main considerations for a foot drop are a common peroneal neuropathy at the fibular head, sciatic neuropathy, and an L4 or L5 radiculopathy. Particularly after hip replacement, a sciatic neuropathy with predominant involvement of the lateral division needs to be considered. In this case, the superficial peroneal SNAP, peroneal–EDB CMAP, and peroneal–TA CMAP were all absent, as would be seen in a lesion of the common peroneal nerve or its proximal extension. However, the sural SNAP is also absent, while normal on the contralateral side, and the patient's postoperative clinical sural territory sensory loss goes along with this finding. The sural is predominantly a branch of the tibial nerve, although it may receive some axons from the communicating sural division of the common peroneal nerve. An absent sural SNAP indicates that the lesion, if there is just one, localizes to the sciatic nerve. The asymmetry of the tibial–AH CMAP amplitudes, although not at a level of abnormality (*i.e.*, 50% side-to-side difference), does add some support to this localization. The needle EMG abnormalities in the short head of the biceps femoris at least tell us that it is not a common peroneal neuropathy at the fibular head. Additional nerve conduction studies that might have been of help would have included bilateral tibial F-waves. These are generally easy to obtain, so normal studies on the left with poor persistence on the right could have provided strong evidence of a sciatic localization.

Several key anatomical points relating to the sciatic nerve include:

- It is formed from the sacral plexus + the lumbosacral trunk.
- The sciatic nerve is separated into lateral and medial trunks; the lateral trunk appears more susceptible to injury.
- In the biceps femoris, the long head is innervated by the sciatic nerve, medial trunk; the short head by the sciatic nerve, lateral trunk.
- The adductor magnus has a dual nerve supply: obturator nerve (L2–L4) and sciatic nerve (L4–L5).

Clinical Pearl

Clinically, many sciatic neuropathies look like common peroneal neuropathies because of apparently increased susceptibility to injury of the lateral division of the sciatic nerve, which gives rise to the common peroneal nerve. Subclinical involvement of portions of the tibial nerve (*i.e.*, reduction of sural SNAP or tibial–AH CMAP amplitude, tibial–AH F-wave abnormalities, needle EMG abnormalities in the long head of the biceps femoris) supports sciatic neuropathy over peroneal neuropathy.

REFERENCES

1. Asnis, S.E., Hanley, S., Shelton, P.D., Sciatic neuropathy secondary to migration of trochanteric wire following total hip arthroplasty, *Clin. Orthop.* 1985; 196:226–228.
2. Edwards, B.N., Tullos, H.S., Noble, P.C., Contributory factors and etiology of sciatic nerve palsy in total hip arthroplasty, *Clin. Orthop.* 1987; 218:136–141.
3. Fischer, S.R., Christ, D.J., Roehr, B.A., Sciatic neuropathy secondary to total hip arthroplasty wear debris, *J. Arthroplasty* 1999; 14:771–774.
4. Yuen, E.C., So, Y.T., Sciatic neuropathy, *Neurol. Clin.* 1999; 17:617–631.
5. Yuen, E.C., So, Y.T., Olney, R.K., The electrophysiologic features of sciatic neuropathy in 100 patients. *Muscle Nerve* 1995; 18:414–420.
6. Yuen, E.C., Olney, R.K., So, Y.T., Sciatic neuropathy: clinical and prognostic features in 73 patients, *Neurology* 1994; 44:1669–1674.
7. Zechmann, J.P., Reckling, F.W., Association of preoperative hip motion and sciatic nerve palsy following total hip arthroplasty, *Clin Orthop.* 1989; 241:197–199

PATIENT 20

A 38-year-old man with left foot weakness and numbness after prior treatment for a posterior thigh sarcoma

This 38-year-old man was treated at the age of 31 for a liposarcoma of the left posterior thigh with surgery and radiation therapy. Seven years later, he developed weakness of ankle plantar flexion and numbness of the lateral foot and sole and the lateral and medial heel, as well as enlargement of his calf muscle. Six months after onset of symptoms, neurological exam showed mild to moderate weakness of gastrocnemius and toe flexion and mild weakness of tibialis anterior and toe extension, with a sensory deficit as described above by the patient's symptoms. Despite gastrocnemius weakness with resulting inability to stand on the ball of his left foot, there was substantial hypertrophy of the left lateral calf (indicated by arrowhead in figure 1). There were frequent fasciculations in the left calf. The superior and lateral portion of the calf demonstrated semirhythmic contractions similar to fasciculations but distinct in having a nearly regular, rhythmic quality. Note the scarring in the distal posterior thigh in figure 1 as well.

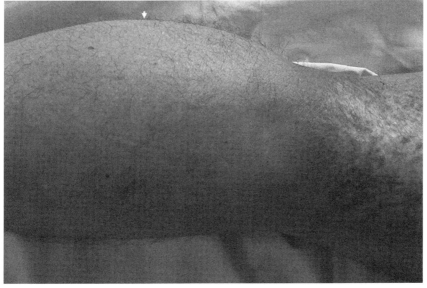

Figure 1

Electrodiagnostic Study:

Sensory NCS

Nerve	Sites	Recording Site	Onset (ms)	Peak (ms)	BP Amplitude (µV)	Distance (cm)	Velocity (m/s)
L. sural–lat mall	1. Mid calf	Ankle	3.45	4.35	8.9	14	40.6
R. sural–lat mall	1. Mid calf	Ankle	3.00	3.50	6.1	14	46.7
L. sup peroneal	1. Lat leg	Ankle	2.70	3.60	7.9	12	44.4

Motor NCS

Nerve	Sites	Recording Site	Latency (ms)	Amplitude (mV)	Distance (cm)	Velocity (m/s)
L. peroneal–EDB	1. Ankle	EDB	5.60	6.5	8	—
	2. Bel FibHd	EDB	13.50	5.7	35	44.3
	3. AbvFibHd	EDB	15.95	5.6	10	40.8
L. tibial–AH	1. Ankle	AH	6.15	14.4	8	
	2. Pop Fossa	AH	16.35	9.5	44	43.1
R. tibial–AH	1. Ankle	AH	5.25	14.5	8	—

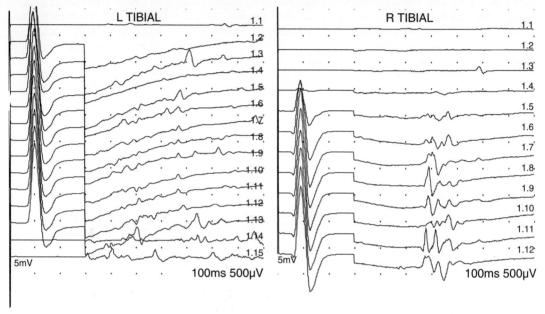

Figure 2

Questions:

1. The patient had marked weakness of toe flexion. How do you explain this in the face of the motor nerve conduction studies above? What additional nerve conduction studies might be of value in testing your hypothesis?
2. The patient had marked numbness in the left sural nerve territory. How do you explain this in the face of the sensory nerve conduction studies above?
3. What sensory nerves appear clinically affected in this patient?
4. What are the potentials seen in the right half of the left tibial nerve study in figure 2? Are they F-waves? (Hint: Look at the bottom two stimulation tracings in the panel)
5. How do you interpret the F-wave results together with the normal tibial-AH CMAP amplitude?
6. What is the electrodiagnostic term for spontaneous activity consisting of semi-rhythmic bursts of grouped motor unit action potentials?

Answers:

1. Focal demyelination and conduction block proximal to stimulation sites; consider F-wave
2. Focal demyelination and conduction block of sensory axons proximal to stimulation sites
3. Sural, lateral plantar, calcaneal nerves
4. Background surface motor unit potentials
5. Focal conduction block proximally
6. Myokymic potentials

Discussion: The sensory territory affected is that of the sural, lateral plantar, and calcaneal nerves, all branches of the tibial nerve. An impressive disturbance of sensation in the sural nerve territory with a preserved SNAP amplitude may be seen in any of the following: hyperacute axonal injury; focal demyelination and conduction block of sensory axons proximal to the point of nerve conduction stimulation; or a lesion proximal to the dorsal root ganglion—root, spinal cord, or brain. Similarly, the marked toe flexion weakness together with robust and symmetric tibial–AH CMAP amplitudes implies the possibilities of hyperacute axonal injury, focal demyelination and conduction block proximal to the stimulation site, or a central nervous system (CNS) lesion. The clinical history excludes hyperacute axonal injury from consideration.

One additional nerve conduction study that might be of help is the tibial F-wave study. Tibial–AH F-waves are generally robust and easy to obtain, unlike peroneal–EDB, which may be bilaterally absent in healthy individuals. Abnormalities in F-wave responses would likely distinguish between conduction block and a CNS lesion. The results are shown in figure 2.

In the left tibial nerve study, the potentials could be F-waves, but they do not look like the typical multiphasic tibial F-waves, as in the right tibial study. The last two tracings do not have a tibial–AH CMAP ("M wave") present; the stimulator was not applied to the patient, yet similar potentials are present. This indicates that the surface electrode is picking up EMG activity, likely motor unit discharges from incomplete relaxation or fasciculations. The marked asymmetry of F-wave responses, absent on the left and robust on the right, with symmetric normal tibial–AH

CMAP amplitudes indicates focal conduction block of motor axons proximal to the ankle. The needle EMG study demonstrated semirhythmic bursts of motor unit action potentials. These are shown in figure 3, where tracing (a) shows three bursts of grouped motor unit discharges; the middle group of motor unit discharges in (a) is enlarged in (b). Examine the figure and then do the following:

1. From tracing (a), calculate the approximate interburst frequency.
2. From tracing (b), calculate the approximate range of interpotential frequencies within a burst (or grouped discharge).

Figure 3A shows myokymic potentials. These typically consist of semirhythmic or rhythmic grouped discharges of motor unit potentials, typically with a significantly longer interburst period than intraburst (*i.e.*, between potentials) period. In the example above, we calculate the interburst frequency using the 325-ms latency between the first and second groups. Thus, 1000 ms divided by 325 ms gives 3 cycles/s, or 3 Hz. The interpotential frequencies within a burst vary; the first two potentials in (b) are 12 ms apart, translating to a frequency of 1000 divided by 12, or 83 Hz. The second and third potentials in (b) are 33 ms apart, translating to a frequency of 1000 divided by 33, or 30 Hz. The range is thus on the order of 30 to 83 Hz. In general, myokymic discharges have interpotential discharge frequencies of less than 100 Hz. Note also two other characteristic, although not universal, features of myokymic discharges: (1) reduction in amplitude of the potentials from start to finish within a given burst, and (2) variation in the number of potentials within each burst. The tabular results of the EMG studies are provided next.

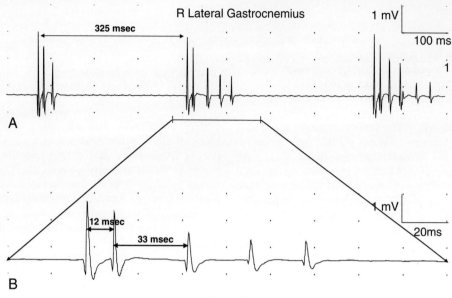

R Lateral Gastrocnemius

325 msec

1 mV
100 ms

A

12 msec

33 msec

1 mV
20ms

B

Figure 3

Needle EMG Summary Table

		SA			Amplitude (MUs)	Duration (MUs)	Activation	Recruitment Pattern
	IA	Fib	Fasc	Other				
L. gastroc med	Inc	0	Occ	Myokymic discharges	Nl	Nl	Full	Sev dec
L. tib ant	Nl	2+	Occ	0	Nl	Nl	Full	Mild dec
L. tib post	Inc	2+	Occ	Myokymic discharges	Nl	Nl	Full	Nl
L. vast med	Nl	0	0	0	Nl	Nl	Full	Nl
L. glut med	Nl	0	0	0	Nl	Nl	Full	Nl
L. L5/S1 paraspinals	Nl	0	0	0	Nl	Nl	Full	Nl

These additional studies show involvement of peroneal-nerve-innervated tibialis anterior. The gastrocnemius does not show any fibrillation potentials despite severely reduced interference pattern, another point supporting conduction block of motor axons supplying this muscle.

In summary, this patient has a sciatic neuropathy with myokymic potentials characteristic of radiation-induced focal neuropathy. A continuous motor unit activity syndrome is also present (see patient 50) with resulting hypertrophy of the calf and clinically visible accompaniment of the myokymic potentials, namely semirhythmic contraction and dimpling of a portion of the gastrocnemius muscle. This later clinical finding does not have a generally accepted name; it is *not* the irregular undulating movements resulting from frequent fasciculations and generally referred to as clinical myokymia. In addition, this patient's syndrome is marked by clinical and electrophysiological evidence of focal demyelination, likely at the site of radiation nerve injury in the posterior thigh.

Clinical Pearls

1. Myokymic potentials are semirhythmic bursts of groups of motor units and are characteristic of radiation-induced nerve injury.

2. Substantial weakness of a muscle with normal bulk or even hypertrophy, in the setting of a peripheral nerve disorder, is likely due to focal demyelination of motor axons.

REFERENCES

1. Daube, J.R., Myokymia and neuromyotonia, *Muscle Nerve* 2001; 24:1711–1712.
2. Gutmann, L., Libell, D., Gutmann, L., When is myokymia neuromyotonia? *Muscle Nerve* 2001; 24:151–153.
3. Gutmann, L., AAEM minimonograph #46: neurogenic muscle hypertrophy, *Muscle Nerve* 1996; 19:811–818.
4. Harper, C.M., Jr., Thomas, J.E., Cascino, T.L., Litchy, W.J., Distinction between neoplastic and radiation-induced brachial plexopathy, with emphasis on the role of EMG, *Neurology* 1989; 39:502–506.
5. Hart, I.K., Maddison, P., Newsom-Davis, J., Vincent, A., Mills, K.R., Phenotypic variants of autoimmune peripheral nerve hyperexcitability. *Brain* 2002; 125:1887–1895.
6. Vincent, A., Understanding neuromyotonia, *Muscle Nerve* 2000; 23:655–657.

PATIENT 21

A 73-year-old man with right leg numbness, weakness, and pain

Four months ago, this 73-year-old man developed mild pain in his right buttock, more moderate pain in his right groin and knee, and tingling paresthesias over the right anterior thigh. He noted his right leg was buckling, and his pain acutely worsened several weeks ago and has gradually improved since. Neurological examination was notable for moderate weakness of right psoas and mild weakness of right adductors and knee extensors. Other leg muscles were normal. On sensory examination, light touch was abnormal at the medial and lateral knee. Reflexes were symmetric at 2+ at the knees.

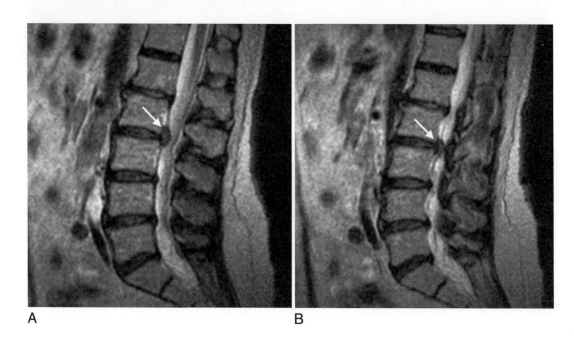

A   B

Electrodiagnostic Study:

Sensory NCS

Nerve	Sites	Recording Site	Onset (ms)	Peak (ms)	BP Amplitude (µV)	Distance (cm)	Velocity (m/s)
R. saphenous	Mid calf	Ankle	Absent	—	—	—	—
L. saphenous	Mid calf	Ankle	Absent	—	—	—	—
R. sural–lat mall	1. Mid calf	Ankle	3.55	4.35	2.8	14	39.4
L. sural–lat mall	1. Mid calf	Ankle	3.50	4.35	3.5	14	40.0

Motor NCS

Nerve	Sites	Recording Site	Latency (ms)	Amplitude (mV)	Distance (cm)	Velocity (m/s)
R. median–APB	1. Wrist	APB	4.30	5.7	7	—
	2. Elbow	APB	9.20	5.9	25.5	52.0
R. peroneal–EDB	1. Ankle	EDB	4.45	3.5	8	—
	2. Fib head	EDB	11.55	3.2	27	38.0
	3. Pop fossa	EDB	13.65	2.7	9.5	45.2

Needle EMG Summary Table

		SA			Amplitude (MUs)	Duration (MUs)	PolyP (MUs)	Activation	Recruitment Pattern
	IA	Fib	Fasc	Other					
R. iliopsoas	Incr	2+	0	0	Nl	Nl	Nl	Full	Nl
R. vast lat	Incr	2+	0	0	Nl	Nl	Nl	Full	Nl
R. tib ant	Nl	0	2+	0	Nl	Nl	Nl	Full	Nl
R. gastroc med	Nl	0	1+	0	Nl	Nl	Nl	Full	Nl
R. add magnus	Incr	2+	0	0	Nl	Nl	Nl	Full	Nl
R. L2 paraspinals	Nl	0	0	0				—	
R. L3 paraspinals	Nl	0	0	0				—	
R. L4 paraspinals	Nl	0	0	0				—	

Question: What is the clinical differential diagnosis?

Answer: L2 or L3 radiculopathy or lumbar plexopathy

Discussion: The electrodiagnostic abnormalities are limited to the needle EMG study (bilateral absence of saphenous SNAPs is a normal finding at any age). Fibrillation potentials are present in the iliopsoas, vastus lateralis, and adductor magnus; the implied localization is to the upper lumbar plexus or the L2 or L3 nerve roots. The figure shows MRI images from the patient; note the large L2–L3 central and right paracentral disc herniation. The clinical diagnosis was an L3 radiculopathy.

Clinical Pearl

Needle EMG abnormalities of paraspinal muscles are not necessarily present in radiculopathy.

PATIENT 22

A 46-year-old woman with right leg pain and intermittent paresthesias

This patient developed right low back and leg pain and intermittent tingling in her right foot 2 years previously and underwent surgical laminectomy for treatment. Acute pain resolved and she has noted more mild chronic pain in her right leg since.

Electrodiagnostic Study:

Sensory NCS

Nerve	Sites	Recording Site	Onset (ms)	Peak (ms)	BP Amplitude (μV)	Distance (cm)	Velocity (m/s)
R. sural–lat mall	1. Mid calf	Ankle	2.70	3.60	10.5	14	51.9
R. sup peroneal	1. Lat leg	Ankle	2.35	3.05	11.5	12	51.1

Motor NCS

Nerve	Sites	Recording Site	Latency (ms)	Amplitude (mV)	Relative Amplitude (%)	Distance (cm)	Velocity (m/s)
R. peroneal–EDB	1. Ankle	EDB	3.65	5.1	100	8	—
	2. Fib head	EDB	9.45	4.5	88.3	29	50.0
	3. Pop fossa	EDB	11.10	4.4	85.6	8.5	51.5
L. tibial–AH	1. Ankle	EDB	3.10	10.5	100	8	—
	2. Fib head	EDB	10.15	9.4	90	36	51.1
R. tibial–AH	1. Ankle	AH	3.55	10.3	100	8	—
	2. Pop fossa	AH	10.10	8.9	86.3	35	53.4

F-Wave

Nerve	F_{min} (ms)	F_{max} (ms)	Max – Min (ms)
R. tibial	43.90	45.30	1.40
L. tibial	44.65	45.90	1.25

H Reflex

Nerve	H Latency (ms)
R. tibial–soleus	Absent
L. tibial–soleus	29.25

EMG Summary Table

	SA				Amplitude (MUs)	Duration (MUs)	PolyP (MUs)	Activation	Recruitment Pattern
	IA	Fib	Fasc	Other					
R. gastroc med	Incr	1+	0	0	Nl	Nl	Nl	Full	Nl
R. bic fem SH	Nl	0	0	0	Nl	Nl	Nl	Full	Nl
R. tib ant	Nl	0	0	0	Nl	Nl	Nl	Full	Nl
R. glut med	Nl	0	0	0	Nl	Nl	Nl	Full	Nl
R. peron ln	Nl	0	0	0	Nl	Nl	Nl	Full	Nl
R. S1 paraspinals	Nl	0	0	0	—	—	—	—	—

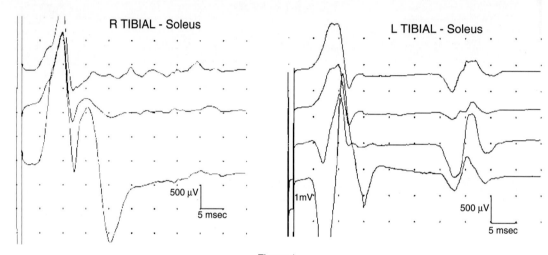

Figure 1

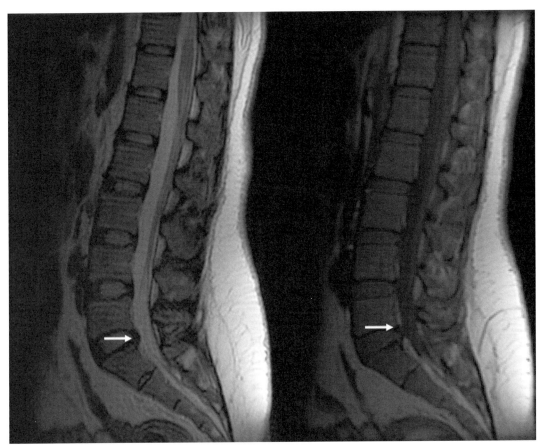

Figure 2

Questions:
1. What abnormality is shown in figure 1?
2. What abnormality is shown in figure 2?

Answers:
1. Absent right tibial H-reflex
2. L5–S1 central and right-sided disc hermination

Discussion: The electrodiagnostic study is abnormal for the inability to obtain H-reflexes from the tibial nerve recording over the soleus on the right and for fibrillation potentials in the right medial gastrocnemius. These findings suggest a right S1 or S2 radiculopathy but are not specific of such and could be seen in a tibial or sciatic neuropathy. However, the radiological findings show an L5–S1 disc central and right-sided herniation; it is likely that the absent H-reflex is a consequence of an S1 root lesion.

Clinical Pearl

Nerve conduction studies are relatively insensitive to detecting radiculopathy, although an H-reflex when available can be informative.

PATIENT 23

A 57-year-old man with right leg weakness after repair of abdominal aortic and internal iliac artery aneurysms

This 57-year-old man underwent surgical repair of an abdominal aortic aneurysm and a right internal iliac artery aneurysm with placement of an aorto-bi-iliac graft. He awoke postoperatively with pain, numbness, and weakness of his right leg and absence of pulses and Doppler flow signal in his foot. He was brought back to the operating room and underwent thrombectomy of an occluded right aorto-iliac graft. His electrodiagnostic study was performed 2 months later.

Electrodiagnostic Study:

Sensory NCS

Nerve	Sites	Recording Site	Onset (ms)	Peak (ms)	Amplitude (µV)	Distance (cm)	Velocity (m/s)
R. sural–lat mall	1. Mid calf	Ankle	Absent	—	—	14	—
R. sup peroneal	1. Lat leg	Ankle	Absent	—	—	12	—
R. saphenous	1. Med leg	Foot	Absent	—	—	10	—
L. sural–lat mall	1. Mid calf	Ankle	3.00	3.75	16.0	14	46.7
L. sup peroneal	1. Lat leg	Ankle	2.60	3.35	8.8	12	46.2
L. saphenous	1. Med leg	Foot	2.40	2.95	4.0	10	41.7

Motor NCS

Nerve	Sites	Recording Site	Latency (ms)	Amplitude (mV)	Distance (cm)	Velocity (m/s)
R. peroneal–EDB	1. Ankle	EDB	Absent	—	8	—
R. peroneal–tib ant	1. Fib head	Tib ant	Absent	—	—	—
R. tibial–AH	1. Ankle	AH	5.90	0.3	8	—
	2. Pop fossa	AH	Absent	—	—	—
R. femoral–rect fem	1. Groin	Rect fem	Absent	—	—	—
L. peroneal–EDB	1. Ankle	EDB	4.20	7.9	8	—
	2. Fib head	EDB	11.40	7.0	32	44.4
	3. Pop fossa	EDB	14.00	6.6	12	46.2
L. tibial–AH	1. Ankle	AH	5.80	7.5	8	—
	2. Pop fossa	AH	13.15	5.9	39	53.1
L. femoral–rect fem	1. Groin	Rect fem	4.95	10.0	—	—

EMG Summary Table

		SA			Amplitude (MUs)	Duration (MUs)	PolyP (MUs)	Activation	Recruitment Pattern
	IA	Fib	Fasc	Other					
R. tib ant	Inc	3+	0	0	Nl	Nl	Nl	Full	Single MU
R. vast lat	Inc	3+	0	0	—	—	—	—	No activity
R. vast med	Inc	3+	0	0	—	—	—	—	No activity
R. psoas	Inc	1+	0	0	Nl	Nl	Nl	Full	Nl

Continued

	SA				Amplitude (MUs)	Duration (MUs)	PolyP (MUs)	Activation	Recruitment Pattern
	IA	Fib	Fasc	Other					
R. med gastroc	Inc	2+	0	0	Nl	Nl	Nl	Full	Mod dec
R. tib post	Inc	2–3+	0	0	Nl	Nl	Nl	Full	Mod dec
R. glut med	Nl	0	0	0	Nl	Nl	Nl	Full	Nl
R. add longus	Inc	3–4+	0	0	—	—	—	—	No activity
R. L3 paraspinal m	Nl	0	0	0	—	—	—	—	—
R. L4 paraspinal m	Nl	0	0	0	—	—	—	—	—
R. L5 paraspinal m	Nl	0	0	0	—	—	—	—	—

Questions:

1. What are the electrodiagnostic abnormalities? Do they favor root, plexus, or more peripheral localization?
2. What is the electrodiagnostic localization?

Answers:
1. They favor a plexous localization
2. Lumbosacral plexopathy

Discussion: The electrodiagnostic abnormalities are (1) inability to record the right sural, superficial peroneal, and saphenous SNAPs, and (2) inability to record the right peroneal–EDB, peroneal–TA, and femoral CMAPs with a severely reduced right tibial–AH CMAP. The results of EMG studies are abnormal for abundant fibrillation potentials and reduction or absence of recruitable motor units in muscles as tabulated above. The absence of right sensory nerve action potentials with normal responses on the left strongly suggests a localization distal to the dorsal root ganglia (*i.e.*, a lumbosacral plexopathy rather than a lumbosacral polyradiculopathy). This patient apparently suffered an ischemic lumbosacral plexopathy related to his vascular disease and its treatment with a surgical procedure. Perioperative ischemic lumbosacral plexopathies do occur uncommonly in vascular procedures of the infrarenal aorta, femoral, and iliac arteries. Lumbosacral plexopathy may be the presenting feature of an iliac artery aneurysm.

Clinical Pearls

1. Sensory nerve studies are generally valuable in distinguishing root from plexus disease; these may need to be performed bilaterally to be confident of their abnormality.
2. Disease of the infrarenal aorta, femoral, and iliac arteries, and its management, may produce ischemic lumbosacral plexopathy.

REFERENCES

1. Dougherty, M.J., Calligaro, K.D., How to avoid and manage nerve injuries associated with aortic surgery: ischemic neuropathy, traction injuries, and sexual derangements, *Semin. Vasc. Surg.* 2001; 14(4):275–281.
2. Gloviczki, P., Cross, S.A., Stanson, A.W., Carmichael, S.W., Bower, T.C., Pairolero, P.C., Hallett, J.W., Jr., Toomey, B.J., Cherry, K.J., Jr., Ischemic injury to the spinal cord or lumbosacral plexus after aorto-iliac reconstruction, *Am. J. Surg.* 1991; 162(2):131–136.
3. Lefebvre, V., Leduc, J.J., Choteau, P.H., Painless ischaemic lumbosacral plexopathy and aortic dissection, *J. Neurol. Neurosurg. Psychiatry* 1995; 58(5):641.
4. Luzzio, C.C., Waclawik, A.J., Gallagher, C.L., Knechtle, S.J., Iliac artery pseudoaneurysm following renal transplantation presenting as lumbosacral plexopathy. *Transplantation* 1999; 67(7):1077–1078.

SECTION II. GENERALIZED NEUROPATHIES

The diversity of presentation of generalized peripheral neuropathies is impressive. This area of clinical neuromuscular practice is one of the most subtle and fascinating. As is always the approach in neurological diagnosis, one focuses on the localization before the differential diagnosis. For generalized neuropathies, we also take the approach of characterizing the neuropathy prior to considering specific causes.

The characterization of peripheral neuropathy by anatomic and physiological involvement is of great value in determining the underlying cause. Neuropathies can be categorized by a combination of anatomical distribution plus extent of physiological involvement. Anatomical distribution is described by terms such as *distal*, *proximal > distal*, *diffuse* (meaning relatively equal proximal and distal involvement), *symmetric*, and *asymmetric*. The physiological involvement is described using terms such as *sensory*, *sensory > motor*, *motor > sensory*, and *autonomic*. Together, we have groupings of specific anatomical and physiological patterns of neuropathy that help to narrow the potential causes to manageable groups (Tables 1 to 6).

Table 1.   Distal Symmetric Purely Sensory or Sensory > Motor Neuropathies

Drug and toxic neuropathies, including alcohol	Toxic
Diabetic distal symmetric polyneuropathy	Paraproteinemic neuropathies
Idiopathic	Amyloidosis
Vitamin deficiency: B_{12}, E, thiamine	Confluent vasculitis

Table 2.   Diffuse Motor > Sensory Neuropathies

Guillain-Barré syndrome	Diphtheria
Chronic inflammatory demyelinating polyneuropathy (CIDP)	Acute arsenic poisoning
Osteosclerotic myeloma	Inherited neuropathies
Drugs: Amiodarone, gold, perhexilene	Acute intermittent porphyria

Table 3.   Diffuse Sensory Neuropathies (Neuronopathies)

Sjögren's syndrome
Anti-Hu paraneoplastic sensory neuronopathy

Table 4.   Neuropathies with Prominent Autonomic Involvement

Diabetes
Guillain-Barré syndrome
Acquired and familial amyloidoses
Paraneoplastic autonomic neuropathy
Hereditary sensory and autonomic neuropathies

Table 5.   Symmetric and Multifocal Sensory and Motor Neuropathies

Multifocal CIDP
Some inherited neuropathies

Table 6. Asymmetric, Multifocal Sensory and Motor Neuropathies

Vasculitis	Hereditary neuropathy with liability to pressure palsies (HNPP)
Multifocal CIDP (MADSAM)	Lyme disease
Neoplastic	HIV-associated CMV multiple mononeuropathy
Diabetic radiculoplexus neuropathy	Sarcoidosis
Nondiabetic radiculoplexus neuropathy	Amyloidosis
Leprosy	Acute brachial neuritis

Accordingly, the electrodiagnostic approach to generalized peripheral neuropathies has the following goals:

- Confirm or reject the presence of a peripheral neuropathy.
- Characterize involvement of sensory or motor nerves or both.
- Establish extent of symmetry.
- Establish length dependence or lack thereof.
- Establish primary physiology as that of axonal degeneration or demyelination.

These goals are achieved by the following approach:

1. Bilateral sural and superficial sensory nerve studies
   a. Abnormalities in the amplitudes of the sural and superficial sensory nerve action potentials (SNAPs) are the most sensitive indicators in most axonal neuropathies.
   b. Bilateral studies are required to establish symmetry or asymmetry of distal sensory involvement and help to distinguish disorders in Table 1 from Table 6.
2. Bilateral peroneal–extensor digitorum brevis (EDB) and tibial–AH motor studies
   a. Amplitudes of the compound muscle action potentials (CMAPs) establish whether involvement includes motor axons and degree of symmetry as in 1(b) above.
3. Unilateral or possibly bilateral median, ulnar, and radial sensory nerve studies
   a. When foot SNAP amplitudes are reduced, determination of hand SNAP amplitudes characterizes the extent of the neuropathy (*i.e.*, limited to the feet or spread to the hands).
   b. When foot SNAP amplitudes are not reduced but hand SNAP amplitudes are, this establishes a non-length-dependent process that may be seen in demyelinating neuropathies and sensory neuronopathies (Tables 2 and 3).
   c. Peripheral neuropathies with superimposed focal neuropathies, such as median at the wrist and ulnar at the elbow, may be demonstrated and further characterize the neuropathy. For example, distal symmetric axonal neuropathies with diabetes often have superimposed bilateral median and ulnar neuropathies.
   d. Same reason as 1(b).
4. Unilateral or bilateral median–abductor pollicis brevis (APB) and ulnar–abductor digiti minimi (ADM) motor studies
   a. When foot CMAP amplitudes are reduced, determination of hand CMAP amplitudes characterizes the extent of the neuropathy (*i.e.*, limited to the feet or spread to the hands), analogous to point 3(a) above.
   b. The median and ulnar forearm motor velocities are more reliable indicators of a primary demyelinating neuropathy than the leg motor velocities and need to be studied, at least unilaterally, in all patients with a generalized peripheral neuropathy.
   c. Same reason as 3(c) above.
   d. Same reason as 3(d) above.
5. F-wave studies
   a. F-wave studies are important when demyelinating neuropathies are a relevant consideration, particularly when acute.
6. Needle EMG studies
   a. Needle EMG studies are valuable in establishing the length dependence of the process. Reduced amplitudes of foot CMAPs should indicate EMG studies in foreleg muscles. Reduced amplitudes of hand CMAPs should indicate EMG studies in hand and forearm muscles and, if the

latter are abnormal, more proximal muscles. For example, finding fibrillation potentials in tibialis anterior, gastrocnemius, and peroneus longus but not hamstrings or gluteus medius localizes the involvement to long motor axons and not roots or a focal cord anterior horn lesion.

b. Needle EMG studies reveal symmetry or asymmetry, multifocality vs. confluence.

REFERENCES

1. Amato, A.A., Approach to peripheral neuropathy, in Dumitru, D., Amato, A., Zwarts, M.J., *Electrodiagnostic Medicine*, Hanley & Belfus, Philadelphia, PA, 2002.
2. Barohn, R.J., Approach to peripheral neuropathy and neuronopathy, *Semin. Neurol.* 1998; 18:7–18.
3. Donofrio, P.D., Albers, J.W., AAEM minimonograph 34: polyneuropathy—classification by nerve conduction studies and electromyography, *Muscle Nerve* 1990; 13:889–903.
4. Dyck, P.J., Dyck, P.J., Grant, I.A., Fealey, R.D., Ten steps in characterizing and diagnosing patients with peripheral neuropathy, *Neurology* 1996; 47:10–17.

PATIENT 24

A 73-year-old man with an IgG-κ paraprotein and several years of progressive numbness and weakness in the feet and hands

This 73-year-old man was referred for electrodiagnostic evaluation because of several years of progressive numbness and weakness that started in his feet and later spread to the hands. Neurological examination demonstrated symmetric paralysis of all toe and ankle movements and moderate weakness and atrophy of intrinsic hand muscles, along with symmetric distal sensory loss in the hands and feet.

Consider the main possibilities for localization and how you would approach the electrodiagnostic study.

Electrodiagnostic Study:

Sensory NCS

Nerve	Sites	Recording Site	Onset (ms)	Peak (ms)	Amplitude (μV)	Distance (cm)	Velocity (m/s)
R. median–dig II	1. Wrist	Dig II	2.50	3.55	5.3	13	52.0
R. ulnar–dig V	1. Wrist	Dig V	2.55	3.45	3.5	11	43.1
R. radial–sn box	1. Forearm	SnBox	2.30	3.05	6.5	10	43.5
R. lat AB cut	1. Elbow	Forearm	Absent	—	—	12	—
R. sural–lat mall	1. Mid-calf	Ankle	Absent	—	—	14	—
L. sural–lat mall	1. Mid-calf	Ankle	Absent	—	—	14	—

Motor NCS

Nerve	Sites	Recording Site	Latency (ms)	Amplitude (μV)	Distance (cm)	Velocity (m/s)
R. median–APB	1. Wrist	APB	4.60	5.5	7	—
	2. Elbow	APB	10.00	4.9	25	46.3
	3. Axilla	APB	12.55	4.8	12	47.1
R. ulnar–ADM	1. Wrist	ADM	3.20	3.0	7	—
	2. B. elbow	ADM	7.55	2.6	22	50.6
	3. A. elbow	ADM	10.65	2.5	15	48.4
R. peroneal–EDB	1. Ankle	EDB	Absent	—	8	—
L. peroneal–EDB	1. Ankle	EDB	Absent	—	8	—
L. peroneal–tib ant	1. Fib head	Tib ant	3.15	0.2	11	—
	2. Pop fossa	Tib ant	5.15	0.2	10	50
R. tibial–AH	1. Ankle	AH	Absent	—	8	—
L. tibial–AH	1. Ankle	AH	Absent	—	8	—

F-Wave

Nerve	F_{min} (ms)	F_{max} (ms)	Max – Min (ms)	%F
R. median	38.50	42.20	3.70	30
R. ulnar	36.85	38.65	1.80	80
R. peroneal	Absent	—	—	—
R. tibial	Absent	—	—	—
L. peroneal	Absent	—	—	—
L. tibial	Absent	—	—	—

EMG Summary Table

		SA			Amplitude (MUs)	Duration (MUs)	PolyP (MUs)	Activation	Recruitment Pattern
	IA	Fib	Fasc	Other					
R. vast med	Inc	2+	0	0	Nl	Nl	Nl	Full	Nl
R. bic fem SH	Inc	2+	0	CRD	Nl	Nl	Nl	Full	Nl
R. tib ant	Inc	3+	0	0	Nl	Nl	Nl	Full	Single MU
R. tib post	Inc	3+	0	0	—	—	Nl	—	No activity
R. gastroc med	Dec	0	0	0	—	—	Nl	—	No activity
R. first dors int	Inc	3+	0	0	Large	Long	Nl	Full	Sev red
R. abd poll br	Inc	3+	0	0	Large	Long	Nl	Full	Sev red
R. biceps	Nl	0	0	0	Nl	Nl	Nl	Full	Nl
R. pron teres	Nl	0	0	0	Nl	Nl	Nl	Full	Nl
R. ext dig comm	Nl	0	0	0	Nl	Nl	Nl	Full	Nl

Questions:

1. Is the process symmetric or asymmetric? What additional electrodiagnostic studies would be valuable in this regard?
2. Is the process length dependent?

Answers:
1. Symmetric; left sensory studies and left leg needle EMG studies
2. Yes

Discussion: The salient electrodiagnostic abnormalities can be grouped in a meaningful way as follows:

- Absent foot (sural) SNAPs and low-amplitude hand SNAPs (median, ulnar, and radial on one side), suggesting length-dependent axonal degeneration of sensory axons in the feet and hands
- Absent foot (bilateral peroneal–EDB and tibial–AH) CMAPs with moderately reduced amplitude of the ulnar–ADM CMAP in the hand, suggesting length-dependent axonal degeneration of motor axons in the hands and feet
- EMG abnormalities with a distal to proximal gradient in the right leg (look at recruitment patterns of foreleg muscles tibialis anterior, medial gastrocnemius, and tibialis posterior, all similar to each other and in contrast to thigh muscles vastus medialis and biceps femoris); similarly, a distal to proximal gradient in the right arm
- Prolongation of the right median–APB minimum F-wave latency in the setting of fibrillation potentials in this muscle

These features establish the presence of a generalized peripheral neuropathy characterized by length-dependent distal degeneration of sensory and motor axons and symmetry in the legs. Further study of left hand SNAPs and bilateral superficial peroneal sensory and needle EMG of left leg and arm muscles could provide even further support of a symmetric process. In this case, this severe axonal neuropathy, with fibrillation potentials present even in thigh muscles, was associated with an IgG-κ paraprotein, although the relationship is unclear. Other potential considerations for this category of neuropathies are listed in the table below. No other definite cause for this particular patient's neuropathy was established after sural nerve biopsy (showing axonal degeneration), bone marrow biopsy, and skeletal survey.

Distal Symmetric Purely Sensory or Sensory > Motor Neuropathies

Drug and toxic neuropathies, including alcohol	Toxic
Diabetic distal symmetric polyneuropathy	Paraproteinemic neuropathies
Idiopathic	Amyloidosis
Vitamin deficiency: B_{12}, E, thiamine	Confluent vasculitis

Paraproteinemic neuropathies are associated with the monoclonal production of a specific population of immunoglobulins or immunoglobulin fragments. In some disorders, the monoclonal protein is highly and specifically directed at nerve antigens and disease is entirely limited to a neuropathy. In other disorders, the neuropathy is one feature of a systemic malignancy of antibody-producing plasma cells. Serum immunofixation (IF) is more sensitive than serum protein electrophoresis (SPEP) and is the essential laboratory test for detection of most of these syndromes. These disorders are summarized in the next table.

Monoclonal gammopathy of undetermined significance (MGUS) is the term applied to the presence of a serum paraprotein without any other identified disease. An IgG or IgA MGUS is associated with neuropathies, although the causal relationship is unclear. The same is true for approximately 50% of IgM MGUS; however, in the other 50% of MGUS patients, the antibody is likely pathogenic and results in the neuropathy syndrome associated with anti-myelin-associated glycoprotein (MAG). MAG-associated peripheral neuropathy appears to result from an IgM-κ antibody directed against the MAG or related components (*e.g.*, sulfatides or sulfoglucuronyl paragloboside [SGPG]) of peripheral nerve. This distinctive syndrome looks clinically like a distal sensory > motor neuropathy, although a greater degree of ataxia is generally present. Electrodiagnostic studies, however, demonstrate a unique picture of sensory and motor demyelination with much greater distal than proximal involvement.

Multiple myeloma (MM) is a plasma cell malignancy, usually but not always producing IgG or IgA and usually but not always a κ light chain. Typical presentation is in middle or late age with fatigue, anemia, and hypercalcemia, with bone pain and renal insufficiency being other prominent aspects. Neuropathy is present in about 10% of patients and may be the presenting feature. It is typically a distal axonal sensory and motor neuropathy. The most common pathogenesis of neuropathy in patients with multiple myeloma results from AL-type amyloidosis, present in at least 30 to 40% of MM neuropathies. Other causes may be related to metabolic and toxic consequences of the disease or its treatment.

Osteosclerotic myeloma is also a plasma cell malignancy and may overlap with multiple myeloma; it is usually but not always due to an IgG or IgA and is almost always a λ light chain. Although much less common than multiple myeloma, the association with neuropathy is much higher (50%) and accordingly neuropathy is a much more common presenting feature. The POEMS syndrome (polyneuropathy, organomegaly, endocrinopathy, M-protein, and skin changes) may result. The associated neuropathy is said to be similar to that of chronic inflammatory demyelinating polyneuropathy (CIDP) with proximal and distal weakness and generalized hypo- or areflexia. Electrodiagnostic studies, however, are those of axonal sensory and motor loss with moderate or marked slowing of nerve conduction velocities, but without the definitive findings of focal conduction block or temporal dispersion more commonly diagnostic of CIDP. Cerebrospinal fluid (CSF) protein is often quite elevated (>100 mg/dl). A skeletal survey is more sensitive than radioisotope bone scans for detection of sclerotic lesions.

Waldenstrom's macroglobulinemia is a plasma cell disorder limited by definition to IgM production; it produces fatigue, anemia, epistaxis, and a hyperviscosity syndrome. The pathogenesis of an associated neuropathy is heterogeneous. For most patients, a distal axonal sensory and motor neuropathy similar to that seen in multiple myeloma is present, sometimes secondary to AL-type amyloidosis. Other patients with an IgM-κ protein with anti-MAG activity and the characteristic features of a MAG-associated neuropathy (see below) have also been described.

Amyloidosis is a group of disorders with a common endpoint: deposition of insoluble fibrillar proteins (termed *amyloid* fibrils) in organs and tissues. In one disorder (AL-amyloidosis), amyloid fibrils consist of fragments of immunoglobulin light chains. For all the other amyloidoses, the amyloid fibrils are not immunoglobulins. Some cases of multiple myeloma may be associated with deposition of amyloid fibrils derived from immunoglobulins but are not classified as principal amyloidoses; this distinction appears to be solely semantic. The neuropathy of AL-type amyloidosis is more distinctive than the generic distal axonal neuropathy seen in multiple myeloma. Early painful sensory and autonomic involvement with concomitant carpal tunnel syndromes is characteristic. Familial amyloidotic polyneuropathy (FAP), when due to mutations in amyloidogenic transthyretin (ATTR), may be diagnosed through sequencing of the transthyretin (TTR) gene.

Cryoglobulinemias are a heterogeneous group of disorders. Type I cryoglobulins are associated with the plasma cell dyscrasias or lymphoproliferative disorders. These are the disorders just discussed above. Type II cryoglobulins consist of a monoclonal immunoglobulin, typically an IgM-κ with anti-IgG activity (rheumatoid factor), and polyclonal IgG. The major cause of type II cryoglobulinemia is chronic hepatitis C infection which produces a confluent distal mononeuritis multiplex, resulting in a distal axonal sensory and motor neuropathy. Type III cryoglobulins are a mixture of only polyclonal immunoglobulins and are more typically present in rheumatoid arthritis and connective tissue diseases.

Paraproteinemic Neuropathies

Disorder	Paraprotein	Systemic Features	Neuropathy	Of Diagnostic Value
MGUS	IgM, IgG, or IgA, usually κ	None	Distal axonal sensory and motor	—
Anti-MAG/SGPG	IgM-κ	None	Sensory > motor with ataxia	Distinctive NCS findings
Multiple myeloma	IgG, IgA, or IgM (usually IgG or IgA)	Bone pain, anemia, renal	Distal axonal sensory and motor	Bone marrow bx Skeletal survey
Osteosclerotic myeloma	IgG or IgA, almost always λ	POEMS	Distal axonal sensory and motor with demyelinating-range nerve conduction velocities	Skeletal survey
Waldenstrom's macroglobulinemia	IgM	Fatigue, hyperviscosity	Distal axonal sensory and motor	—
Amyloidosis	AL—light chains λ or κ (3:1) AA—not paraprotein Familial ATTR	Heart and kidney	Autonomic + axonal sensory and motor neuropathy; + carpal tunnel syndrome	AL—fat pad bx + serum/urine AA—fat pad bx + stain AA protein ATTR—fat pad bx + TTR mutation
Lymphoma	Any	Systemic, hematologic	Distal axonal sensory and motor; mononeuritis multiplex from nerve invasion	Chest/Abd CT
Cryoglobulinemia Hepatitis C	IgM-κ	Complement-mediated immune complex deposition vasculitis	Confluent mononeuritis multiplex	HepC Ab, RF

Clinical Pearls

1. Establishing length dependence and symmetry are important principles in the electrodiagnostic assessment of peripheral neuropathies.
2. The relationship between paraproteins in MGUS and neuropathy is uncertain.

REFERENCES

1. Falk, R.H., Comenzo, R.L., Skinner, M., The systemic amyloidoses, *N. Engl J. Med.* 1997; 337:898–909.
2. Gorson, K.C., Ropper, A.H., Axonal neuropathy associated with monoclonal gammopathy of undetermined significance, *J. Neurol. Neurosurg. Psychiatry* 1997; 63:163–168.
3. Notermans, N.C., Wokke, J.H.J., Lokhorst, H.M., Franssen, H., van der Graaf, Y., Jennekens, F.G.I., Polyneuropathy associated with monoclonal gammopathy of undetermined significance: a prospective study of the prognostic value of clinical and laboratory abnormalities, *Brain* 1994; 117:1385–1393.
4. Notermans, N.C., Wokke, J.H.J., van den Berg, L.H. et al., Chronic idiopathic axonal polyneuropathy:comparison of patients with and without monoclonal gammopathy, *Brain* 1996; 119:421–427.
5. Ropper, A.H., Gorson, K.C., Neuropathies associated with paraproteinemia, *N. Engl. J. Med.* 1998; 338:1601–1607.
6. Simovic, D., Gorson, K.C., Ropper, A.H., Comparison of IgM–MGUS and IgG–MGUS polyneuropathy, *Acta Neurol. Scand.* 1998; 97:194–200.
7. Van den Berg, L.H., Hays, A.P., Nobile-Orazio, E. *et al.*, Anti-MAG and anti-SGPG antibodies in neuropathy, *Muscle Nerve* 1996; 19:63–143.

PATIENT 25

A 43-year-old man with diabetes and multiple neurologic symptoms

This 43-year-old businessman with a history of diabetes for 7 years presented in August 2000 with a history summarized as follows:

- Summer 1999—right lower abdominal pain and a bulge in the right lower abdomen
- Late 1999—multiple postprandial gastrointestinal complaints (fullness, belching)
- January 2000—constant tingling paresthesias in left thigh and deep aching pain
- March to May 2000—progressive weakness of left leg
- June 2000—HbA$_{1C}$ 12.1%; initiation of insulin therapy
- July 2000—Right thigh weakness and pain; left leg strength starting to improve
- February to August 2000—40-lb weight loss
- Exam in August 2000:

Strength

Legs	Psoas	Quads	Adductor	TA	Hams	Toe Flex	Toe Ext	Glut Max	Glu Med
Right	2	2	2	5–	4–	4	4	5	5
Left	3	4	2	4	4–	4	4	5	5

- Reflexes—Absent bilateral knees and ankles.
- Sensory—Absent vibration in toes bilaterally; light touch abnormal in right saphenous n. territory; decreased pin prick up to the ankles bilaterally and in the right saphenous n. territory.
- Gait—Walk with a walker only.

Electrodiagnostic Study:

Sensory NCS

Nerve	Sites	Recording Site	Onset (ms)	Peak (ms)	Amplitude (μV)	Distance (cm)	Velocity (m/s)
R. median–dig II	1. Wrist	Dig II	3.4	4.5	7.4	13	38
R. ulnar–dig V	1. Wrist	Dig V	Absent	—	—	11	—
R. radial–sn box	1. Forearm	Sn box	2.5	3.3	7.8	10	43.5
R. sural–lat mall	1. Mid Calf	Ankle	Absent	—	—	14	—
L. sural–lat mall	1. Mid Calf	Ankle	Absent	—	—	14	—

Motor NCS

Nerve	Sites	Recording Site	Latency (ms)	Amplitude (mV)	Distance (cm)	Velocity (m/s)
R. median–APB	1. Wrist	APB	4.5	7.8	7	
	2. Elbow	APB	10.7	6.4	25	40
R. ulnar–ADM	1. Wrist	ADM	3.9	7.0	7	—
	2. B. elbow	ADM	8.1	4.8	18	43
	3. A. elbow	ADM	12.5	6.5	18	41
R. peroneal–EDB	1. Ankle	EDB	Absent	—	—	—
L. peroneal–EDB	1. Ankle	EDB	6.1	0.3	8	—
	2. Bel fib hd	EDB	18.0	0.2	33.5	28

Continued

Motor NCS—cont'd

Nerve	Sites	Recording Site	Latency (ms)	Amplitude (mV)	Distance (cm)	Velocity (m/s)
	3. Abv fib hd	EDB	21.6	0.2	11	31
R. peroneal–tib ant	1. Fib head	Tib ant	4.2	4.0	8	—
	2. Pop fossa	Tib ant	6.4	3.6	8	36
L. peroneal–tib ant	1. Fib head	Tib ant	2.6	2.5	8	—
	2. Pop fossa	Tib ant	6.9	1.8	11	26
R. tibial–AH	1. Ankle	AH	Absent	—	—	—
L. tibial–AH	1. Ankle	AH	Absent	—	—	—

EMG Summary Table

	IA	SA			Amplitude (MUs)	Duration (MUs)	PolyP (MUs)	Activation	Recruitment Pattern
		Fib	Fasc	Other					
R. vast med	Inc	1+	0	0	Nl	Nl	Nl	Full	Sev dec
R. add long	Inc	1+	0	0	Nl	Nl	Nl	Full	Sev dec
L. vast lat	Inc	1+	0	0	Inc	Inc	Nl	Full	Mod dec
L. tib ant	Inc	1+	0	0	Nl	Nl	Nl	Full	Mod dec
L. gastroc med	Inc	1+	0	0	Inc	Inc	Nl	Full	Normal
L. L3 paraspinals	Nl	0	0	0	—	—	—	—	—
L. L4 paraspinals	Nl	0	0	0	—	—	—	—	—

Questions:

1. Does the electrodiagnostic study support the clinical characterization of this syndrome?
2. How would you characterize this syndrome, assuming it is a neuropathy?

Discussion: This syndrome is clinically classified as a neuropathy with multifocal asymmetric sensory and motor involvement. The electrodiagnostic studies support this view and further characterize the physiology as that of axonal degeneration. These findings put this disorder in the category represented by Table 6 in the introduction to this section. Additional noteworthy clinical characteristics are that it is painful and has a subacute progression, and the multifocality is present in time as well, with worsening involvement in one leg while the other is in fact improving.

Several specific and separate disorders associated with diabetes are present in this patient:
- Proximal diabetic neuropathy (diabetic radiculoplexus neuropathy, diabetic amyotrophy)
- Thoracoabominal neuropathy
- Diabetic gastroparesis
- Distal symmetric polyneuropathy

Diabetic neuropathies other than the distal symmetric polyneuropathy (DSP) are of several types and may occur independently of DSP.

Autonomic involvement is common in diabetes, and a separate form of neuropathy, termed *autonomic neuropathy*, may be present and exist independently of, or together with, distal symmetric neuropathy. Diabetic gastroparesis is a common manifestation of diabetic autonomic neuropathy. Postural lightheadedness and erectile dysfunction in men are other less common features.

Focal cranial neuropathies with diabetes are well described and relatively common for the third and sixth cranial nerves. These palsies are typically acute and painful but have excellent prognosis for full recovery.

Other multifocal diabetic neuropathies include *thoracoabdominal neuropathy* and *diabetic proximal neuropathy*. Diabetic thoracoabdominal neuropathy is a curious syndrome of acute or subacute pain and paresthesias, typically in the distribution of one or several adjacent unilateral thoracic dermatomes. As the pain resolves, a bulging of the abdominal musculature may appear and is likely due to focal abdominal muscle weakness. Thoracoabdominal neuropathy may occur bilaterally.

Diabetic proximal neuropathy (diabetic radiculoplexus neuropathy) is an even more curious entity. Subacute proximal thigh pain, paresthesias, and weakness (unilateral or bilateral) may progress for several months before stabilizing. Pain is often severe and the major component of this syndrome, leading to poor appetite and depression. Involvement can be bilateral from the start or can be on one side for months before the other side becomes involved. The initial side may be improving when the other side is evolving. Although predominant involvement in the quadriceps suggesting a femoral neuropathy is the rule, involvement of a wider territory is universal, localizing this disorder to the lumbosacral plexus more commonly. Weakness of adductor muscles and medial thigh numbness (obturator nerve) and sometimes portions of the lateral trunk of the sciatic nerve (common peroneal nerve, foot drop) are common and suggest specific localization to the lumbar plexus or lumbosacral trunk, with involvement of the sacral plexus less common. The cause is unknown, but it is often associated with weight loss. It may be a result of a vasculitis of small or microscopic vessels. The syndrome has been attributed to both poor diabetic control as well as institution of good diabetic control (*i.e.,* initial use of insulin); as the latter usually occurs because of the former, it may be more reasonable to assume that poor diabetic control is the cause. The major emphasis of treatment is on weight stabilization and pain control. The syndrome is often protracted but has an excellent prognosis for good recovery of motor function, even in wheelchair-bound patients, over 6 to 24 months after symptoms stabilize.

For this patient, treatment was directed at emphasizing weight gain, pain control, and tighter diabetic control. Over the ensuing 9 months, the pain resolved and there was continued gradual improvement in strength. By April 2002, the patient had regained all weight and was walking without a walker. His strength was as follows:

						Toe	Toe	Glut	Glu
Legs	Psoas	Quads	Adductor	TA	Hams	Flex	Ext	Max	Med
Right	5	4	5	5–	5	4	4	5	5
Left	5	4	5	5–	5	4	4	5	5

Strength

Clinical Pearls

1. Diabetic neuropathies comprise a number of distinct syndromes.
2. Diabetic proximal neuropathy generally has an excellent long-term prognosis for recovery.

REFERENCES

1. Asbury, A.K., Proximal diabetic neuropathy, *Ann. Neurol.* 1977; 2:179–180.
2. Barohn, R.J., Sahenk, Z., Warmolts, J.R., Mendell, J.R., The Bruns-Garland syndrome (diabetic amyotrophy): revisited 100 years later, *Arch. Neurol.* 1991; 48:1130–1135.
3. Dyck, P.J., Windebank, A.J., Diabetic and nondiabetic lumbosacral radiculoplexus neuropathies: new insights into pathophysiology and treatment, *Muscle Nerve* 2002; 25:477–491.
4. Dyck, P.J., Norell, J.E., Dyck, P.J., Microvasculitis and ischemia in diabetic lumbosacral radiculoplexus neuropathy, *Neurology* 1999; 53:2113–2121.

PATIENT 26

A 73-year-old man with diabetes and several months of chest pain

This 73-year-old man with diabetes for several years developed right-sided, lower chest and upper abdominal continuous burning pain and tingling paresthesias 9 months prior to this study. He noted that a light touch, such as his clothes or a bed sheet, over the area provoked pain.

Electrodiagnostic study:

Sensory NCS

Nerve	Sites	Recording Site	Onset (ms)	Peak (ms)	Amplitude (μV)	Distance (cm)	Velocity (m/s)
R. median–dig II	1. Wrist	Dig II	3.85	4.75	11.5	13	33.8
L. median–dig II	1. Wrist	Dig II	3.10	3.95	16.3	13	41.9
R. ulnar–dig V	1. Wrist	Dig V	2.60	3.45	9.9	11	42.3
L. ulnar–dig V	1. Wrist	Dig V	2.65	3.50	13.4	11	41.5
R. radial–sn box	1. Forearm	Sn box	1.70	2.45	16.9	10	58.8
R. sural–lat mall	1. Mid-calf	Ankle	3.65	4.40	4.9	14	38.4

Motor NCS

Nerve	Sites	Recording Site	Latency (ms)	Amplitude (mV)	Distance (cm)	Velocity (m/s)
R. median–APB	1. Wrist	APB	5.20	6.5	7	—
	2. Elbow	APB	9.80	5.4	22	47.8
L. median–APB	1. Wrist	APB	4.80	4.8	7	—
	2. Elbow	APB	9.45	4.5	21	45.2
R. ulnar–ADM	1. Wrist	ADM	3.65	8.2	7	—
	2. B. elbow	ADM	7.30	7.1	19	52.1
	3. A. elbow	ADM	10.05	5.6	12	43.6
L. ulnar–ADM	1. Wrist	ADM	3.55	8.3	7	—
	2. B. elbow	ADM	7.45	7.7	19.5	50.0
	3. A. elbow	ADM	10.50	6.8	12.5	41.0
R. ulnar–FDI	1. Wrist	FDI	5.20	9.5	—	—
	2. B. elbow	FDI	9.15	8.5	19	48.1
	3. A. elbow	FDI	11.65	7.7	12	48.0
R. peroneal–EDB	1. Ankle	EDB	5.00	5.4	8	—
	2. Fib head	EDB	12.90	4.6	29	36.7
	3. Pop fossa	EDB	15.25	4.6	9	38.3

EMG Summary Table

	IA	SA Fib	SA Fasc	SA Other	Amplitude (MUs)	Duration (MUs)	PolyP (MUs)	Activation	Recruitment Pattern
R. thoracic PSP mid	Nl	2+	0	0	—	—	—	—	—
R. thoracic PSP lower	Nl	2+	0	0	—	—	—	—	—
R. thoracic PSP upper	Nl	0	0	0	—	—	—	—	—
L. thoracic PSP mid	Nl	1+	0	0	—	—	—	—	—

Question: What is the clinical diagnosis?

Answer: Diabetic thoracoabdominal neuropathy

Discussion: The nerve conduction studies show mild abnormalities in the reduction of the right median distal sensory velocity (33.8 m/s) and prolongation of the right median–APB distal motor latency (5.2 ms), both suggestive of a right carpal tunnel syndrome. In addition, there is mild or borderline slowing of the ulnar–ADM across-elbow motor velocities (43.6 and 41 m/s) suggesting subclinical ulnar neuropathies at the elbow. These findings are commonly seen in patients with diabetes and are often asymptomatic. There is no evidence of a distal symmetric polyneuropathy in this patient (normal right sural SNAP and peroneal–EDB CMAP amplitudes). The study is most remarkable for the presence of fibrillation potentials in bilateral mid-thoracic and right lower thoracic paraspinal muscles. The ideal study would have included further demonstration of the limits of these abnormalities (such as needle EMG of cervical and lumbosacral paraspinal muscles and several arm and leg muscles).

This patient has diabetic thoracoabdominal neuropathy. This syndrome is typically that of subacute progressive pain and paresthesias in the distribution of several contiguous thoracic dermatomes on one side or sometimes bilaterally. Sometimes only the sensory territories of the ventral ramus are involved. The pain may last for weeks to months before it plateaus and then typically resolves spontaneously. Many patients with proximal diabetic neuropathy (diabetic amyotrophy) have a preceding history of diabetic thoracoabdominal neuropathy. Sometimes there is a unilateral bulge in the abdominal wall from weakness of abdominal musculature. The authors have seen several patients thought to have an abdominal mass. One patient underwent ultrasound of this apparent mass; gallstones were seen in the gall bladder, and he underwent cholecystectomy (without benefit). It is noteworthy that the anatomic distribution of this syndrome is typically wide and not due to a disorder of a single thoracic root.

Clinical Pearl

Diabetic thoracoabdominal neuropathy is a poorly understood disorder that is not confined to a single root or spinal nerve territory and may be mistaken for an internal thoracic or abdominal disorder.

REFERENCES
1. Brown, M.J., Asbury, A.K., Diabetic neuropathy, *Ann. Neurol.* 1984; 15:2–12.
2. Simmons, Z., Feldman, E.L., Update on diabetic neuropathy, *Curr. Opin. Neurol.* 2002; 15:595–603.
3. Sun, S.F., Streib, E.W., Diabetic thoracoabdominal neuropathy: clinical and electrodiagnostic features, *Ann. Neurol.* 1981; 9:75–79.

PATIENT 27

A 55-year-old woman with 6 months of progressive numbness in her feet

A 55-year-old woman complains that six months ago she began to experience a constant mild numbness and tingling paresthesias in the toes of her left foot with a gradual progression since that time. Several months later, she is experiencing similar numbness in the toes of her right foot with gradual progression since. Over the last month, some mild numbness and tingling in her left thumb has also been noted.

Physical Examination: Normal strength; light touch, pinprick, and vibration sense in toes, left more than right; normal ankle reflexes.

Stop and Consider: Using the approach of characterizing the neuropathy, characterize this patient's neuropathy clinically.

Electrodiagnostic Study: Relevant electrodiagnostic studies follow (all motor studies were normal).

Sensory

Nerve	Sites	Recording Site	Onset (ms)	Peak (ms)	Amplitude (μV)
R. median–dig I	1. Wrist	Dig I	2.2	2.7	20.1
L. median–dig I	1. Wrist	Dig I	2.1	2.5	9.7
R. sup peroneal	1. Lat leg	Ankle	Absent	—	—
L. sup peroneal	1. Lat leg	Ankle	3.0	3.3	5.7
R. sural–lat mall	1. Mid-calf	Ankle	3.2	3.5	3.7
L. sural–lat mall	1. Mid-calf	Ankle	3.1	3.4	2.6

Questions:
1. Does the electrodiagnostic study support your characterization of this patient's neuropathy?
2. Why is this *not* a distal symmetric axonal sensory neuropathy?

Answers:

1. Yes
2. Asymmetric involvement of left thumb and asymmetric onset in left foot

Discussion: The clinical features and the electrodiagnostic study both suggest characterization as a multifocal asymmetric sensory neuropathy. A distal asymmetric neuropathy could also be considered, although the lateral thumb numbness makes the term *distal* less preferable compared to *multifocal*. The reduction in the left median–D1 and right superficial peroneal SNAP amplitudes compared to the other sides are important clues to avoiding a mistaken label as a symmetric axonal sensory neuropathy. A brief differential diagnosis of multifocal asymmetric neuropathies should include vasculitis, neoplastic, Lyme disease, and sarcoidosis.

This patient's laboratory studies showed an IgM-κ monoclonal protein with quantitative IgM of 2190 mg/dl (normal < 230 mg/dl), a negative skeletal survey, and a bone marrow biopsy with 30% cellularity with small lymphoid cells, lymphoplasmacytic forms, and plasma cells. Flow cytometry confirmed a B-cell lymphoproliferative disorder with pathological diagnosis of lymphoplasmacytic lymphoma. As nerve biopsy was not indicated, it is difficult to determine the pathophysiology in this case, although the main considerations would be amyloid deposition or lymphomatous infiltration.

Clinical Pearl

The symmetry and possible multifocality of a distal axonal neuropathy should be closely examined through the study of bilateral sural and superficial peroneal sensory studies at a minimum. Asymmetries or multifocality should prompt evaluation for disorders including vasculitis, neoplastic infiltration of nerves, Lyme disease, and sarcoidosis.

REFERENCES

1. Kraus, M.D., Lymphoplasmacytic lymphoma/Waldenstrom macroglobulinemia: one disease or three?, *Am. J. Clin. Pathol.* 2001; 116(6):799–801.
2. Pangalis, G.A., Angelopoulou, M.K., Vassilakopoulos, T.P., Siakantaris, M.P., Kittas, C., B-chronic lymphocytic leukemia, small lymphocytic lymphoma, and lymphoplasmacytic lymphoma, including Waldenstrom's macroglobulinemia: a clinical, morphologic, and biologic spectrum of similar disorders, *Semin. Hematol.* 1999; 36(2):104–114.

PATIENT 28

A 71-year-old woman with several years of progressive numbness in her hands and feet

A 71-year-old woman developed numbness in her left hand. Nine months later she developed numbness in her left foot, followed a month later with right foot numbness. Over the ensuing 2 years, numbness came to involve the right hand and increased in intensity in the other limbs, and burning dysesthesias in her feet became prominent. She then developed an anterior uveitis, and workup including chest CT demonstrated diffuse reticular nodular disease throughout both lungs and scattered mediastinal, pretracheal, and aortopulmonic window lymph nodes.

Electrodiagnostic Study:

Sensory NCS

Nerve	Sites	Recording Site	Onset (ms)	Peak (ms)	BP Amplitude (μV)	Distance (cm)	Velocity (m/s)
L. median–dig II	1. Wrist	Dig II	Absent	—	—	13	—
L. ulnar–dig V	1. Wrist	Dig V	3.05	4.55	15.5	11	36.1
L. radial–sn box	1. Forearm	Sn box	1.60	2.50	18.5	10	62.5
L. sural–lat mall	1. Mid-calf	Ankle	Absent	—	—	14	—
L. sup peroneal	1. Lat leg	Ankle	Absent	—	—	12	—
R. sural–lat mall	1. Mid-calf	Ankle	Absent	—	—	14	—
R. sup peroneal	1. Lat leg	Ankle	Absent	—	—	12	—

Motor NCS

Nerve	Sites	Recording Site	Latency (ms)	Amplitude (mV)	Distance (cm)	Velocity (m/s)
L. median–APB	1. Wrist	APB	4.40	9.0	7	—
	2. Elbow	APB	8.65	8.7	21	49.4
L. ulnar–ADM	1. Wrist	ADM	3.35	7.2	7	—
	2. B. elbow	ADM	7.65	7.0	20.5	47.7
	3. A. elbow	ADM	10.20	6.7	13	51.0
L. peroneal–EDB	1. Ankle	EDB	Absent	—	8	—
	2. Fib head	EDB	Absent	—	—	—
L. tibial–AH	1. Ankle	AH	Absent	—	8	—
	2. Pop fossa	AH	Absent	—	—	—

EMG Summary Table

		SA			Amplitude (MUs)	Duration (MUs)	PolyP (MUs)	Activation	Recruitment Pattern
	IA	Fib	Fasc	Other					
L. tib ant	Inc	1+	0	0	Nl	Nl	Nl	Full	Nl
L. gastroc med	Nl	0	0	0	Nl	Nl	Nl	Full	Nl
R. tib ant	Nl	0	0	0	Nl	Nl	Nl	Full	Nl
R. gastroc med	Nl	0	0	0	Nl	Nl	Nl	Full	Nl
L. pronator teres	Nl	0	0	0	Nl	Nl	Nl	Full	Nl
L. abd pollicis brevis	Nl	0	0	0	Nl	Nl	Nl	Full	Nl

1. What is the possible relationship of the eye and lung disease to the neurological syndrome?
2. How would you proceed with management of this patient?

Answers:
1. Suggestive of sarcoidosis
2. Nerve and muscle biopsy

Discussion: The electrodiagnostic study demonstrates a polyneuropathy with symmetric distal degeneration of sensory and motor axons in the feet and possibly multifocal involvement given the absence of the left median SNAP with normal amplitudes for the left ulnar and radial SNAPs. The left ulnar distal sensory segment does have reduced velocity, also possibly another indication of multifocal involvement. Although the median SNAP may be absent because of a carpal tunnel syndrome, the normal median–APB distal motor latency argues somewhat against this, as a carpal tunnel syndrome severe enough to result in an absent median SNAP will usually have a prolonged distal motor latency. Accordingly, this is probably not best classified as a distal symmetric neuropathy but rather as an asymmetric sensory and motor neuropathy, with differential diagnosis that of Table 6 in the introduction of Section II. This electrodiagnostic interpretation would by highly supported by the clinical history of asymmetric onset and evolution of her symptoms.

The history of uveitis and pulmonary and mediastinal lymphadenopathy suggest sarcoidosis, and this is a potential cause of a neuropathy of this type. Sarcoid neuropathy requires long-term treatment with steroids with often less than satisfactory outcomes. Because of this, we were not comfortable embarking on therapy without a tissue diagnosis, so the patient underwent superficialperoneal nerve and peroneus brevis muscle biopsy. Muscle biopsy is done because of the possibility of detecting granulomas in muscle tissue in patients with sarcoidosis, regardless of the presence or absence of a myopathy. Nerve biopsy demonstrated granulomas.

Peripheral neuropathy from sarcoidosis is rare. Non-caseating granulomas in nerve are the pathological hallmark. In a recent series of 11 patients with biopsy-proven sarcoid neuropathy,[4] the neuropathy was focal or multifocal in 6 patients. Only 2 patients had elevated serum angiotensin converting enzyme, reflecting the limited value of this test in this diagnosis. All patients improved somewhat with steroid treatment, but 2 developed severe complications of steroids, including 1 death.

Clinical Pearl

As noted in case 27, multifocality (in this case, preferential involvement of one nerve over another in the same anatomic region) should prompt consideration for some less common causes of peripheral neuropathy.

REFERENCES
1. Gainsborough, N., Hall, S.M., Hughes, R.A., Leibowitz, S., Sarcoid neuropathy, *J. Neurol.* 1991; 238(3):177–180.
2. Heck, A.W., Phillips, L.H., Sarcoidosis and the nervous system, *Neurol. Clin.* 1989; 7(3):641–654.
3. Nemni, R., Galassi, G., Cohen, M., Hays, A.P., Gould, R., Singh, N., Bressman, S., Gamboa, E.T., Symmetric sarcoid polyneuropathy: analysis of a sural nerve biopsy, *Neurology* 1981; 31(10):1217–1223.
4. Said, G., Lacroix, C., Plante-Bordeneuve, V., Le Page, L., Pico, F., Presles, O., Senant, J., Remy, P., Rondepierre, P., Mallecourt, J., Nerve granulomas and vasculitis in sarcoid peripheral neuropathy: a clinicopathological study of 11 patients, *Brain* 2002; 125(pt. 2):264–275.

PATIENT 29

A 38-year-old man with numbness and weakness in the hands and feet and a skin rash

A 38-year-old man developed progressive numbness and weakness in all four limbs over a 3-year period. He was an immigrant to Boston from Cape Verde and had not left the United States for 10 years. He was treated by a physician with monthly doses of Chinese herbal medicine, which was activated by boiling it in water. The patient spilled the boiling water on his right arm and was hospitalized with a third-degree burn of his right arm, requiring a skin graft from his thigh. During hospitalization, a rash was noticed as well as hand weakness, and both dermatology and neurology consultants were asked to see him. The figures show his hand deformities and one of his skin lesions.

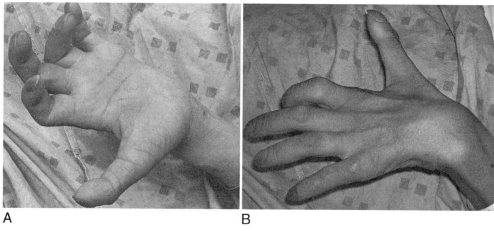

A   B

Figure 1

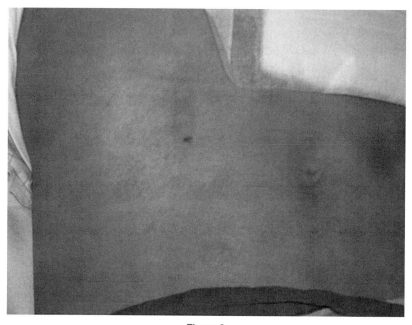

Figure 2

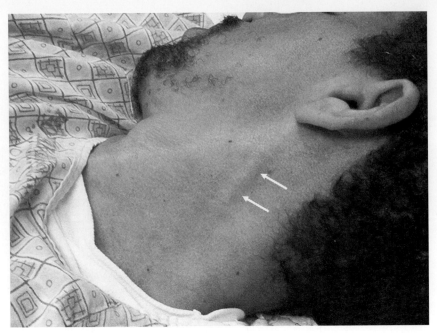

Figure 3

Electrodiagnostic Study:

Sensory NCS

Nerve	Sites	Recording Site	Onset (ms)	Peak (ms)	BP Amplitude (μV)	Distance (cm)	Velocity (m/s)
L. median–dig II	1. Wrist	Dig II	Absent	—	—	13	—
L. ulnar–dig V	1. Wrist	Dig V	Absent	—	—	11	—
L. radial–sn box	1. Forearm	Sn box	Absent	—	—	10	—
R. sural–lat mall	1. Mid-calf	Ankle	Absent	—	—	14	—
L. sup peroneal	1. Lat leg	Ankle	Absent	—	—	12	—
L. sural–lat mall	1. Mid-calf	Ankle	Absent	—	—	14	—

Motor NCS

Nerve	Sites	Recording Site	Latency (ms)	Amplitude (mV)	Distance (cm)	Velocity (m/s)
L. median–APB	1. Wrist	APB	Absent	—	7	—
L. ulnar–ADM	1. Wrist	ADM	Absent	—	7	—
R. peroneal–EDB	1. Ankle	EDB	Absent	—	8	—
L. peroneal–EDB	1. Ankle	EDB	Absent	—	8	—
R. tibial–AH	1. Ankle	AH	Absent	—	8	—
L. tibial–AH	1. Ankle	AH	4.45	3.7	8	—
	2. Pop fossa	AH	12.90	2.8	40	47.3
R. peroneal–tib ant	1. Fib head	Tib ant	4.15	1.3	—	—
	2. Pop fossa	Tib ant	7.00	0.6	—	—
L. peroneal–tib ant	1. Fib head	Tib ant	7.05	0.3	8	—
	2. Pop fossa	Tib ant	9.20	0.1	10	46.5

Questions:

1. The right hand could not be studied because of bandaging from his burn. What potential value might there have been to studying it?
2. What is the most likely diagnosis?

Answers:
1. Further establishment of a multifocal, asymmetric process
2. Lepromatous neuropathy

Discussion: The patient's left hand (see figure 1) is notable for marked atrophy of the dorsal and palmar interossei muscles. The electrodiagnostic studies show absent sensory nerve action potentials and absent or variously reduced CMAP amplitudes, suggesting a peripheral neuropathy. This peripheral neuropathy is characterized by multifocality and asymmetry. For asymmetry, note the absent right tibial–AH response with normal amplitude for the left tibial–AH CMAP and the much greater reduction in amplitude of the left peroneal–TA compared to the right peroneal–TA CMAPs. For multifocality, note the absence of the left peroneal–EDB and severe reduction of the left peroneal–TA CMAPs with normal amplitude of the left tibial–AH response, suggesting a peroneal neuropathy with relatively spared tibial nerve function. Further studies of the right hand might possibly have provided further evidence of asymmetry and multifocality. Accordingly, this neuropathy is best characterized as an asymmetric multifocal motor and sensory axonal neuropathy with causes listed in Table 6 in the introduction to Section II. Of these causes, the one most associated with a large erythematous skin lesion with patchy hypopigmentation, as shown in figure 2, is leprosy. Skin biopsy indeed showed acid-fast bacilli in this patient with lepromatous neuropathy. Figure 3 shows an additional finding characteristic of this disease—nerve enlargement (in this case, the greater auricular nerve).

Although uncommon in developed countries, leprosy is estimated to be the most common cause of a peripheral neuropathy worldwide. Leprosy is caused by the acid-fast bacillus *Mycobacterium leprae*. The bacteria reproduce maximally at temperatures of 27 to 30° which accounts for its predilection for cooler regions of the body (*e.g.*, pinnae of the ears, bridge of the nose, distal extremities). The clinical and pathological spectrum of leprosy is dependent on the host's immune response to *M. leprae* and reflects the relative balance between Th1 (helper) and Th2 (suppressor) T cells. Tuberculoid leprosy and lepromatous leprosy represent the two extremes of disease manifestation. In tuberculoid leprosy, the cell-mediated immune response is intact, leading to focal, circumscribed, inflammatory lesions involving the skin or nerves. The skin lesions appear as well-defined, scattered hypopigmented patches and plaques with central anesthesia and raised, erythematous borders. Pathologically, the tuberculoid form is characterized by granuloma formed by macrophages and Th1 cells that are surrounded by Th2 cells. Of note, bacilli cannot be demonstrated. The more superficial nerves in the vicinity of the skin lesions may also be affected. In addition, there is a predilection for involvement of specific nerve trunks. Typical sites include the ulnar nerve at the medial epicondyle, the median nerve at the distal forearm, the peroneal nerve at the fibular head, the sural nerve, the greater auricular nerve, and the superficial radial nerve at the wrist. These nerves can become encased within granulomas, causing them to become thickened and easily palpable. The most common neurological manifestation of tuberculoid leprosy is mononeuropathy or mononeuropathy multiplex.

In lepromatous leprosy, cell-mediated immunity is significantly impaired, resulting in an extensive infiltration of bacilli. Histologically, the lesions in lepromatous leprosy demonstrate large number of infiltrating bacilli, Th2 lymphocytes, and organism-laden, foamy macrophages with minimal granulomatous infiltration. Clinical manifestations tend to be more severe in the lepromatous subtype, but as in the tuberculoid form cooler regions of the body are more susceptible. The organisms multiply virtually unchecked and hematogenously disseminate, producing confluent and symmetrical areas of rash, anesthesia, and anhidrosis. Typically, a slowly progressive symmetric sensorimotor polyneuropathy develops over time. In early phases of the disease, the superficial cutaneous nerves of the pinnae and distal extremities are affected. The continued multiplication and infiltration of the organism into the epi-, peri-, and endoneurium results in sensory loss of the ears, dorsum of the feet and hands, dorsal medial aspect of the forearms, and anterior–lateral aspects of the lower legs. Although superficially similar to the stocking-glove pattern of involvement of most other types of distal symmetric axonal polyneuropathies (*e.g.*, idiopathic, toxic, diabetic) that are length dependent, the pattern of involvement in lepromatous leprosy is temperature dependent and distinct from other forms of neuropathy. Distal weakness ensues as the motor nerves become involved in the infiltrative process. Large sensory fiber modalities are relatively spared as are muscle stretch reflexes. As with the tuberculoid subtype, nerve trunks may be affected with time, leading to superimposed mononeuropathies. In advanced disease, facial neuropathies can occur.

Patients with borderline leprosy have the highest incidence of neurologic complications. These patients may show clinical and histological features of both the lepromatous and tuberculoid forms of leprosy. Although impaired cellular immunity of borderline patients results in mycobacterial spread, the immune system is still active enough to generate an inflammatory response. Patients may develop generalized symmetric sensorimotor polyneuropathy, mononeuropathies, and mononeuropathy multiplex, including multiple mononeuropathies in atypical locations, such as the brachial plexus.

Rarely, patients with leprosy present with isolated peripheral neuropathy without skin lesions. Lepromatous neuropathy should be suspected in individuals without skin lesions who live in endemic areas. Virtually all cases of pure neuritic leprosy have the tuberculoid or borderline tuberculoid subtypes of the disease.

Electrodiagnostic studies can demonstrate a mononeuropathy, mononeuropathy multiplex, or generalized sensorimotor polyneuropathy. Nerve conduction studies reflect a primarily axonal or mixed axonal and demyelinating process. Electromyography can demonstrate active denervation and decreased recruitment of large polyphasic motor unit potentials in the affected nerve distributions.

Multidrug therapy with dapsone, rifampin, and clofazimine is the mainstay of treatment, although other agents, including thalidomide, perfloxacin, ofloxacin, sparfloxacin, minocycline, and clarithromycin are also effective. Treatment typically requires two years of therapy in order to achieve full eradication of the organism. A potential complication of therapy, particularly in the borderline leprosy, is the reversal reaction, which can occur at any time during treatment of the disease. The reversal reaction occurs as a result of a shift to the tuberculoid end of the spectrum with an increase in cellular immunity. Upregulation of the cellular response is characterized by excessive release of tumor necrosis factor-alpha, gamma-interferon, and interleukin-2 with new granuloma formation. This may result in an exacerbation of the rash and the neuropathy and in the appearance of new lesions. High-dose corticosteroids appear to blunt this adverse reaction and may even be used prophylactically in high-risk patients at treatment onset.

A second type of reaction to treatment is erythema nodosum leprosum (ENL), which occurs in patients at the lepromatous end of the disease spectrum. ENL is associated with the appearance of multiple erythematous, sometimes painful, subcutaneous nodules; exacerbation of the neuropathy may also occur. The reaction of ENL is due to the slow degradation of antigens (bacterial debris) resulting in antigen–antibody complex formation and complement deposition in affected tissue. ENL may be treated with corticosteroids or, if available, thalidomide.

Clinical Pearls

1. As in the previous two cases, multifocality is an important clue to the cause of a peripheral neuropathy when present.
2. Look for enlargement of nerves when considering leprosy as a diagnosis

REFERENCES

1. Altman, D., Amato, A.A., Lepromatous neuropathy, *J. Clin. Neuromusc. Dis.* 1999; 1:68–73.
2. Nations, S.P., Barohn, R.J., Peripheral neuropathy due to leprosy, *Curr. Treat. Options Neurol.* 2002; 4(3):189–196.

PATIENT 30

**A 64-year-old woman with severe left shoulder pain and weakness
of shoulder abduction for 3 days, followed by progressive
neurologic deficits**

This 64-year-old retired nurse developed increasing headaches over a 6-week period in August and September followed by severe left shoulder blade pain for several days and then sudden onset of complete paralysis of left shoulder abduction. She had electrophysiological studies 3 days after her shoulder paralysis occurred.

Initial Electrodiagnostic Study:

Sensory NCS

Nerve	Sites	Recording Site	Onset (ms)	Peak (ms)	BP Amplitude (μV)	Distance (cm)	Velocity (m/s)
L. median–dig II	1. Wrist	Dig II	2.10	3.00	37.6	13	61.9
L. median–dig III	1. Wrist	Dig II	2.50	3.25	32.8	13	52.0
L. ulnar–dig V	1. Wrist	Dig V	2.05	2.90	39.7	11	53.7
L. radial–sn box	1. Forearm	Sn box	1.65	2.40	26.2	10	60.6
L. med AB cut	1. Elbow	Forearm	2.15	2.55	15.5	12	55.8
L. lat AB cut	1. Elbow	Forearm	2.05	2.50	32.8	12	58.5
R. lat AB cut	1. Elbow	Forearm	1.15	1.65	21.0	12	104.3

Motor NCS

Nerve	Sites	Recording Site	Latency (ms)	Amplitude (mV)	Distance (cm)	Velocity (m/s)
L. median–APB	1. Wrist	APB	3.10	10.0	7	—
	2. Elbow	APB	7.00	9.2	21	53.8
L. ulnar–ADM	1. Wrist	ADM	2.85	9.0	7	—
	2. B. elbow	ADM	6.30	8.2	20.5	59.4
	3. A. elbow	ADM	7.80	8.1	8	53.3

F-Wave

Nerve	F_{min} (ms)	F_{max} (ms)	Max – Min (ms)	%F
L. ulnar	29.25	33.70	4.45	—

EMG Summary Table

	IA	SA Fib	Fasc	Other	Amplitude (MUs)	Duration (MUs)	PolyP (MUs)	Activation	Recruitment Pattern
L. infra spinat	Nl	0	0	0	Nl	Nl	Nl	Full	SingleMU
L. deltoid	Nl	0	0	0	Nl	Nl	Nl	Full	MarkRed
L. biceps	Nl	0	0	0	Nl	Nl	Nl	Full	ModRed

EMG Summary Table—cont'd

	IA	SA Fib	SA Fasc	SA Other	Amplitude MUs	Duration MUs	PolyP MUs	Activation	Recruitment Pattern
L. triceps	Nl	0	0	0	Nl	Nl	Nl	Full	Nl
L. pron teres	Nl	0	0	0	Nl	Nl	Nl	Full	Nl
L. first dors int	Nl	0	0	0	Nl	Nl	Nl	Full	Nl
L. C4 para-spinal	Nl	0	0	0	—	—	—	—	—
L. C5 para-spinal	Nl	0	0	0	—	—	—	—	—
L. C6 para-spinal	Nl	0	0	0	—	—	—	—	—

Second Electrodiagnostic Study (8 Days After Initial Study):

Sensory NCS

Nerve	Sites	Recording Site	Onset (ms)	Peak (ms)	BP Amplitude (μV)	Distance (cm)	Velocity (m/s)
R. median–dig II	1. Wrist	Dig II	2.50	3.40	27.5	13	52.0
L. median–dig II	1. Wrist	Dig II	2.20	3.10	40.2	13	59.1
R. ulnar–dig V	1. Wrist	Dig V	2.40	3.05	18.2	11	45.8
L. ulnar–dig V	1. Wrist	Dig V	2.10	2.95	33.7	11	52.4
R. radial–sn box	1. Forearm	Sn box	1.90	2.40	35.4	10	52.6
R. med AB cut	1. Elbow	Forearm	2.05	2.65	1.8	12	58.5
R. Lat AB cut	1. Elbow	Forearm	2.10	2.65	12.3	12	57.1
L. Lat AB cut	1. Elbow	Forearm	2.10	2.55	28.4	12	57.1
R. sural–lat mall	1. Mid-calf	Ankle	3.10	3.75	10.9	14	45.2
L. sural–lat mall	1. Calf	Lat mall	2.85	3.75	11.0	14	49.1
R. sup peroneal	1. Lat leg	Ankle	2.95	3.85	4.2	12	40.7
L. sup peroneal	1. Lat leg	Ankle	3.40	4.25	4.0	12	35.3

Motor NCS

Nerve	Sites	Recording Site	Latency (ms)	Amplitude (mV)	Distance (cm)	Velocity (m/s)
R. median–APB	1. Wrist	APB	3.15	6.1	7	—
	2. Elbow	APB	7.45	5.9	23	53.5
L. median–APB	1. Wrist	APB	2.70	8.3	7	—
	2. Elbow	APB	6.80	7.1	21.5	52.4
R. ulnar–ADM	1. Wrist	ADM	2.60	9.9	7	—
	2. B. elbow	ADM	6.05	9.0	20	58.0
	3. A. elbow	ADM	7.95	8.5	10	52.6
L. ulnar–ADM	1. Wrist	ADM	2.55	9.6	7	—
	2. B. elbow	ADM	5.65	8.5	18	58.1
	3. A. elbow	ADM	7.65	8.9	10	50.0
R. peroneal–EDB	1. Ankle	EDB	3.80	7.9	8	—
	2. Fib head	EDB	11.15	5.4	30	40.8
	3. Pop fossa	EDB	13.55	4.1	9.5	39.6
L. peroneal–EDB	1. Ankle	EDB	4.60	7.3	8	—
	2. Fib head	EDB	12.20	6.4	31	40.8
	3. Pop fossa	EDB	15.00	2.3	7.5	26.8
L. peroneal–tib ant	1. Fib head	Tib ant	3.85	6.4	13.5	—
	2. Abv fib hd	Tib ant	6.45	4.3	8	30.8
R. tibial–AH	1. Ankle	AH	5.20	18.3	8	—
	2. Pop fossa	AH	14.60	10.0	43	45.7
L. tibial–AH	1. Ankle	AH	4.70	18.1	8	—
	2. Pop fossa	AH	14.35	11.5	40	41.5

EMG Summary Table

		SA			Amplitude (MUs)	Duration (MUs)	PolyP (MUs)	Activation	Recruitment Pattern
	IA	Fib	Fasc	Other					
L. tib ant	Nl	0	0	0	Nl	Nl	Few	Full	Mod red
L. peron ln	Nl	0	0	0	Nl	Nl	Nl	Full	Mod red
L. tib post	Nl	0	0	0	Nl	Nl	Nl	Full	Nl
L. vast lat	Nl	0	0	0	Nl	Nl	Nl	Full	Nl
L. bic fem SH	Nl	0	0	0	Nl	Nl	Nl	Full	Nl
L. thoracic PSP lower	Incr	0	0	0	—	—	—	—	—
L. deltoid	Nl	0	0	0	Nl	Nl	Few	Full	Mod red
L. ext dig comm	Nl	0	0	0	Nl	Nl	Nl	Full	Mild red
L. triceps	Nl	0	0	0	Nl	Nl	Nl	Full	Nl
R. pron teres	Nl	0	0	0	Nl	Nl	Nl	Full	Nl
R. flex dig pr I	Nl	0	0	0	Nl	Nl	Nl	Full	Nl
R. abd poll br	Nl	0	0	0	Nl	Nl	Nl	Full	Mod red
R. first dors int	Nl	0	0	0	Nl	Nl	Nl	Full	Nl

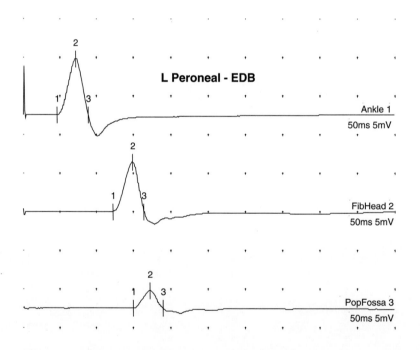

Questions:

1. The initial electrodiagnostic study is suggestive of either of two different localizations; what are they?
2. How might one best distinguish between them?
3. Suggest two alternative explanations for the absence of fibrillation potentials.

1. Upper trunk brachial plexopathy or C5 radiculopathy
2. Relevent sensory potentials and paraspinal muscle needle EMG
3. Pure demyelination or insufficient time for wallerian degeneration

Discussion: This patient has normal nerve conduction studies. Needle EMG studies show marked reduction in recruitment of motor units in the left infraspinatus, deltoid, and biceps. This is a pattern suggestive of either an upper trunk brachial plexopathy or a C5 radiculopathy, as these three muscles share different nerves and cords but the same trunk and root. In general, the best way to distinguish between root and more peripheral localizations is by examination of relevant sensory potentials and paraspinal muscle needle EMG. The SNAPs potentially affected by an upper trunk lesion are the lateral antebrachial cutaneous, the radial–webspace or radial–D1, and the median–D1 (see Table 1). Two of these were studied and are normal, although the short history could explain this. One reason fibrillation potentials may be absent is the short history of symptoms and insufficient time for Wallerian degeneration of axons to have occurred; fibrillation potentials can take up to 3 weeks to develop after acute axonal nerve injury. An alternative explanation for reduction in motor unit recruitment in the absence of fibrillation potentials is a pure demyelinating lesion. The electrodiagnostic interpretation was an acute C5 radiculopathy.

One week later, this patient developed a left mid-thoracic radiculopathy and a left foot drop. Examination showed weakness in the right proximal median nerve territory including flexor pollicis longus (FPL) and APB, weakness of left tibialis anterior and peroneus longus but not tibialis posterior with decreased sensation in the left lateral leg from the ankle to halfway up the leg, and weakness of left finger extensors but not wrist extensors or triceps. There was an area of sensory disturbance corresponding to approximately the complete left T9 dermatome, including the most posterior and anterior extent. She underwent repeat electrodiagnostic studies, now 11 days after onset of the shoulder weakness and 1 day after the foot drop. Over the ensuing week, she developed hoarseness (suggestive of a recurrent laryngeal nerve palsy) and mild bilateral asymmetric facial weakness and had a generalized tonic-clonic seizure with a post-ictal right hemiparesis.

Clinically, her peripheral nerve involvement is characterized as a multifocal neuropathy; there are features of a polyradiculopathy, peripheral multiple mononeuropathy, and cranial neuropathies. This is an asymmetric multifocal motor and sensory process whose differential diagnosis is that listed in

Table 6 in the introduction to Section II. The repeat electrodiagnostic studies should emphasize sensory potentials (root versus more distal involvement), although preservation of them could still reflect a very acute process distal to the dorsal root ganglia. In addition, repeating the previous needle EMG studies of the deltoid and biceps and studying the left peroneal and right median nerves and innervated muscles could potentially be valuable.

The important findings in the repeat study are:
- Mild relative but not definite reduction in the right median and ulnar SNAPs (27 and 18 μV, respectively, compared with left side of 40 and 33 μV)
- Definite reduction in the right lateral antebrachial cutaneous SNAP amplitude (12.3 μV compared to left of 28.4 mV; also reduced compared to previous study's right side value of 21 μV)
- Definite reduction in the right medial antebrachial cutaneous SNAP amplitude (1.8 μV) compared to the left side studied 8 days earlier (15.5 μV)
- Apparent conduction block (amplitude 6.4 to 2.3 mV) and focal slowing of the left peroneal–EDB across-fibular-head segment (see figure)
- Needle EMG abnormalities limited to decreased recruitment in the left common peroneal distribution, right APB but not first dorsal interosseous (FDI) and left extensor digitorum communis (EDC) but not FDI, suggesting peripheral lesions of the left common peroneal nerve, right distal median, and left posterior interosseous nerves

These findings support the clinical impression discussed earlier. The conduction block for the peroneal nerve could represent true injury to myelin or might reflect the *pseudo-conduction block* seen with acute axonal injury (further discussion of this concept can be found in case 31).

The patient's CSF showed 250 WBC (all mononuclear), protein of 150 mg/dl, and normal glucose. Serum Lyme ELISA and Western blot were positive. CSF Lyme Western blot was positive and CSF/serum Lyme IgG indices were markedly elevated. This is a case of early disseminated Lyme disease with a polyradiculopathy as well as more peripheral involvement. Her only known potential exposure was a trip 4 to 6 weeks before onset of symptoms to Cape Cod for 2 days, during which she spent almost all of her time indoors in an ice-skating rink. She was never aware of a skin rash. She was treated with intravenous ceftriaxone and has made a remarkably full recovery over several months.

Lyme disease is caused by the spirochete *Borrelia burgdorferi*, transmitted by tick bite except in very rare congenital cases. It is characterized by three stages of infection: early local (with skin manifestations only), early disseminated (with skin, peripheral, and central nervous system; heart; and eye manifestations), and late infection. The neurological manifestations of early disseminated infection are those of meningitis, cranial neuropathies, and *radiculoneuritis*, a term that reflects the combination of a polyradiculopathy and a more peripheral mononeuritis multiplex. Severe intrascapular pain has been noted as a frequent early symptom,[2] as in this case. Thoracic radiculopathy has also been commented on.[8] Asymmetrical dermatomal and myotomal abnormalities may be present, also as in this case, although this presentation is said to be common in Europe (where it has been referred to as lymphocytic meningoradiculitis or Bannwarth's syndrome) and is unusual in North America.

Clinical Pearls

1. Early disseminated Lyme disease may present with a polyradiculopathy; particularly when a thoracic radiculopathy is present, a high index of suspicion should be maintained.

2. Focal slowing and apparent conduction block may occur in acute axonal injury.

REFERENCES

1. Avanzi, S., Messa, G., Marbini, A., Pavesi, G., Granella, F., Isolated neuritis of the sciatic nerve in a case of Lyme disease, *Ital. J. Neurol. Sci.* 1998; 19:81–85.
2. Coyle, P.K., Schutzer, S.E., Neurologic aspects of Lyme disease, *Med. Clin. North Am.* 2002; 86:261–284.
3. Deltombe, T., Hanson, P., Boutsen, Y., Laloux, P., Clerin, M., Lyme borreliosis neuropathy: a case report, *Am. J. Phys. Med. Rehabil.* 1996; 75(4):314–316.
4. Gilchrist, J.M., AAEM case report 26: seventh cranial neuropathy, *Muscle Nerve* 1993; 16(5):447–452.
5. Krishnamurthy, K.B., Liu, G.T., Logigian, E.L., Acute Lyme neuropathy presenting with polyradicular pain, abdominal protrusion, and cranial neuropathy. *Muscle Nerve* 1993; 16(11):1261–1264.
6. Logigian, E.L., Peripheral nervous system Lyme borreliosis, *Semin. Neurol.* 1997; 17:25–30.
7. Logigian, E.L., Steere, A.C., Clinical and electrophysiological findings in chronic neuropathy of Lyme disease, *Neurology* 1992; 42:303–311.
8. Mormont, E., Esselinckx, W., De Ronde, T., Hanson, P., Deltombe, T., Laloux, P., Abdominal wall weakness and lumboabdominal pain revealing neuroborreliosis: a report of three cases, *Clin. Rheumatol.* 2001; 20:447–450.
9. Pachner, A.R., Steere, A.C., The triad of neurological manifestations of Lyme disease: meningitis, cranial neuritis, and radiculoneuritis, *Neurology* 1985; 35:47–53.
10. Scelsa, S.N., Herskovitz, S., Berger, A.R., A predominantly motor polyradiculopathy of Lyme disease, *Muscle Nerve* 1996; 19:780–783.
11. Steere, A.C., Lyme disease, *N. Engl. J. Med.* 2001; 345:115–125.

PATIENT 31

A 38-year-old man with fever and acute generalized weakness and distal numbness

This 38-year-old man developed fever to 102° and myalgias. Over the subsequent 5 days, he developed numbness of the medial hands and feet bilaterally. He then developed weakness in his legs and underwent electrodiagnostic testing within 3 days of the onset of weakness. He was admitted to the hospital, where examination showed fever to 101.5° and symmetric diffuse (proximal and distal) weakness (generally grade 4/5) and distal sensory loss in the arms and legs.

Initial Electrodiagnostic Study:

Sensory NCS

Nerve	Sites	Recording Site	Onset (ms)	Peak (ms)	Amplitude (μV)	Distance (cm)	Velocity (m/s)
L. median–dig II	1. Wrist	Dig II	2.40	3.10	43.9	13	54.0
L. ulnar–dig V	1. Wrist	Dig V	2.10	2.80	22.1	11	52.0
R. sural–lat mall	1. Mid-calf	Ankle	Absent	—	—	—	—

Motor NCS

Nerve	Sites	Recording Site	Latency (ms)	Amplitude (mV)	Distance (cm)	Velocity (m/s)
L. median–APB	1. Wrist	APB	3.2	14.6	7	—
	2. Elbow	APB	7.1	5.9	24	62
L. ulnar–ADM	1. Wrist	ADM	2.6	11.3	7	—
	2. B. elbow	ADM	6.7	2.2	20.5	50
	3. A. elbow	ADM	8.8	2.5	14	67
R. peroneal–EDB	1. Ankle	EDB	3.7	4.6	8	—
	2. Fib head	EDB	10.9	2.0	34	47
	3. Pop fossa	EDB	13.7	0.8	12	43
R. tibial–AH	1. Ankle	AH	4.8	11.0	8	—
	2. Pop fossa	AH	14.7	3.4	44	44

F-Wave

Nerve	F_{min} (ms)	%F
R. peroneal	Absent	—
R. tibial	53.1	60
L. ulnar	26.2	80
L. median	26.3	80

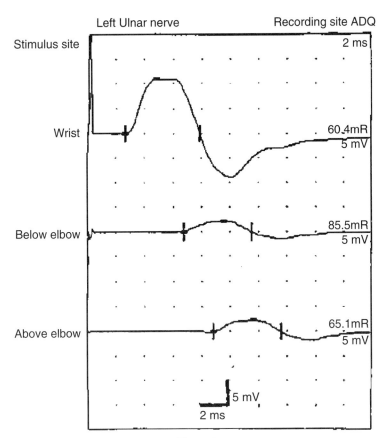

Figure 1

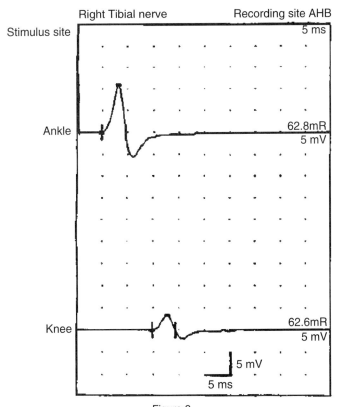

Figure 2

Repeat Electrodiagnostic Studies 5 Days Later:

Sensory NCS

Nerve	Sites	Recording Site	Onset (ms)	Peak (ms)	Amplitude (μV)	Distance (cm)	Velocity (m/s)
L. median–dig II	1. Wrist	Dig II	2.40	3.00	26.1	13	54.0
L. ulnar–dig V	1. Wrist	Dig V	2.00	2.50	4.1	11	55.0

Motor NCS

Nerve	Sites	Recording Site	Latency (ms)	Amplitude (mV)	Distance (cm)	Velocity (m/s)
L. median–APB	1. Wrist	APB	3.1	4.8	7	—
	2. Elbow	APB	7.3	4.5	24	57
L. ulnar–ADM	1. Wrist	ADM	3.0	1.2	7	—
	2. B. elbow	ADM	7.2	1.0	23.5	56
	3. A. elbow	ADM	8.9	1.1	10	59
R. peroneal–EDB	1. Ankle	EDB	5.6	0.3	8	—
	2. Fib head	EDB	12.5	0.3	34	50
R. tibial–AH	1. Ankle	AH	5.1	2.0	8	—
	2. Pop fossa	AH	14.7	1.0	44	43

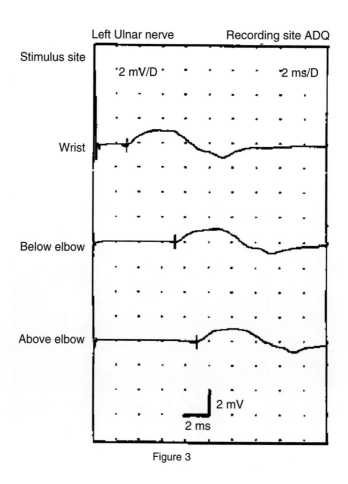

Figure 3

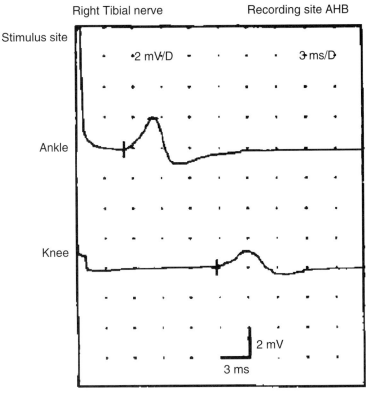

Right Tibial nerve

Recording site AHB

Stimulus site

•2 mV/D

3 ms/D

Ankle

Knee

2 mV

3 ms

Figure 4

Questions:
1. In the initial electrodiagnostic study, what are the major electrodiagnostic abnormalities?
2. Look at the waveforms in figures 1 and 2. What do they demonstrate? What is your clinical and electrodiagnostic diagnosis?
3. What clinical feature of this case is highly unusual? What additional tests should be considered?
4. What do the repeat electrodiagnostic studies show?
5. Is there still evidence of conduction block?

Answers:
1. Absent sural SNAP and amplitude drops of CMAPs with proximal stimulation
2. Amplitude drops in CMAPs with proximal stimulation—possible conduction block
3. Fever; consider nerve biopsy
4. The previously apparent "conduction block" was actually "pseudoconduction block"
5. No

Discussion: The electrodiagnostic abnormalities in the initial study are the absent sural SNAP and the drop in amplitudes of all CMAPs with proximal compared to distal stimulation. The waveforms in figures 1 and 2 demonstrate the amplitude drops without temporal dispersion and suggest conduction block

The patient was diagnosed with Guillain–Barré syndrome and treated with intravenous immunoglobulin (IVIg). Guillain–Barré syndrome is associated with infections and the patient had fever and myalgias. Guillain–Barré syndrome is associated with infections, although as a *post-infectious* sequela. The presence of continued fever during active progression of the neurological symptoms is highly atypical and raises the possibility of other diagnoses. Repeat electrodiagnostic studies and nerve biopsy were performed, both 5 days after the initial electrodiagnostic study.

The repeat electrodiagnostic studies show evolution of reduction in distal evoked SNAP and CMAP amplitudes and the loss of the previous apparent conduction block, with proximal stimulation resulting in similar amplitudes as distal stimulation (see figures). The findings are now those of degeneration of sensory and motor axons. This patient has a vasculitic neuropathy. Laboratory evaluation was notable for elevated erythrocyte sedimentation rate of 69, negative hepatitis C antibodies and hepatitis B surface antigen, negative ANA and ANCA, and serum lyme. Nerve biopsy showed necrotizing vasculitis with true fibrinoid necrosis of medium-sized epineurial arterioles and mild patchy axonal loss. He was treated with prednisone and gradually improved. Long-term follow-up is not known.

As we have emphasized previously, acute axonal nerve injury, from any cause, may produce apparent conduction block and this condition has been termed *pseudo-conduction block*. As Wallerian degeneration proceeds and neuromuscular transmission failure occurs, the distal evoked CMAP amplitudes drop as well. In this case, the evolution of changes clearly defines this process as not that of conduction block from focal demyelination. The repeat ulnar nerve study shows the distal wrist evoked CMAP becoming the same size and shape as the initial study's proximal evoked CMAPs (see figures 1 and 2).

Clinical Pearls

1. Apparent conduction block is sometimes pseudo-conduction block, demonstrable through repeat nerve conduction studies several days to weeks afterward. Therefore, in acute neuropathies, keep in mind that apparent conduction block may be acute axonal injury and consider a follow-up diagnostic study.

2. Guillain–Barré syndrome is a *post-infectious* process; the presence of fever should raise suspicion of an alternative diagnosis.

REFERENCES

1. Briemberg, H.R., Levin, K., Amato, A.A., Multifocal conduction block in peripheral nerve vasculitis, *J. Clin. Neuromusc. Dis.* 2002; 3(4):153–158.
2. Dyck, P.J., Benstead, T.J., Conn, D.L. *et al.*, Non-systemic vasculitic neuropathy, *Brain* 1987; 110: 843–854.
3. Greenberg, S.A., P-ANCA vasculitic neuropathy with 12 year latency from onset to systemic symptoms, *BMC Neurol.* 2002; 2:10–13.
4. Hawke, S.H., Davies, L., Pamphlett, R., Guo, Y.P., Pollard, J.D., McLeod, J.G., Vasculitic neuropathy: a clinical and pathological study, *Brain* 1991; 114:2175–2190.
5. Kissel, J.T., Slivka, A.P., Warmolts, J.R., Mendell, J.R., The clinical spectrum of necrotizing angiopathy of the peripheral nervous system, *Ann. Neurol.* 1985; 18:251–257.
6. Magistris, M.R., Kohler, A., Estade, M., Conduction block in vasculitic neuropathy, *Eur. Neurol.* 1994; 34:283–285.
7. McCluskey, L., Feinberg, D., Cantor, C., Bird, S., "Pseudo-conduction block" in vasculitic neuropathy, *Muscle Nerve* 1999; 22:1361–1366.
8. Nadeau, S.E., Neurological manifestations of systemic vasculitis, *Neurol. Clin.* 2002; 20:123–150.
9. Sandbrink, F., Klion, A.D., Floeter, M.K., "Pseudo-conduction block" in a patient with vasculitic neuropathy, *Electromyogr. Clin. Neurophysiol.* 2001; 41:195–202.

PATIENT 32

A 66-year-old woman with numbness in her hands and feet and progressive generalized weakness

This 66-year-old woman developed mild numbness in her hands and feet 9 months prior and over the last month has developed progressive severe generalized weakness. She was hospitalized because she was unable to sit up in bed unsupported and had severe generalized weakness and areflexia, as well as distal sensory loss.

Electrodiagnostic Study:

Sensory NCS

Nerve	Sites	Recording Site	Onset (ms)	Peak (ms)	Amplitude (µV)	Distance (cm)	Velocity (m/s)
L. median–dig II	1. Wrist	Dig II	Absent	—	—	13	—
L. ulnar–dig V	1. Wrist	Dig V	2.60	3.45	7.1	11	42.3
L. radial–sn box	1. Forearm	Sn box	1.55	2.10	28.1	10	64.5
L. sural–lat mall	1. Mid-calf	Ankle	3.30	4.20	36.3	14	42.4

Motor NCS

Nerve	Sites	Recording Site	Area mVms	Latency (ms)	Amplitude (mV)	Distance (cm)	Velocity (m/s)
L. median–APB	1. Wrist	APB	14.9	16.95	3.7	7	—
	2. Elbow	APB	18.0	22.85	3.7	16	27.1
R. median–APB	1. Wrist	APB	20.2	17.55	5.5	7	—
	2. Elbow	APB	20.8	21.85	5.2	20	46.5
	3. Axilla	APB	24.5	25.35	5.3	19	54.3
L. ulnar–ADM	1. Wrist	ADM	19.1	4.25	3.7	7	—
	2. B. elbow	ADM	17.4	6.90	3.6	16.5	62.3
	3. A. elbow	ADM	12.4	9.40	2.4	9	36.0
R. ulnar–ADM	1. Wrist	ADM	18.9	4.20	3.3	7	—
	2. B. elbow	ADM	14.9	8.35	3.0	15	36.1
	3. A. elbow	ADM	3.5	19.10	1.2	11	10.2
L. peroneal–EDB	1. Ankle	EDB	17.4	11.35	3.5	8	—
	2. Fib head	EDB	18.6	17.80	3.4	25.5	39.5
	3. Pop fossa	EDB	16.8	19.95	3.0	9.5	44.2
L. tibial–AH	1. Ankle	AH	7.3	14.30	1.0	8	—
	2. Pop fossa	AH	5.2	22.95	1.1	35	40.5

F-Wave

Nerve	F_{min} (ms)	F_{max} (ms)	Max – Min (ms)	%F
L. peroneal	72.20	75.45	3.25	30
L. ulnar	Absent	—	—	—
R. median	47.95	52.65	4.70	20
R. ulnar	28.10	33.20	5.10	20

Nerve	H Latency (ms)
R. tibial–soleus	Absent
L. tibial–soleus	Absent

EMG Summary Table

		SA			Amplitude (MUs)	Duration (MUs)	PolyP (MUs)	Activation	Recruitment Pattern
	IA	Fib	Fasc	Other					
L. vast lat	Nl	0	0	0	Nl	Nl	Nl	Full	Nl
L. tib ant	Incr	0	0	0	Nl	Nl	Nl	Full	Mod red
L. gastroc med	Incr	0	0	0	Nl	Nl	Nl	Full	Mild red
L. flex hall ln	Incr	2+	0	0	Nl	Nl	Nl	Full	Mod red
L. deltoid	Nl	0	0	0	Nl	Nl	Nl	Full	Nl
L. biceps	Nl	0	0	0	Nl	Nl	Nl	Full	Nl
L. triceps	Nl	0	0	0	Nl	Nl	Nl	Full	Mod red
L. first dors int	Incr	3+	2+	0	Nl	Nl	Nl	Full	Mod red
L. pron teres	Nl	0	0	0	Nl	Nl	Nl	Full	Nl

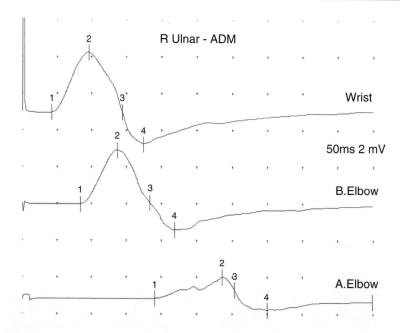

Questions:

1. The sensory studies show a pattern of abnormalities referred to by the abbreviation AMNS. What does this stand for and what does it imply?
2. Look at the right and left median distal motor latencies and velocities. Do you think the left median forearm motor velocity represents primary demyelination?
3. The left tibialis anterior muscle was MRC grade 2 in strength and had been this weak for 1 month. Do you think the weakness was due to loss of motor axons or conduction block of motor axons supplying this muscle?

Answers:

1. "Abnormal median normal sural," suggestive of a demyelinating neuropathy
2. Yes
3. Conduction block

Discussion: This case illustrates an issue central to many studies of patients with suspected peripheral neuropathy: the characterization of the physiology as predominantly axonal or demyelinating. The electrodiagnostic literature supports the use of several concepts in this regard:

- The abnormal median normal sural pattern of SNAPs
- Focal demyelination: focal slowing, partial conduction block, or temporal dispersion
- Reduced needle EMG interference patterns without fibrillation potentials or positive waves in muscles that are chronically weak

The first is a pattern of sensory abnormalities referred to as AMNS, which stands for *abnormal median normal sural* and is a characteristic feature of chronic inflammatory demyelinating neuropathies. Of course, isolated carpal tunnel syndrome can also produce this picture, but in the particular setting of patients with a neuropathy, reduced hand (not necessarily just median) but normal sural SNAP amplitudes are highly specific for a demyelinating neuropathy.

The second concept reflects the electrophysiological correlates of focal demyelination of a nerve: focal conduction slowing, partial conduction block, and temporal dispersion. These three electrodiagnostic findings may occur together or independently in a nerve segment, but all provide evidence of focal demyelination. Abnormalities in nerve segments that are common sites of compression (*i.e.*, median at the wrist, ulnar at the elbow, and peroneal at the fibular head) need to be interpreted cautiously and are not sufficient in general for the diagnosis of a generalized demyelinating neuropathy. There are also occasional circumstances, particularly acute ischemic injury of a nerve, when these findings are present without demyelination as the cause. Furthermore, some demyelinating neuropathies preferentially produce one of these findings but not others; the lack of partial conduction block with anti-MAG neuropathies and CMT1a are examples.

What constitutes electrodiagnostic criteria for focal conduction slowing sufficient to conclude demyelination is the cause? A large body of literature and criteria has evolved. There is no *a priori* reason to assume that criteria accurate for diagnosis applies to all demyelinating neuropathies; in fact, criteria for demonstrating demyelination in acute inflammatory demyelinating polyneuropathies (AIDP), such as Guillain–Barré syndrome, is likely different than that for chronic inflammatory demyelinating polyneuropathy (CIDP). Some of the differences in criteria referenced below reflect different diseases to which they are optimized. There is consensus, nevertheless, of one broad principle. The lower limit of normal of velocities is not sufficiently accurate as a cutoff for demyelinating neuropathies. Clearly, axonal neuropathies commonly produce mild slowing, and the characterization of a neuropathy as primarily demyelinating on the basis of mild slowing is one of the most frequent and detrimental mistakes made by electrodiagnostic practitioners. As slowing in axonal neuropathy correlates with reduction in CMAP amplitudes, the latter is generally used in the interpretation of the abnormal cutoff for the velocity. Sample proposed research criteria for both AIDP and CIDP are shown below.

Suggestive of Demyelination in AIDP (Albers and Kelly[3])

At least 3 of the following:
In 2 or more nerves,
  Amplitude > 50% lower limit of normal (LLN) → conduction velocity < 90% LLN
  Amplitude < 50% LLN → conduction velocity < 80% LLN
In 2 or more nerves,
  Amplitude normal → distal latency > 110% upper limit of normal (ULN)
  Amplitude < normal → distal latency > 120% ULN
In 1 or more nerves,
  Conduction block as defined by amplitude reduction > 30%, *or*
  Temporal dispersion as defined by proximal–distal duration increase of 30% or more
In 1 or more nerves,
  Minimum F response latency > 120% ULN

Suggestive of Demyelination in CIDP (Albers and Kelly[3])

At least 3 of the following:
In 2 or more nerves,
  Conduction velocity < 75% LLN
In 2 or more nerves,
  Distal latency > 130% ULN
In 1 or more nerves,
  Conduction block as defined by amplitude reduction > 30%, *or*
  Temporal dispersion as defined by proximal–distal duration increase of 30% or more
In 1 or more nerves,
  Minimum F response latency > 130% ULN

Suggestive of Demyelination for Both AIDP and CIDP (Cornblath,[8] AAN AIDS Task Force[4])

At least 3 of the following:
In 2 or more nerves,
  Amplitude > 80% LLN → conduction velocity < 80% LLN
  Amplitude < 80% LLN → conduction velocity < 70% LLN
In 2 or more nerves,
  Amplitude > 80% LLN → distal motor latency > 125% ULN
  Amplitude < 80% LLN → distal motor latency > 150% ULN
In 1 or more nerves,
  Conduction block as defined by amplitude reduction > 20%, *or*
  Temporal dispersion as defined by proximal–distal duration increase of 15% or more
  (Conduction block is considered possible only if temporal dispersion abnormal.)
In 2 or more nerves,
  Amplitude > 80% LLN → minimum F-wave latency > 120% ULN
  Amplitude < 80% LLN → minimum F-wave latency > 150% ULN

Other criteria, the same for both AIDP and CIDP, have been proposed:

Suggestive of Demyelination for Both AIDP and CIDP (Saperstein et al.[13])

Similar to AAN criteria above, except 2 out of 4 (instead of 3 out of 4) criteria are required, and the definition of conduction block is per AAEM consensus criteria:

For example, to provide evidence of primary demyelination, for a median–APB motor nerve study with CMAP amplitude of 3.6 (=75% of LLN), the forearm motor velocity would have to be less than 70% of 44 m/s, which is 30.8 m/s. Its distal latency would have to be at least 150% of 4.5 ms, which is 6.8 msec.

These criteria are complex, and those for CIDP were reviewed by Bromberg.[7] Both Albers and the AAN criteria were found to be approximately 50% sensitive and 100% specific in a population that included patients with distal symmetric polyneuropathy and motor neuron disease; however, a single criterion—one nerve with a conduction velocity of less than 70% the LLN—had a sensitivity of 66% and specificity of 100%. This finding suggests that the criteria listed above are too cumbersome and can be improved upon for clinical use. In particular, a nerve with conduction velocity of less than 70% the LLN was not seen in patients with strictly motor axonal degeneration, such as motor neuron disease, or patients with distal symmetric axonal neuropathies and is a powerful indicator of a primary demyelinating disorder. This roughly translates into the following conservative rule: *Motor conduction velocities of <30 m/s in the forearm or <25 m/s in the leg reliably indicate the presence of primary demyelination.*

Regarding question 2 above and this case, the left median motor forearm segment has a velocity of 27 m/s. We think this is sufficiently abnormal to consider as reflective of primary demyelination.

Question 3 deals with criteria for partial conduction block of motor nerves. The above criteria use variously 20% or 30% reduction in CMAP amplitudes as indicative of conduction block. This is likely too liberal and does not factor in such considerations as distal CMAP amplitude reduction; that is, if distal CMAP is already very small, such as 0.4, then proximal CMAPs will commonly meet this degree of reduction (in this example, 0.3 is a 25% drop). Criteria have been devised and published as consensus criteria of the American Association of Electrodiagnostic Medicine (AAEM).[11] These criteria are shown in the table below. They are much more conservative and are noteworthy in the following regards:

(1) definite conduction block cannot be judged present if the distal CMAP is less than 20% the LLN or if temporal dispersion is greater than 30%; (2) definite conduction block can never be judged present in the radial nerve or the tibial nerve in the leg; and (3) definite conduction block should not be concluded based on Erb's point or cervical root stimulation studies.

Amplitude Reduction Criteria for Partial Conduction Block (AAEM Conduction Block Criteria[11])

Nerve/Segment	Temporal Dispersion < 30%		Temporal Dispersion 31–60%	
	Definite	Probable	Definite	Probable
Median				
Forearm	>50%	40–50%	—	>50%
Arm	>50%	40–50%	—	>50%
Proximal (Erb's point)	—	>40%	—	>50%
Ulnar				
Forearm	>50%	40–50%	—	>50%
Across Elb	>50%	40–50%	—	>50%
Arm	>50%	40–50%	—	>50%
Proximal (Erb's point)	—	>40%	—	>50%
Radial				
Forearm	—	>50%	—	>60%
Arm	—	>50%	—	>60%
Proximal (Erb's point)	—	>50%	—	>60%
Peroneal				
Leg	>60%	50–60%	—	>60%
Across Fib	>50%	40–50%	—	>50%
Thigh (sciatic notch)	—	>50%	—	>60%
Tibial				
Leg	>60%	50–60%	—	>60%
Thigh (sciatic notch)	—	>50%	—	>60%

Note: Criteria for area reduction are always of magnitude 10% less than amplitude (*i.e.*, amp/area = 50%/40%). Applicable to CMAP ≥ 20% LLN. Erb's point and sciatic notch stimulation are controversial. Nerve root stimulation is not accepted.

With regard to this specific case study, the right ulnar–ADM across-elbow segment shows a 60% reduction in amplitude, from 3.0 to 1.2. Inspection of the waveforms in the figure allows for a rough calculation of the degree of temporal dispersion, calculated as the duration of the negative phase of the CMAP (time between markers 1 and 3). For the below-elbow site, this is ~100 msec, and for the above-elbow site, this is ~120 ms, indicating temporal dispersion of ~20% and meeting the criteria for definite conduction block in the table. Of course, this is a common compression site and, although reflective of conduction block, should not be taken by itself as convincing evidence of a generalized demyelinating neuropathy.

Question 4 aims to emphasize the fourth concept relating to the electrodiagnosis of demyelination—namely, that reduced ("neurogenic") interference patterns in weak muscles without fibrillation potentials is a likely indicator of demyelination of motor axons. The main exception is the acute setting, whereby acute axonal injury may immediately result in a reduced interference pattern, while fibrillation potentials may take up to 3 weeks to appear. Profound chronic denervation with partial and incomplete reinnervation may often give this pattern but will almost always have clear abnormalities of motor unit morphology (*i.e.*, increased duration and amplitude) to distinguish itself from the above findings of pure motor nerve demyelination.

Clinical Pearls

Electrodiagnostic support of a demyelinating neuropathy may come from any of the following:

1. The abnormal median normal sural (AMNS) pattern of SNAPs
2. Focal demyelination: focal slowing, partial conduction block, or temporal dispersion
3. Reduced needle EMG interference patterns without fibrillation potentials or positive waves in muscles that are chronically weak
4. Definitive and highly conservative criteria for focal slowing representative of demyelination: motor conduction velocities of <30 m/s in the arms and <25 m/s in the legs

REFERENCES

1. Alam, T.A., Chaudhry, V., Cornblath, D.R., Electrophysiological studies in the Guillain–Barré syndrome: distinguishing subtypes by published criteria, *Muscle Nerve* 1998; 21(10):1275–1279.
2. Albers, J.W., Donofrio, P.D., McGonagle, T., Sequential electrodiagnostic abnormalities in acute inflammatory demyelinating polyradiculoneuropathy, *Muscle Nerve* 1985; 8:528–539.
3. Albers, J.W., Kelly, J.J., Jr., Acquired inflammatory demyelinating polyneuropathies: clinical and electrodiagnostic features, *Muscle Nerve* 1989; 12(6):435–451.
4. American Academy of Neurology, Research criteria for diagnosis of chronic inflammatory demyelinating polyneuropathy (CIDP): report from an Ad Hoc Subcommittee of the American Academy of Neurology AIDS Task Force, *Neurology* 1991; 41(5):617–618.
5. Asbury, A.K., Cornblath, D.R., Assessment of current diagnostic criteria for Guillain–Barré syndrome, *Ann. Neurol.* 1990; 27(suppl.):S21–S24.
6. Barohn, R.J., Kissel, J.T., Warmolts, J.R., Mendell, J.R., Chronic inflammatory demyelinating polyradiculoneuropathy: clinical characteristics, course, and recommendations for diagnostic criteria, *Arch. Neurol.* 1989; 46:878–884.
7. Bromberg, M.B., Comparison of electrodiagnostic criteria for primary demyelination in chronic polyneuropathy, *Muscle Nerve* 1991; 14(10):968–976.
8. Cornblath, D.R., Electrophysiology in Guillain–Barré syndrome, *Ann. Neurol.* 1990; 27(suppl.):S17–S20.
9. Cornblath, D.R., Sumner, A.J., Daube, J., Gilliat, R.W., Brown, W.F., Parry, G.J., Albers, J.W., Miller, R.G., Petajan, J., Conduction block in clinical practice, *Muscle Nerve* 1991; 14(9):869–871.
10. Meulstee, J., van der Meche, F.G., Electrodiagnostic criteria for polyneuropathy and demyelination: application in 135 patients with Guillain–Barré syndrome, Dutch Guillain–Barré Study Group. *J. Neurol. Neurosurg. Psychiatry* 1995; 59(5):482-6.
11. Olney, R.K., Consensus criteria for the diagnosis of partial conduction block, *Muscle Nerve* 1999; 22(suppl. 8):S225–S229.
12. Olney, R.K., Aminoff, M.J., Electrodiagnostic features of the Guillain–Barré syndrome: the relative sensitivity of different techniques, *Neurology* 1990; 40:471–475.
13. Sander, H.W., Latov, N., Research criteria for defining patients with CIDP, *Neurology* 2003; 60(8, suppl. 3):S8–S15.
14. Saperstein, D.S., Katz, J.S., Amato, A.A., Barohn, R.J., Clinical spectrum of chronic acquired demyelinating polyneuropathies. *Muscle Nerve* 2001; 24:311–324.
15. Taylor, P.K., CMAP dispersion, amplitude decay, and area decay in a normal population, *Muscle Nerve* 1993; 16(11):1181–1187.

PATIENT 33

A 43-year-old woman with progressive generalized weakness and numbness for 5 months

This 43-year-old woman with rheumatoid arthritis since age 37 developed difficulty walking upstairs, getting out of a low chair, and raising her arms up when hanging clothes or washing her hair. Within one month, she then developed constant bilateral perioral, tongue, and lower facial numbness and tingling paresthesias, as if these areas were "waking up from Novocain." Tingling and numbness in her hands, left more than right, then developed. Neurological examination was remarkable for diffuse generalized weakness with moderate asymmetries (*i.e.*, tibialis anterior right 4+, left 4−; infraspinatus right 4+, left 3), sensory disturbances on the lower face and anterior neck and all fingertips, and complete areflexia.

Electrodiagnostic Study:

Sensory NCS

Nerve	Sites	Recording Site	Onset (ms)	Peak (ms)	BP Amplitude (μV)	Distance (cm)	Velocity (m/s)
L. median–dig II	1. Wrist	Dig II	2.25	3.15	6.7	13	57.8
L. ulnar–dig V	1. Wrist	Dig V	2.45	3.20	6.0	11	44.9
L. radial–sn box	1. Forearm	Sn box	1.75	2.45	6.8	10	57.1
R. ulnar–dig V	1. Wrist	Dig V	2.80	4.00	10.4	11	39.3
R. median–dig II	1. Wrist	Dig II	4.35	5.75	6.0	13	29.9
R. radial–sn box	1. Forearm	Sn box	2.05	2.85	14.8	10	48.8
L. median–ulnar	1. Median–palm	Wrist	1.70	2.30	4.9	8	47.1
(palmar)	2. Ulnar–palm	Wrist	Absent	—	—	8	—
L. sural–lat mall	1. Mid-calf	Ankle	3.85	4.75	9.4	14	36.4
R. sural–lat mall	1. Mid-calf	Ankle	3.75	4.70	11.2	14	37.3
L. sup peroneal	1. Lat leg	Ankle	3.10	4.05	11.1	12	38.7
R. sup peroneal	1. Lat leg	Ankle	2.80	3.90	14.3	12	42.9

Motor NCS

Nerve	Sites	Recording Site	Latency (ms)	Amplitude (mV)	Distance (cm)	Velocity (m/s)
R. median–APB	1. Wrist	APB	5.85	9.4	7	—
	2. Elbow	APB	10.70	9.6	21	43.3
	3. Axilla	APB	12.90	9.1	12	54.5
L. median–APB	1. Wrist	APB	3.60	6.9	7	—
	2. Elbow	APB	7.90	6.6	19.5	45.3
	3. Axilla	APB	10.80	6.8	12	41.4
R. ulnar–ADM	1. Wrist	ADM	3.20	8.1	7	—
	2. B. elbow	ADM	6.20	8.3	16.5	55.0
	3. A. elbow	ADM	8.05	8.5	10	54.1
	4. Axilla	ADM	9.75	7.9	10	58.8
L. ulnar–ADM	1. Wrist	ADM	2.55	8.3	7	—
	2. B. elbow	ADM	5.95	7.6	18	52.9
	3. A. elbow	ADM	7.50	8.0	10	64.5
	4. Axilla	ADM	9.25	7.8	10	57.1
R. peroneal–EDB	1. Ankle	EDB	6.60	4.5	8	—
	2. Fib head	EDB	15.35	4.8	33.5	38.3
	3. Pop fossa	EDB	17.90	4.3	8	31.4
R. tibial–AH	1. Ankle	AH	5.65	6.2	8	—
	2. Pop fossa	AH	14.65	5.1	39.5	43.9

F-Wave

Nerve	F_{min} (ms)	F_{max} (ms)	Max – Min (ms)	%F
R. peroneal	58.15	63.00	4.85	70
R. median	34.20	36.65	2.45	80
R. ulnar	29.80	33.65	3.85	80
L. median	29.35	32.75	3.40	80
L. ulnar	27.20	30.30	3.10	70

Needle EMG Summary Table

		SA			Amplitude (MUs)	Duration (MUs)	PolyP (MUs)	Activation	Recruitment Pattern
	IA	Fib	Fasc	Other					
L. deltoid	Nl	0	0	0	Nl	Brief	Nl	Full	Mild red
L. triceps	Incr	2+	0	0	Nl	Nl	Nl	Full	Sev red
L. biceps	Nl	0	0	0	Small	Brief	Nl	Full	Mod red
L. ext dig comm	Nl	0	0	0	Nl	Nl	Nl	Full	Mod red
L. infra spinat	Nl	0	0	0	Nl	Nl	Nl	Full	Mod red
L. first dors int	Inc	2+	0	0	Nl	Nl	Nl	Full	Mod red
L. tib ant	Inc	2+	0	0	Nl	Nl	Nl	Full	Mild red
L. vast med	Nl	0	0	0	Nl	Nl	Nl	Full	Nl

Questions:
1. What pattern of abnormalities is present in the sensory nerve conduction studies? What does this suggest?
2. Is there evidence of primary demyelination with this electrodiagnostic study?
3. What clinical diagnoses should be considered?

1. The abnormal median normal sural pattern suggests a demyelinating neuropathy.
2. No
3. Chronic inflammatory demyelinating polyneuropathy, vasculitic neuropathy

Discussion: This patient has the AMNS (abnormal median normal sural) pattern of abnormalities on sensory nerve conduction studies (see case 32). More generally, she has low amplitudes for bilateral median, left ulnar, and left radial SNAPs. The right ulnar and radial SNAPs are probably reduced as well, especially given the well above normal size of the sural and superficial peroneal SNAPs. This pattern suggests chronic inflammatory demyelinating polyneuropathy (CIDP).

Is there evidence of primary demyelination to support the diagnosis of CIDP? The right median distal motor latency and distal sensory latency are prolonged, but this may be due to carpal tunnel syndrome; the other distal motor and sensory latencies are normal. The motor segments have normal velocities with the exception of the peroneal–EDB across the fibular head, which is mildly reduced at 31 m/s, although the temperature in the leg was only 27°C. The peroneal–EDB minimum F-wave response is prolonged at 56 ms, but again the finding is discounted because of the temperature in the leg; the other F-waves are normal or explained, in the case of the median at 34 ms, by the carpal tunnel syndrome. Accordingly, the nerve conduction studies do not provide any definitive evidence of primary demyelination.

The needle EMG study does provide such evidence, however. The presence of moderately reduced recruitment patterns in several arm muscles (biceps, extensor digitorum communis, infraspinatus) without fibrillation potentials to suggest acute denervation or motor units with increased duration or amplitude to suggest reinnervation is best explained by proximal demyelination of motor nerves.

This patient was diagnosed with CIDP, although a vasculitic neuropathy could not be completely excluded. The CSF protein was normal. She was treated with prednisone (60 mg/day) and at follow-up at 3 weeks she noted "marked" improvement. The right hand numbness for digits 2 to 4 had resolved completely, her arm strength had improved, and her left foot drop had resolved. Long-term follow-up of over 1 year has shown sustained improvement on low doses of prednisone (5 to 10 mg/day).

Clinical Pearls

1. The spectrum of CIDP is wide and includes multifocal variants.
2. The abnormal median normal sural (AMNS) pattern of nerve conduction abnormalities is an important indicator of a demyelinating neuropathy.

PATIENT 34

A 48-year-old man with acute progressive numbness and paresthesias in his hands and feet and generalized weakness

This 48-year-old man with AML underwent bone marrow transplant. He developed low-grade fever to 100.5°F a month later. Two days later he noted paresthesias in his hands and feet; on the following day, he noted weakness; and one day later he was unable to walk. The electrodiagnostic study was performed 7 days after onset of the paresthesias.

Electrodiagnostic Study:

Sensory NCS

Nerve	Sites	Recording Site	Onset (ms)	Peak (ms)	Amplitude (μV)	Distance (cm)	Velocity (m/s)
L. median–dig II	1. Wrist	Dig II	Absent	—	—	13	—
L. ulnar–dig V	1. Wrist	Dig V	Absent	—	—	11	—
L. radial–sn box	1. Forearm	SnBox	1.85	2.30	5.4	10	54.1
R. median–dig V	1. Wrist	Dig II	Absent	—	—	11	—
R. ulnar–dig V	1. Wrist	Dig V	Absent	—	—	11	—
L. sural–lat mall	1. Mid-calf	Ankle	2.50	3.30	5.5	14	56.0
R. sural–lat mall	1. Mid-calf	Ankle	2.95	3.85	9.6	14	47.5

Motor NCS

Nerve	Sites	Recording Site	Latency (ms)	Amplitude (mV)	Distance (cm)	Velocity (m/s)
L. median–APB	1. Wrist	APB	6.65	1.6	7	—
	2. Elbow	APB	12.70	1.3	23	38.0
L. ulnar–ADM	1. Wrist	ADM	4.85	1.8	7	—
	2. B. elbow	ADM	8.50	1.5	21	57.5
	3. A. elbow	ADM	11.45	1.2	15	50.8
L. peroneal–EDB	1. Ankle	EDB	7.70	0.3	8	—
	2. Fib head	EDB	14.05	0.2	26	40.9
	3. Pop fossa	EDB	17.00	0.1	10	33.9
R. median–APB	1. Wrist	APB	10.00	1.2	7	—
	2. Elbow	APB	14.55	0.9	22	48.4
	3. Axilla	APB	17.70	0.9	12	38.1

F-Wave

Nerve	F_{min} (ms)
R. median	Absent
L. median	Absent
L. ulnar	Absent
L. peroneal	Absent
R. median	Absent

EMG Summary Table

| | | SA | | Amplitude | Duration | PolyP | | Recruitment |
	IA	Fib	Fasc	Other	(MUs)	(MUs)	(MUs)	Activation	Pattern
L. deltoid	Nl	0	0	0	Nl	Nl	Nl	Full	Nl
L. triceps	Nl	0	0	0	Nl	Nl	Nl	Full	Mild red
L. first dors int	Nl	0	0	0	Nl	Nl	Nl	Full	Mod red
L. tib ant	Nl	0	0	0	Nl	Nl	Nl	Sub max	Mod red
L. gastroc med	Inc	3+	0	0	Nl	Nl	Nl	Full	Sev red
L. vast med	Nl	0	0	0	Nl	Nl	Nl	Sub max	Nl

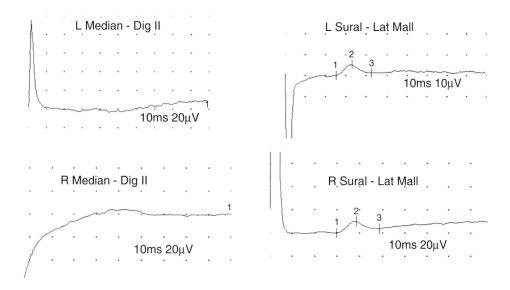

Questions:
1. What is the clinical differential diagnosis?
2. Assuming the study suggests a generalized peripheral neuropathy, how would you characterize the process? (See case 32 for an explanation of characterization of neuropathies.)
3. Is there any evidence for a demyelinating neuropathy from the sensory studies? What finding is illustrated in the figure? Is there any evidence of a demyelinating neuropathy in the EMG studies?

1. Guillain-Barré syndrome, vasculitic neuropathy
2. Diffuse symmetric motor and sensory
3. Yes. The abnormal median normal sural pattern is present.

Discussion: The electrodiagnostic study shows low amplitudes or absent SNAPs for bilateral median and ulnar and one radial sensory nerve, but normal sural SNAP amplitudes. The motor studies are notable for reduced amplitudes of all CMAPs studied, prolongation of bilateral right > left median, left ulnar, and left peroneal–EDB distal motor latencies. All F-waves are unobtainable, although CMAP amplitudes are markedly reduced. Needle EMG studies show mostly reduced recruitment patterns without fibrillation potentials, although they are seen in the gastrocnemius. The neuropathy is best characterized clinically and electrophysiologically as diffuse, symmetric, motor, and sensory. The electrophysiological study gives support, although is not definitive, for a demyelinating neuropathy. The figure demonstrates the typical abnormal median normal sural (AMNS) pattern of sensory abnormalities seen in acute and chronic acquired demyelinating neuropathies (see cases 32 and 33). The needle EMG recruitment patterns without fibrillation potentials suggest demyelination, although they are not definitive. Perhaps the most compelling evidence for primary demyelination comes from the combination of small hand CMAPs but no fibrillation potentials in FDI, suggesting distal conduction block. Needle EMG of APB or ADM would have been valuable in this regard, as we did not actually record an ulnar–FDI CMAP to compare to the ulnar needle EMG study.

This patient has Guillain–Barré syndrome. The CSF WBC cell count was 1 and the protein was 166 mg/dl (normal, <50). He was treated with IVIg (0.4 gm/kg/day for 5 days) and rapidly stabilized despite this initial aggressive course (time from onset of paresthesias to inability to walk of only 2 days). Electrodiagnostic studies 2 weeks later, terminated prematurely by the patient's respiratory difficulties, were as follows:

Sensory NCS

Nerve	Sites	Recording Site	Onset (ms)	Peak (ms)	Amplitude (μV)	Distance (cm)
L. radial–sn box	1. Forearm	Sn box	Absent	—	—	—

Motor NCS

Nerve	Sites	Recording Site	Latency (ms)	Amplitude (mV)	Distance (cm)
L. median–APB	1. Wrist	APB	Absent		7
L. ulnar–ADM	1. Wrist	ADM	12.5	0.9	7

There has been further progression of axonal loss and now very clear-cut focal demyelination of the ulnar–ADM across-wrist segment, with a distal motor latency of 12.5. Clinical follow-up 6 months later showed marked recovery of motor function with independent ambulation.

Clinical Pearls

1. The electrophysiology of Guillain-Barré syndrome was discussed in case 32 in the setting of CIDP and shares similar features; however, there are also important differences.

2. The acute presentation of patients with Guillain-Barré syndrome results more often in less substantial electrophysiological abnormalities, and a significant number of patients with GBS have no electrophysiological abnormalities.

3. It is likely that F-wave abnormalities are in general the earliest abnormal and most sensitive studies in the diagnosis of Guillain-Barré syndrome.

4. Sequential studies demonstrating evolution of initially mild abnormalities can be helpful in confirming the diagnosis.

REFERENCES

1. Alam, T.A., Chaudhry, V., Cornblath, D.R., Electrophysiological studies in the Guillain–Barré syndrome: distinguishing subtypes by published criteria, *Muscle Nerve* 1998; 21(10):1275–1279.
2. Albers, J.W., Donofrio, P.D., McGonagle, T., Sequential electrodiagnostic abnormalities in acute inflammatory demyelinating polyradiculoneuropathy, *Muscle Nerve* 1985; 8:528–539.
3. Albers, J.W., Kelly, J.J., Jr., Acquired inflammatory demyelinating polyneuropathies: clinical and electrodiagnostic features, *Muscle Nerve* 1989; 12(6):435–451.
4. Asbury, A.K., Cornblath, D.R., Assessment of current diagnostic criteria for Guillain–Barré syndrome, *Ann. Neurol.* 1990; 27(suppl.):S21–S24.
5. Cornblath, D.R., Electrophysiology in Guillain–Barré syndrome, *Ann. Neurol.* 1990; 27(suppl.):S17–S20.
6. Meulstee, J., van der Meche, F.G., Electrodiagnostic criteria for polyneuropathy and demyelination: application in 135 patients with Guillain–Barré syndrome, Dutch Guillain–Barré Study Group, *J. Neurol. Neurosurg Psychiatry* 1995; 59(5):482–486.
7. Olney, R.K., Aminoff, M.J., Electrodiagnostic features of the Guillain–Barré syndrome: the relative sensitivity of different techniques, *Neurology* 1990; 40:471–475.

PATIENT 35

A 49-year-old woman with numbness in her right hand and both feet

This 49-year-old woman noted episodes 3 years ago of continuous numbness in her right hand lasting days to weeks and progressing to continuous numbness in digits 2 to 4 and lateral palm. Two years ago she developed numbness in her feet limited to the ventral surfaces of digits 2 and 3 bilaterally and in the right medial leg from the ankle to the knee. Symptoms have remained unchanged for the last year.

Neurological examination was notable for mild weakness of right APB and otherwise normal strength. Light touch sensation was impaired in the right median, saphenous, and bilateral distal medial plantar nerves. Reflexes are listed below:

Side	Biceps	Triceps	Knees	Ankles
R	2+	2+	Absent	Absent
L	2+	Absent	2+	Absent

Try to determine the clinical differential diagnosis. Consider the appropriate initial electrodiagnostic plan.

Electrodiagnostic Study:

Sensory NCS

Nerve	Sites	Recording Site	Onset (ms)	Peak (ms)	Amplitude (µV)	Distance (cm)	Velocity (m/s)
R. median–dig II	1. Wrist	Dig II	2.4	3.3	2.4	13	54
L. ulnar–dig V	1. Wrist	Dig V	1.8	2.5	27.1	11	61
R. sural–lat mall	1. Mid-calf	Ankle	2.8	3.65	7.4	14	50
L. sural–lat mall	1. Mid-calf	Ankle	2.9	3.60	8.9	14	48

Motor NCS

Nerve	Sites	Recording Site	Latency (ms)	Amplitude (mV)	Distance (cm)	Velocity (m/s)
R. median–APB	1. Wrist	APB	3.2	6.6	7	—
	2. Elbow	APB	8.9	2.2	19	33
	3. Axilla	APB	14.9	0.8	12	20
L. median–APB	1. Wrist	APB	3.2	9.6	7	—
	2. Elbow	APB	7.0	9.2	21	55
	3. Axilla	APB	8.7	9.0	12	71
R. ulnar–ADM	1. Wrist	ADM	2.5	7.5	7	—
	2. B. elbow	ADM	5.5	6.5	18	60
	3. A. elbow	ADM	7.7	6.0	15	68
R. peroneal–EDB	1. Ankle	EDB	4.1	5.2	8	—
	2. Fib head	EDB	9.9	4.9	28	48
	3. Pop fossa	EDB	12.1	2.4	10	46

F-Wave

Nerve	F_{min} (ms)	F_{max} (ms)	%F
R. median	Absent	—	—
L. median	27.4	29.0	100
L. peroneal	42.5	45.0	100

EMG Summary Table

	IA	SA Fib	SA Fasc	SA Other	Amplitude (MUs)	Duration (MUs)	PolyP (MUs)	Activation	Recruitment Pattern
R. abd poll brev	Inc	2+	2+	0	Nl	Nl	Nl	Full	MildRed
R. pron teres	Nl	0	0	0	Nl	Nl	Nl	Full	Normal
R. flex poll long	Nl	0	0	0	Nl	Nl	Nl	Full	Normal
R. flex dig supf	Nl	0	0	0	Nl	Nl	Nl	Full	Normal
R. first dors inteross	Nl	0	0	0	Nl	Nl	Nl	Full	Normal
R. vast med	Nl	0	0	0	Nl	Nl	Nl	Full	Normal

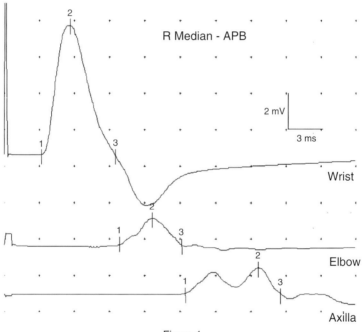

Figure 1

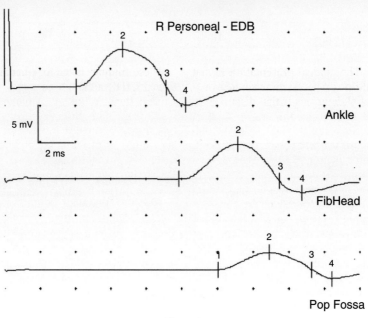

Figure 2

Questions:
1. What do the figures show?
2. How would you interpret the electrodiagnostic study?

Answers:
1. Conduction block
2. It suggests chronic inflammatory demyelinating polyneuropathy (CIDP).

Discussion: The clinical presentation is that of a chronic multifocal and asymmetric neuropathy. The differential diagnosis is that discussed in the introduction to this section in Table 6. It includes vasculitis, multifocal CIDP (also referred to as multifocal acquired demyelinating sensory and motor neuropathy, or MADSAM), and a variety of other causes.

The first figure shows conduction block of the right median–APB motor nerve in the forearm, temporal dispersion in the upper arm, and focal slowing in both locations. As the patient's median distribution hand numbness developed 3 years prior and she has not noted any change in her symptoms for 1 year, it is unlikely to be due to acute nerve infarction (pseudo-conduction block; see case 31). The second figure shows conduction block of the right peroneal–EDB motor nerve across the fibular head.

The electrodiagnostic study is abnormal for the conduction block and focal slowing in the right median and peroneal nerves noted above, as well as absent median F-wave responses despite preserved distal CMAP amplitude, a corroborative finding of demyelination proximal to the wrist. In addition, the median–D2 SNAP is reduced.

These findings taken together are those of multifocal CIDP, although conceivably the inherited neuropathy X-linked Charcot–Marie–Tooth (CMT-X) could produce this picture as well. Vasculitic neuropathy would not likely produce the finding of presumably long-standing conduction block in the median nerve as in this case. Follow-up electrodiagnostic studies 2 months later were unchanged, with continued right median forearm conduction block.

It should be emphasized that CIDP may be strikingly asymmetric and multifocal despite generally accepted criteria for symmetry. Such multifocal forms of CIDP are important to recognize as such because they share the excellent treatment responsiveness to prednisone that symmetric and confluent CIDP typically has and should thus be treated the same way. This stands in marked contrast to the syndrome of multifocal motor neuropathy (MMN), which does not respond to prednisone and is best not classified or confused with CIDP and its variants. MMN is discussed in greater detail through several cases in Section IV on motor neuropathies and motor neuron diseases.

Clinical Pearl

CIDP may be strikingly asymmetric and multifocal despite generally accepted criteria for symmetry

REFERENCES

1. Lewis, R.A., Sumner, A.J., Brown, M.J., Asbury, A.K., Multifocal demyelinating neuropathy with persistent conduction block, *Neurology* 1982; 32(9):958–964.
2. Saperstein, D.S., Amato, A.A., Wolfe, G.I., Katz, J.S., Nations, S.P., Jackson, C.E., Bryan, W.W., Burns, D.K., Barohn, R.J., Multifocal acquired demyelinating sensory and motor neuropathy: the Lewis Sumner syndrome, *Muscle Nerve* 1999; 22:560–566.
3. Saperstein, D.S., Katz, J.S., Amato, A.A., Barohn, R.J., Clinical spectrum of chronic acquired demyelinating neuropathies, *Muscle Nerve* 2001; 24:311–324.
4. Van den Berg-Vos, R.M., Van den Berg, L.H., Franssen, H. *et al.*, Multifocal inflammatory demyelinating neuropathy: a distinct clinical entity?, *Neurology* 2000; 54:26–32.

PATIENT 36

A 35-year-old woman with numbness in her hands and feet for 3 weeks and a right facial palsy for several days

Electrodiagnostic Study:

Sensory NCS

Nerve	Sites	Recording Site	Onset (ms)	Peak (ms)	BP Amplitude (µV)	Distance (cm)	Velocity (m/s)
R. sup peroneal	1. Lat leg	Ankle	2.85	3.60	8.9	12	42.1
R. sural–lat mall	1. Mid-calf	Ankle	3.30	3.90	11.7	14	42.4
L. sural–lat mall	1. Mid-calf	Ankle	3.50	4.05	15.8	14	40.0
R. median–dig II	1. Wrist	Dig II	2.25	2.95	36.9	13	57.8
R. ulnar–dig V	1. Wrist	Dig V	2.15	2.85	28.5	11	51.2

Motor NCS

Nerve	Sites	Recording Site	Latency (ms)	Amplitude (mV)	Distance (cm)	Velocity (m/s)
R. median–APB	1. Wrist	APB	3.85	7.3	7	—
	2. Elbow	APB	8.10	6.8	21	49.4
R. ulnar–ADM	1. Wrist	ADM	3.00	9.5	7	—
	2. B. elbow	ADM	6.35	8.8	18	53.7
	3. A. elbow	ADM	9.75	5.9	12.5	36.8
R. ulnar–FDI	1. Wrist	FDI	5.30	8.7	—	—
	2. B. elbow	FDI	8.45	7.3	19	60.3
	3. A. elbow	FDI	10.75	5.2	11	47.8
R. ulnar–inching	1. Wrist	ADM	3.40	9.6	7	—
	2. Elb − 5	ADM	6.60	9.1	17	53.1
	3. Elb − 2.5	ADM	6.95	9.0	2.5	71.4
	4. Elb	ADM	7.80	7.8	2.5	29.4
	5. Elb + 2.5	ADM	9.05	6.2	2.5	20.0
	6. Elb + 5	ADM	9.55	6.1	2.5	50.0
L. ulnar–ADM	1. Wrist	ADM	3.10	8.3	7	—
	2. B. elbow	ADM	6.85	7.2	21	56.0
	3. A. elbow	ADM	10.55	5.6	11	29.7
R. peroneal–EDB	1. Ankle	EDB	10.55	4.9	7	—
	2. Fib head	EDB	16.50	4.1	30	50.4
	3. Pop fossa	EDB	19.70	4.1	9	28.1
R. tibial–AH	1. Ankle	AH	7.10	6.6	8	—
	2. Pop fossa	AH	16.25	5.2	38	41.5
L. peroneal–EDB	1. Ankle	EDB	15.85	2.2	8	—
	2. Fib head	EDB	23.80	2.1	30	37.7
	3. Pop fossa	EDB	26.05	2.1	10	44.4
L. tibial–AH	1. Ankle	AH	7.00	8.5	8	—
	2. Pop fossa	AH	15.95	5.5	44	49.2

F-Wave

Nerve	F_{min} (ms)	F_{max} (ms)	Max – Min (ms)	%F
R. median	28.05	31.65	3.60	80
R. ulnar	33.10	35.20	2.10	80
L. peroneal	48.50	50.10	1.60	30
R. peroneal			A-waves present	
R. tibial			A-waves present	
L. tibial			A-waves present	

EMG Summary Table

		SA			Amplitude		Duration				
	IA	Fib	Fasc	Other	(MUs)	—	(MUs)	—	PolyP (MUs)	Activation	Recruitment Pattern
R. first dors int	Nl	0	0	0	Nl	—	Nl	—	Nl	Full	Nl
R. tib ant	Nl	0	0	0	Nl	—	Nl	—	Nl	Full	Nl

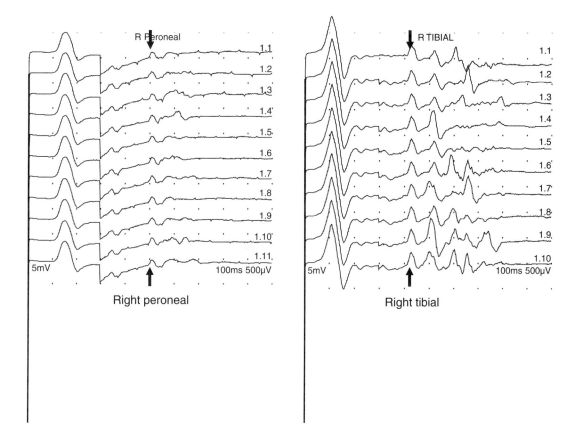

R Peroneal

1.1
1.2
1.3
1.4
1.5
1.6
1.7
1.8
1.9
1.10
1.11

5mV   100ms 500µV

Right peroneal

R TIBIAL

1.1
1.2
1.3
1.4
1.5
1.6
1.7
1.8
1.9
1.10

5mV   100ms 500µV

Right tibial

Question: What do the arrows demonstrate in the figure, and what is the significance of this finding?

Answer: A-waves suggest a demyelinating neuropathy.

Discussion: The results of nerve conduction studies are abnormal for: (1) prolongation of bilateral peroneal–EDB distal motor latencies, (2) focal slowing of bilateral ulnar–ADM across-elbow motor segments, (3) focal slowing of the right peroneal–EDB across-fibular-head motor segment, (4) prolongation of the right ulnar–ADM minimum F-wave latency, and (5) the presence of A-waves during F-wave studies. The results of limited EMG studies were normal. The figure shows the presence of A-waves in the right peroneal and tibial nerves, and the table indicates that they are present in the left tibial nerve as well.

The sensory and motor nerve conduction studies alone suggest a demyelinating neuropathy. There is focal slowing not just at the common compression sites but also for the peroneal–EDB segments at the ankles, with markedly increased distal motor latencies of 10.55 and 15.85 ms.

The nomenclature of late responses being termed *A-waves* is not well established. There are several distinct phenomena. Rare afterdischarges that occur at submaximal stimulation of motor nerves and disappear with increasing stimulus intensity have been called an *axon reflex*; these afterdischarges are better viewed as delayed components of the M-response and not as late responses. The motor axon loop is another A-wave attributed to collateral axonal branches and a resulting reentrant electrical impulse at submaximal stimulation. The most common use of the term *A-wave*, however, is to describe late responses that appear at supramaximal stimulation with constant shape and latency (unlike F-waves). Although the presence of A-waves in a single nerve may occur in up to 5% of asymptomatic individuals, multiple A-waves have diagnostic relevance. The electrodiagnostic significance of multiple, supramaximally stimulated A-waves has received recent attention,[1,4] and demyelinating neuropathies, both acquired and inherited, are highly associated with them. The presence of A-waves in multiple nerves, especially if the waveforms are complex, supports the electrodiagnosis of a primary demyelinating neuropathy. The mechanism is unknown, but ephaptic connection of neighboring demyelinated axons is one possible mechanism.

The patient's clinical diagnosis was Guillain-Barré syndrome; cerebrospinal fluid protein was normal (36 mg/dl), and she was not treated because she was almost 4 weeks into the illness with findings limited to numbness and paresthesias in her hands and a right facial palsy. However, she continued to progress over the ensuing weeks and returned with progressive generalized weakness at 10 weeks since onset of hand numbness. Results of follow-up studies 3 weeks later follow:

Sensory NCS

Nerve	Sites	Recording Site	Onset (ms)	Peak (ms)	BP Amplitude (μV)	Distance (cm)	Velocity (m/s)
R. ulnar–dig V	1. Wrist	Dig V	2.55	3.65	12.8	11	43.1
L. sural–lat mall	1. Mid-calf	Ankle	3.05	3.75	14.6	14	45.9
R. median–dig II	1. Wrist	Dig II	2.65	3.65	16.3	13	49.1
R. sural–lat mall	1. Mid-calf	Ankle	2.75	3.65	17.2	14	50.9

Motor NCS

Nerve	Sites	Recording Site	Latency (ms)	Amplitude (mV)	Distance (cm)	Velocity (m/s)
R. median–APB	1. Wrist	APB	6.85	5.0	7	—
	2. Elbow	APB	11.00	4.7	24	57.8
	3. Axilla	APB	13.80	4.1	17	60.7
L. median–APB	1. Wrist	APB	7.70	4.3	7	—
	2. Elbow	APB	13.10	4.3	23	42.6
	3. Axilla	APB	15.45	4.2	17.5	74.5

Nerve	Sites	Recording Site	Latency (ms)	Amplitude (mV)	Distance (cm)	Velocity (m/s)
R. ulnar–ADM	1. Wrist	ADM	5.05	7.0	7	—
	2. B. elbow	ADM	8.45	6.4	18	52.9
	3. A. elbow	ADM	12.60	5.1	10	24.1
	4. Axilla	ADM	15.50	4.8	13.5	46.6
L. ulnar–ADM	1. Wrist	ADM	5.85	5.4	7	—
	2. B. elbow	ADM	8.95	4.2	17	54.8
	3. A. elbow	ADM	13.95	3.7	10	20.0
	4. Axilla	ADM	15.95	3.5	13	65.0
R. peroneal–EDB	1. Ankle	EDB	14.45	2.6	8	—
	2. fib head	EDB	22.65	1.9	30	36.6
	3. Abv fib H	EDB	25.10	2.0	8.5	34.7
L. peroneal–EDB	1. Ankle	EDB	22.85	0.3	8	—
	2. Fib head	EDB	29.75	0.2	30.5	44.2
	3. Abv fib H	EDB	32.20	0.2	9	36.7
R. tibial–AH	1. Ankle	AH	6.70	1.4	8	—
	2. Pop fossa	AH	15.50	1.1	40	45.5
L. tibial–AH	1. Ankle	AH	8.90	2.0	8	—
	2. Pop fossa	AH	18.95	1.6	38	37.8

F-Wave

Nerve	F_{min} (ms)	F_{max} (ms)
R. peroneal	A-wave at 68.10	
R. tibial	A-wave at 30.10	
L. tibial	Absent	
L. peroneal	A-wave at 35.10	
R. median	34.40	39.20
R. ulnar	35.85	39.95
L. median	35.75	38.10
L. ulnar	35.55	45.15

EMG Summary Table

	IA	Fib	Fasc	Other	Amplitude (MUs)	Duration (MUs)	PolyP (MUs)	Activation	Recruitment Pattern
		SA							
L. first dors int	Nl	0	0	0	Nl	Nl	Nl	Full	Mild red
L. ext dig comm	Nl	0	0	0	Nl	Nl	Nl	Full	Mild red
L. vast med	Nl	0	0	0	Nl	Nl	Nl	Full	Nl
L. tib ant	Nl	0	0	0	Nl	Nl	Nl	Full	Nl
L. tib post	Nl	0	0	0	Nl	Nl	Nl	Full	Nl
L. gastroc med	Nl	0	0	0	Nl	Nl	Nl	Full	Nl
L. flex dig long	Nl	0	0	0	Nl	Nl	Nl	Full	Nl
L. ext dig brev	Nl	0	0	0	Nl	Nl	Nl	Full	Nl

In comparison to the prior studies, this study is remarkable for: (1) reduction in right median–D2 and ulnar–D5 SNAP amplitudes, (2) prolongation of all distal motor latencies (*i.e.*, left ulnar 3.10 → 5.85 ms, right median 3.85 → 6.85 ms, left peroneal 15.85 → 22.85 ms), (3) increased focal slowing of bilateral ulnar–ADM across-elbow motor segments (right 48 → 24 m/s, left 30 → 20 m/s), and (4) further prolongation and reduced persistence of median and ulnar minimum F-wave latencies. The results of EMG studies showed mild reductions in motor unit recruitment as tabulated.

The patient's CSF protein was now 51 mg/dl (normal, <44 mg/dl). Her continued progression of disease at 10 weeks led to revision of her diagnosis as CIDP, and treatment with IVIg was followed by oral prednisone, with sustained substantial improvement. CIDP may present acutely[2] and is difficult if not impossible to distinguish from Guillain–Barré syndrome at onset; however, continued disease progression past 4 weeks is uncommon for Guillain–Barré, and past 8 weeks is highly unusual.

Clinical Pearls

1. The presence of A-waves in multiple nerves, especially if the waveforms are complex, supports the electrodiagnosis of a primary demyelinating neuropathy.

2. CIDP may present acutely and is difficult if not impossible to distinguish from Guillain-Barré syndrome at onset.

REFERENCES

1. Kornhuber, M.E., Bischoff, C., Mentrup, H., Conrad, B., Multiple A waves in Guillain-Barré syndrome, *Muscle Nerve* 1999; 22:394–399.
2. Mori, K., Hattori, N., Sugiura, M., Koike, H., Misu, K., Ichimura, M., Hirayama, M., Sobue, G., Chronic inflammatory demyelinating polyneuropathy presenting with features of GBS, *Neurology* 2002; 58(6):979–982.
3. Roth, G., Egloff-Baer, S., Motor axon loop: an electroneurographic response, *Muscle Nerve* 1984; 7:294–297.
4. Rowin, J., Meriggioli, M.N., The electrodiagnostic significance of supramaximally stimulated A-waves, *Muscle Nerve* 2000; 23:1117–1120.

PATIENT 37

A 74-year-old woman with progressive weakness in her hands

This 74-year-old woman was referred by an orthopedic surgeon who noted diffuse atrophy and weakness of her hands. She complained of increasing weakness and atrophy for several years without paresthesias or reduction in sensation. She reported a mother and sister with high arches in their feet and atrophy of their hands similar to hers.

Electrodiagnostic Study:

Sensory NCS

Nerve	Sites	Recording Site	Onset (ms)	Peak (ms)	BP Amplitude (μV)	Distance (cm)	Velocity (m/s)
R. median–dig II	1. Wrist	Dig II	5.75	8.40	3.6	13	22.6
L. median–dig II	1. Wrist	Dig II	7.55	8.70	2.3	13	17.2
R. ulnar–dig V	1. Wrist	Dig V	Absent	—	—	11	—
L. ulnar–dig V	1. Wrist	Dig V	11.05	13.65	1.3	11	10.0
R. radial–sn box	1. Forearm	Digit 1	Absent	—	—	13	—
L. radial–sn box	1. Forearm	Digit 1	8.90	10.60	1.8	13	14.6
L. sural–lat mall	1. Mid-calf	Ankle	10.40	12.70	1.4	14	13.5

Motor NCS

Nerve	Sites	Recording Site	Latency (ms)	Amplitude (μV)	Distance (cm)	Velocity (m/s)
R. median–APB	1. Wrist	APB	9.30	1.9	7	—
	2. Elbow	APB	21.15	1.2	21.5	18.1
L. median–APB	1. Wrist	APB	11.20	0.9	7	—
	2. Elbow	APB	20.40	0.6	20	21.7
	3. Axilla	APB	25.30	0.7	12	24.5
R. ulnar–ADM	1. Wrist	ADM	8.15	1.2	7	—
	2. A. elbow	ADM	23.70	0.9	26	16.7
L. ulnar–ADM	1. Wrist	ADM	6.45	4.2	7	—
	2. B. elbow	ADM	17.05	4.2	16.5	15.6
	3. A. elbow	ADM	22.10	4.0	10	19.8
	4. Axilla	ADM	27.95	3.5	12.5	21.4
L. peroneal–EDB	1. Ankle	EDB	Absent		8	—
L. peroneal–tib ant	1. Fib head	Tib ant	7.30	2.5	7	—
	2. Pop fossa	Tib ant	10.95	2.1	9	24.7
L. tibial–AH	1. Ankle	AH	17.50	0.1	8	—
	2. Pop fossa	—	—	Absent	—	—

F-Wave

Nerve	F$_{min}$ (ms)	F$_{max}$ (ms)	Max – Min (ms)	%F
R. median	Absent	—	—	—
R. ulnar	Absent	—	—	—
L. median	Absent		Reproducible A-waves	
L. ulnar	Absent		Reproducible A-waves	

Questions:
1. Would you characterize this neuropathy as primarily axonal or demyelinating?
2. Does the electrophysiology support an acquired or inherited disorder? Why?

Answers:

1. Demyelinating
2. Inherited disorder

Discussion: These studies are notable for diffusely reduced sensory nerve and compound muscle action potential amplitudes and marked slowing of conduction velocities. Every nerve segment examined has marked slowing, with distal sensory velocities ranging from 10 to 23 m/s, motor conduction velocities ranging from 16 to 25 m/s, and distal motor latencies of 6.5 to 9.3 ms in the hands (the 17.5 ms in the tibial–AH study could reflect the difficulty in measuring an accurate take-off of a very small potential). In addition, there are multiple A-waves (present in more than 1 nerve; see case 36). These features are those of a demyelinating neuropathy, and the relatively uniform slowing of nerve conduction velocities is a characteristic feature of inherited neuropathies.

Dyck and Lambert in 1968 classified dominantly inherited neuropathies as axonal or demyelinating based on a single parameter: the ulnar forearm motor conduction velocity, with 38 m/s being the cutoff for demyelinating versus axonal. Refinements in the 1970s identified patients with intermediate conduction velocities of 30 to 40 m/s, with velocities of 15 to 30 m/s classified as demyelinating type I and velocities of >40 m/s as axonal type II.

A publication of Lewis and Sumner in 1982[5] has been influential in emphasizing the electrodiagnostic distinction of inherited versus acquired demyelinating neuropathy. This paper emphasized the characteristic features of inherited demyelinating neuropathies: uniform conduction slowing and the absence of conduction block. The presence of nonuniform slowing (substantial differences in segmental conduction velocities, with a mixture of normal and abnormal segments) or of conduction block is instead characteristic of an acquired demyelinating neuropathy. Two exceptions to this rule have required a revision of this view[36]: X-linked Charcot–Marie–Tooth disease (CMT-X) and hereditary neuropathy with liability to pressure palsies (HNPP) may have nonuniform slowing and conduction block. Other exceptions may occur as well (see case 38).

Clinical Pearl

Inherited demyelinating neuropathies, with the exception of CMT-X and HNPP, are partially distinguishable from acquired demyelinating neuropathies by their uniform conduction slowing and absence of conduction block; however, exceptions do occur, and the advent of molecular genetics is increasingly invalidating this basic principle of electrodiagnostic medicine.

REFERENCES

1. Boerkoel, C.F., Takashima, H., Garcia, C.A., Olney, R.K., Johnson, J., Berry, K., Russo, P., Kennedy, S., Teebi, A.S., Scavina, M., Williams, L.L., Mancias, P., Butler, I.J., Krajewski, K., Shy, M., Lupski, J.R., Charcot–Marie–Tooth disease and related neuropathies: mutation distribution and genotype-phenotype correlation, *Ann. Neurol.* 2002; 51:190–201.
2. Dyck, P.J., Lambert, E.H., Lower motor and primary sensory neuron diseases with peroneal muscular atrophy. I Neurologic, genetic, and electrophysiolgical findings in hereditary polyneuropathies, *Arch. Neurol.* 1968; 18:603–618.
3. Kaku, D.A., Parry, G.J., Malamut, R., Lupski, J.R., Garcia, C.A., Uniform slowing of conduction velocities in Charcot–Marie–Tooth polyneuropathy type 1. *Neurology* 1993; 43:2664–2667.
4. Kaku, D.A., Parry, G.J., Malamut, R., Lupski, J.R., Garcia, C.A., Nerve conduction studies in Charcot–Marie–Tooth polyneuropathy associated with a segmental duplication of chromosome 17, *Neurology* 1993; 43:1806–1808.
5. Lewis, R.A., Sumner, A.J., The electrodiagnostic distinctions between chronic familial and acquired demyelinative neuropathies, *Neurology* 1982; 32:592–596.
6. Lewis, R.A., Sumner, A.J., Shy, M.E., Electrophysiological features of inherited demyelinating neuropathies: a reappraisal in the era of molecular diagnosis, *Muscle Nerve* 2000; 23:1472–1487.
7. Pareyson, D., Charcot–Marie–Tooth disease and related neuropathies: molecular basis for distinction and diagnosis, *Muscle Nerve* 1999; 22:1498–1509.

PATIENT 38

**A 68-year-old woman with slowly progressive weakness in her legs
without paresthesias**

Electrodiagnostic Study:

Sensory NCS

Nerve	Sites	Recording Site	Response	Onset (ms)	Peak (ms)	Amplitude (μV)	Distance (cm)	Velocity (m/s)
R. radial–sn box	1. Forearm	SnBox	—	1.8	2.6	21.5	10	56
R. sural–lat mall	1. Mid-calf	Ankle	Absent	—	—	—	14	—

Motor NCS

Nerve	Sites	Recording Site	Latency (ms)	Amplitude (mV)	Distance (cm)	Velocity (m/s)
L. ulnar–ADM	1. Wrist	ADM	3.2	8.4	7	—
	2. B. elbow	ADM	6.5	7.6	15	45
	3. A. elbow	ADM	8.3	7.3	10	56
	4. Axilla	ADM	9.8	7.9	10	67
L. median–APB	1. Wrist	APB	4.7	5.7	7	—
	2. Elbow	APB	8.3	4.8	—	53
R. peroneal–EDB	1. Ankle	EDB	8.7	0.3	8	—
	2. Fib head	EDB	17.3	0.3	28	32
	3. Pop fossa	EDB	20.7	0.2	10	29
L. peroneal–EDB	1. Ankle	EDB	4.0	0.3	8	—
	2. Fib head	EDB	11.6	0.4	26	34
	3. Pop fossa	EDB	16.1	0.4	10	22
R. peroneal–TA	1. Fib head	TA	2.7	3.6	8	—
	2. Pop fossa	TA	6.2	2.5	28	32
L. tibial–AH	1. Ankle	AH	6.1	0.5	8	—
	2. Pop fossa	AH	20.4	0.5	34	24

EMG studies were limited to right tibialis anterior, showing 2+ fibrillation potentials, large amplitude and long-duration motor unit action potentials, and moderately reduced recruitment.

Question: Do the electrodiagnostic studies suggest an inherited or an acquired demyelinating neuropathy?

Answer: Acquired

Discussion: This study shows axonal degeneration of sensory and motor axons in the feet, with an absent sural SNAP and reduced amplitudes of bilateral peroneal–EDB and left tibial–AH CMAPs; however, the motor velocities in some of the leg segments (left tibial leg, 24 m/sec; right peroneal leg, 32 m/sec; left peroneal across fibular head, 22 m/s) are slower than one would feel comfortable with attributing to the axonal degeneration alone. The motor velocities in nerves eliciting preserved CMAP amplitudes, such as the median and ulnar, show a borderline reduced ulnar forearm velocity (45 m/s) but normal other segments. In fact, the range of motor velocities is 22 to 67 m/s, suggesting that this patient has an acquired demyelinating neuropathy (see discussion for case 37).

Genetic testing in this patient revealed a point mutation in the myelin protein zero (MPZ or P0) gene. Accordingly, by genetic classification, this patient has CMT1b (mutations in MPZ), a demyelinating neuropathy. As noted in the forthcoming discussion for case 40, some patients previously classified electrodiagnostically as axonal CMT (CMT2) in fact have mutations in the MPZ gene.

Clinical Pearl

Some patients with MPZ mutations have borderline ulnar nerve conduction velocities not readily classified as axonal or demyelinating neuropathies.

REFERENCES

1. Marrosu, M.G., Vaccargiu, S., Marrosu, G., Vannelli, A., Cianchetti, C., Muntoni, F., Charcot–Marie–Tooth disease type 2 associated with mutation of the myelin protein zero gene, *Neurology* 1998; 50:1397–1401.
2. Mastaglia, F.L., Nowak, K.J., Stell, R., Phillips, B.A., Edmondston, J.E., Dorosz, S.M., Wilton, S.D., Hallmayer, J., Kakulas, B.A., Laing, N.G., Novel mutation in the myelin protein zero gene in a family with intermediate hereditary motor and sensory neuropathy, *J. Neurol. Neurosurg. Psychiatry* 1999; 67(2):174–179.

PATIENT 39

A 32-year-old woman with a severe neuropathy since childhood

This 32-year-old woman had significant developmental delay; she learned to walk with help at the age of 3 but then required a wheelchair within several years and remained stable into her 20s. At the age of 15, the ulnar motor nerve conduction velocity was 11 m/s (CMAP amplitude not known). Nerve biopsy was abnormal with proliferation of Schwann cells in an onion bulb appearance. Marked thoracolumbar scoliosis led to surgery with placement of Harrington rods. Over the last 5 to 10 years, she has noticed increasing weakness in her hands. There was no family history of a neuropathy in either parent or several siblings.

Neurological examination showed severe weakness of distal and mild weakness of proximal muscles in all limbs. There was marked loss of position sense, and the patient was unsteady sitting in her wheelchair with eyes closed.

Electrodiagnostic Study:

Sensory NCS

Nerve	Sites	Recording Site	Response	Onset (ms)	Amplitude (mV)	Distance (cm)	Velocity (m/s)
L. median–dig II	1. Wrist	Dig II	No	—	—	13	—
L. ulnar–dig V	1. Wrist	Dig V	No	—	—	11	—
L. radial–sn box	1. Forearm	Sn box	No	—	—	10	—
L. sural	1. Mid-calf	Ankle	No	—	—	14	—
R. median–dig V	1. Wrist	Dig II	No	—	—	13	—
R. ulnar–dig V	1. Wrist	Dig V	No	—	—	11	—
R. radial–sn box	1. Forearm	Sn box	No	—	—	10	—

Motor NCS

Nerve	Sites	Recording Site	Response	Latency (ms)	Amplitude (mV)	Distance (cm)	Velocity (m/s)
L. median–APB	1. Wrist	APB	No	—	—	7	—
L. ulnar–ADM	1. Wrist	ADM	No	—	—	7	—
R. median–APB	1. Wrist	APB	No	—	—	7	—
R. ulnar–ADM	1. Wrist	ADM	No	—	—	7	—

Question: Assuming this patient has an inherited neuropathy, do you think it is dominantly or recessively inherited?

Answer: It cannot be determined.

Discussion: The complete absence of sensory and motor responses indicates a severe generalized neuropathy but gives little other information. The previous history of an ulnar motor nerve conduction velocity of 11 m/s suggests that previously there was evidence of primary demyelination, as did the nerve biopsy. Could this patient have chronic inflammatory demyelinating polyneuropathy, which is treatable? The definitive answer came from sequencing of her PMP-22 gene, which demonstrated a point mutation (C264T). This patient has a PMP-22 point mutation with a CMT3 phenotype.

The severe phenotype of CMT-3, known as Dejerine–Sottas disease or congenital hypomyelination neuropathy, was once classified as a recessive demyelinating disorder. It has since become clearer that most cases are dominant *de novo* mutations. Patients with a broad range of affected genes have been reported with this phenotype, including point mutations of PMP22, MPZ, EGR2, and PRX (periaxin).

Clinical Pearls

1. Severe slowing of nerve conduction velocities is characteristic of CMT-3, which may result from a variety of mutations in different genes. The disorder is mostly autosomal dominant, although a high spontaneous mutation rate results in *de novo* cases with no previous family history.

2. The availability of genetic testing for this disorder should replace the use of nerve biopsy for diagnosis.

REFERENCES

1. Boerkoel, C.F., Takashima, H., Stankiewicz, P., Garcia, C.A., Leber, S.M., Rhee-Morris, L., Lupski, J.R., Periaxin mutations cause recessive Dejerine–Sottas neuropathy, *Am. J. Hum. Genet.* 2001; 68:325–333.
2. Fabrizi, G.M., Simonati, A., Taioli, F., Cavallaro, T., Ferrarini, M., Rigatelli, F., Pini, A., Mostacciuolo, M.L., Rizzuto, N., PMP22 related congenital hypomyelination neuropathy, *J. Neurol. Neurosurg. Psychiatry* 2001; 70:123–126.
3. Fabrizi, G.M., Cavallaro, T., Morbin, M., Simonati, A., Taioli, F., Rizzuto, N., Novel mutation of the P0 extracellular domain causes a Dejerine–Sottas syndrome, *J. Neurol. Neurosurg. Psychiatry* 1999; 66:386–389.
4. Ionasescu, V.V., Ionasescu, R., Searby, C., Neahring, R., Dejerine–Sottas disease with *de novo* dominant point mutation of the PMP22 gene, *Neurology* 1995; 45:1766–1767.
5. Ionasescu, V.V., Searby, C., Greenberg, S.A., Dejerine–Sottas disease with sensorineural hearing loss, nystagmus, and peripheral facial nerve weakness: *de novo* dominant point mutation of the PMP22 gene, *J. Med. Genet.* 1996; 33:1048–1049.
6. Warner, L.E., Shohat, M., Shorer, Z., Lupski, J.R., Multiple *de novo* MPZ (P0) point mutations in a sporadic Dejerine–Sottas case, *Hum Mutat.* 1997; 10:21–24.

PATIENT 40

A 33-year-old woman with long-standing asymmetric weakness in all four limbs and a family history of neuropathy

This 33-year-old woman has noticed weakness of all limbs, greater in the right foot and hand than the left, since her early 20s with gradual progression since. Her family history is remarkable for a neuropathy affecting males considerably more severely than females and a lack of male–male transmission. In particular, her mother developed a neuropathy in her 20s and is still ambulatory while her mother's brother (M.) was severely affected at age 5. M. has a healthy son and an affected daughter (S.). S. has 3 boys, one of whom is known to be affected. The patient has a severely affected brother who was diagnosed at age 8, 3 normal sisters, and 4 other normal brothers. The neurological exam for strength in several muscles is noted below:

Legs	APB	FDI	TA
Right	0	3	0
Left	4	4	4–

Electrodiagnostic Study:

Sensory NCS

Nerve	Sites	Recording Site	Onset (ms)	Peak (ms)	Amplitude (µV)	Distance (cm)	Velocity (m/s)
R. median–dig II	1. Wrist	Dig II	Absent	—	—	—	—
L. median–dig V	1. Wrist	Dig II	Absent	—	—	—	—
R. ulnar–dig V	1. Wrist	Dig V	Absent	—	—	—	—
L. ulnar–dig V	1. Wrist	Dig V	Absent	—	—	—	—
R. radial–sn box	1. Forearm	Sn box	Absent	—	—	—	—
L. radial–sn box	1. Forearm	Sn box	Absent	—	—	—	—
R. sural–lat mall	1. Mid-calf	Ankle	Absent	—	—	—	—
L. sural–lat mall	1. Mid-calf	Ankle	Absent	—	—	—	—

Motor NCS

Nerve	Sites	Recording Site	Latency (ms)	Amplitude (mV)	Distance (cm)	Velocity (m/s)
R. median–APB	1. Wrist	APB	6.0	1.1	7	—
	2. Elbow	APB	14.1	1.1	23	28
L. median–APB	1. Wrist	APB	5.5	4.2	7	—
	2. Elbow	APB	12.0	3.6	21	32
R. ulnar–ADM	1. Wrist	ADM	3.4	3.0	7	—
	2. B. elbow	ADM	7.3	2.4	19	49
	3. A. elbow	ADM	9.8	2.3	10	38
L. ulnar–ADM	1. Wrist	ADM	4.0	4.4	7	—
	2. B. elbow	ADM	8.7	4.0	19	40
	3. A. elbow	ADM	11.2	3.9	10	40
R. peroneal–EDB	1. Ankle	EDB	Absent	0.0	8	—

Nerve	Sites	Recording Site	Latency (ms)	Amplitude (mV)	Distance (cm)	Velocity (m/s)
L. peroneal–EDB	1. Ankle	EDB	Absent	0.0	8	—
R. peroneal–TA	1. Fib head	TA	4.7	0.2	8	—
	2. Pop fossa	TA	6.0	0.2	8.5	57
L. peroneal–TA	1. Fib head	TA	3.0	2.1	7	—
	2. Pop fossa	TA	5.3	0.8	8	35
R. tibial–AH	1. Ankle	AH	6.0	0.1	8	—
	2. Pop fossa	AH	Absent	0.0	—	—
L. tibial–AH	1. Ankle	AH	Absent	0.0	—	—

F-Wave

Nerve	F_{min} (ms)
R. median	Absent
L. median	25.9
R. ulnar	30.2
L. ulnar	30.2

Question: What are the clinical diagnostic considerations?

Answer: Inherited neuropathy, X-linked dominant

Discussion: The patient has an inherited neuropathy with greater severity of males and absence of male–male transmission. This pattern of inheritance suggests an X-linked dominant disorder with partial expression in female carriers. The remarkable aspects of the limited motor strength testing exam results are the marked asymmetry and multifocality. Certainly, the right TA and APB are dramatically different than the left, establishing the asymmetry. Furthermore, the right median-innervated APB muscle is also more severely affected than the right ulnar-innervated FDI, suggesting multifocality as well. Clinically, these features together suggest an asymmetric multifocal X-linked dominantly inherited neuropathy.

The electrodiagnostic study provides further information. There is evidence for primary demyelination in the right median–APB forearm motor segment, with a velocity of 28 m/s, less than 70% the lower limit of normal of 44 m/s (=31 m/s; see case 32 for discussion of criteria for primary demyelination). The left median–APB forearm motor segment velocity of 32 m/s meets such criteria as well (the relative preservation of the distal evoked CMAP amplitude would lead to application of an 80% LLN factor). In addition, there is conduction block of the right peroneal–TA across-fibular-head motor segment (amplitude drop > 50%). There clearly is distal axonal loss as well, but the presence of any clear-cut demyelination establishes this as a demyelinating neuropathy.

The nerve conduction studies also support the notion of a multifocal and asymmetric process. The range of velocities is 28 to 57 m/s. As noted previously (see case 37), this generally suggests an acquired demyelinating neuropathy, although there are exceptions, this being one of them. It is not clear whether to characterize this neuropathy as having a predilection for compression sites. There is conduction block at one fibular head, but the other peroneal across fibular head segment and neither ulnar across-elbow segment demonstrates focal demyelination. The median–APB distal motor latencies are not dramatically increased either.

Given the above views, two inherited neuropathies should be considered: CMT-X (X-linked Charcot–Marie–Tooth) and HNPP (hereditary neuropathy with liability to pressure palsies). These disorders are largely due, respectively, to mutations of the connexin 32 (Cx32) gene and deletions of the peripheral myelin protein 22 (PMP-22) gene. These two inherited neuropathies may show a significant range of motor conduction velocities and be characterized as having asymmetric and multifocal involvement. The greater severity in males and lack of male–male transmission in this case strongly suggest CMT-X. Genetic testing of this patient showed intact PMP-22 genes with normal sequences and a point mutation in the coding region of Cx32 (832delT).

The history of classification of CMT-X reflects its unusual inheritance pattern. Premolecular classification of CMT looked something like the first figure. The CMT dominant intermediate velocities (ulnar motor forearm velocities of 30 to 40 m/s) category fell between the strict criteria for demyelinating versus axonal neuropathies of the 1970s. Subsequent discoveries, particularly in molecular genetics, have made it clear that most of these CMT dominant intermediate families were indeed CMT-X, and most of the remainder of these patients have point mutations of myelin protein zero (MPZ; CMT1-b), as shown in the second figure.

Pre-Molecular Genetic
Classification of CMT

Demyelinating Dominant	Axonal Dominant
1 HNPP	2

CMT-Dominant Intermediate

Demyelinating Recessive	Axonal Recessive
3	"AR-2"

CMT-X

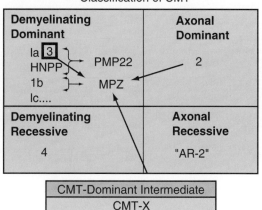

Molecular Genetic
Classification of CMT

Connexin-32, also called gap junction protein B1 (GJB1), is believed to form gap junctions within non-compact myelin. At least 264 mutations were reported in molecular mutation databases as of November 2003 (http://molgen-www.uia.ac.be/ CMTmutations), mostly point mutations. A wide range of severity exists, with null or truncation mutations causing a severe phenotype, similar to CMT3 (Dejerine–Sotas disease).

Clinical Pearl

Although uniform slowing of nerve conduction studies and absence of conduction block have classically been used to distinguish acquired from inherited demyelinating neuropathies, there are two exceptions: CMT-X and HNNP, both of which may have nonuniform slowing and conduction block.

REFERENCES

1. Birouk, N., LeGuern, E., Maisonobe, T., Rouger, H., Gouider, R., Tardieu, S., Gugenheim, M., Routon, M.C., Leger, J.M., Agid, Y., Brice, A., Bouche, P., X-linked Charcot–Marie–Tooth disease with Connexin 32 mutations: clinical and electrophysiologic study, *Neurology* 1999; 52:432–433.
2. Dubourg, O., Tardieu, S., Birouk, N., Gouider, R., Leger, J.M., Maisonobe, T., Brice, A., Bouche, P., LeGuern, E., Clinical, electrophysiological and molecular genetic characteristics of 93 patients with X-linked Charcot–Marie–Tooth disease, *Brain* 2001; 124:1958–1967.
3. Gutierrez, A., England, J.D., Sumner, A.J., Ferer, S., Warner, L.E., Lupski, J.R., Garcia, C.A., Unusual electrophysiological findings in X-linked dominant Charcot–Marie–Tooth disease, *Muscle Nerve* 2000; 23:182–188
4. Hahn, A.F., Ainsworth, P.J., Naus, C.C., Mao, J., Bolton, C.F., Clinical and pathological observations in men lacking the gap junction protein connexin 32, *Muscle Nerve* 2000; 999(9):S39–S48.
5. Hahn, A.F., Ainsworth, P.J., Bolton, C.F., Bilbao, J.M., Vallat, J.M., Pathological findings in the X-linked form of Charcot–Marie–Tooth disease: a morphometric and ultrastructural analysis, *Acta Neuropathol. (Berlin)* 2001; 101:129–139.
6. Lewis, R.A., The challenge of CMTX and Connexin 32 mutations, *Muscle Nerve* 2000; 23:147–149.
7. Nicholson, G., Nash, J., Intermediate nerve conduction velocities define X-linked Charcot–Marie–Tooth neuropathy families, *Neurology* 1993; 43:2558–2564.
8. Pareyson, D., Charcot–Marie–Tooth disease and related neuropathies: molecular basis for distinction and diagnosis, *Muscle Nerve* 1999; 22:1498–1509.
9. Tabaraud, F., Lagrange, E., Sindou, P., Vandenberghe, A., Levy, N., Vallat, J.M., Demyelinating X-linked Charcot–Marie–Tooth disease: unusual electrophysiological findings, *Muscle Nerve* 1999; 22:1442–1447.
10. Vital, A., Ferrer, X., Lagueny, A., Vandenberghe, A., Latour, P., Goizet, C., Canron, M.H., Louiset, P., Petry, K.G., Vital, C., Histopathological features of X-linked Charcot–Marie–Tooth disease in 8 patients from 6 families with different Connexin 32 mutations, *J. Peripher. Nerv. Syst.* 2001; 6:79–84.

PATIENT 41

A 72-year-old woman with 12 years of progressive numbness and paresthesias in her hands and feet and mild gait ataxia

At the age of 60, this woman developed numbness and tingling paresthesias in her feet and her fingertips which have gradually progressed since. The tingling paresthesias in the legs go up to just below the knees and in the hands remain confined to the fingertips. Her balance is mildly impaired.
Electrodiagnostic Study:

Sensory NCS

Nerve	Sites	Recording Site	Onset (ms)	Peak (ms)	Amplitude (μV)	Distance (cm)	Velocity (m/s)
R. median–dig II	1. Wrist	Dig II	5.15	6.75	3.0	13	25.2
L. median–dig II	1. Wrist	Dig II	4.80	7.15	3.7	13	27.1
R. ulnar–dig V	1. Wrist	Dig V	Absent	—	—	11	—
L. ulnar–dig V	1. Wrist	Dig V	5.00	6.90	3.3	11	22.0
R. radial–sn box	1. Forearm	Sn box	2.80	3.60	6.2	10	35.7
R. sural–lat mall	1. Mid-calf	Ankle	Absent	—	—	14	—
L. sural–lat mall	1. Mid-calf	Ankle	Absent	—	—	14	—

Motor NCS

Nerve	Sites	Recording Site	Latency (ms)	Amplitude (mV)	Distance (cm)	Velocity (m/s)
R. median–APB	1. Wrist	APB	8.95	5.2	7	—
	2. Elbow	APB	14.25	5.3	20	37.7
L. median–APB	1. Wrist	APB	9.30	4.5	7	—
	2. Elbow	APB	15.15	3.3	22	37.6
R. ulnar–ADM	1. Wrist	ADM	6.30	6.6	7	—
	2. B. elbow	ADM	10.00	5.3	17.5	47.3
	3. A. elbow	ADM	14.40	5.1	10	22.7
L. ulnar–ADM	1. Wrist	ADM	6.40	7.3	7	—
	2. B. elbow	ADM	10.10	7.2	17.5	47.3
	3. A. elbow	ADM	14.15	6.8	9.5	23.5
R. Peroneal–EDB	1. Ankle	EDB	Absent	—	8	—
R. Peroneal–tib ant	1. Fib head	Tib ant	4.95	3.3	8	—
	2. Pop fossa	Tib ant	10.15	2.2	7.5	14.4
R. tibial–AH	1. Ankle	AH	Absent	—	8	—

F-Wave

Nerve	F_{min} (ms)	F_{max} (ms)	Max – Min (ms)	%F
R. median	40.70	43.70	3.00	80
R. ulnar	39.80	43.25	3.45	80
L. median	41.60	46.25	4.65	80
L. ulnar	39.25	45.00	5.75	80

Questions:

1. The electrodiagnostic studies demonstrate a generalized peripheral neuropathy. Should it be characterized as primarily axonal or demyelinating?
2. Does the study suggest an inherited or an acquired neuropathy?

Answers:
1. Demyelinating
2. Acquired

Discussion: The electrodiagnostic features are those of an acquired demyelinating neuropathy. There is nonuniform slowing of motor nerve conduction velocities (range, 14.4 to 47.3 m/s). The distal latencies and some of the motor segment velocities are definitively in the demyelinating range, while other segments have normal velocities (ulnar–ADM forearm). As a rule, inherited demyelinating neuropathies have uniform slowing (with some exceptions, notably CMT-X and HNPP), while nonuniform slowing indicates an acquired demyelinating neuropathy. The study shows a predilection for greater slowing at common compression sites (median at the wrist, ulnar at the elbow, and peroneal at the fibular head), but other sites are also significantly involved, such as the ulnar across the wrists for both motor and sensory fibers.

One can also argue from this study that, except for the compression sites, the slowing is preferentially distal. All distal motor latencies are significantly prolonged, and to a greater extent than the velocity reductions in the other non-compression site segments. For example, the ulnar distal latencies are at least 70% increased above the upper limit of normal, with normal forearm velocities. The median distal motor latencies are at least 100% increased, with forearm motor velocities that are not more than 10 to 20% reduced. The distal sensory velocities are similarly substantially reduced, beyond what would be expected from axonal loss alone. Note the absence of conduction block, characteristic of this particular neuropathy.

The clinical features of distal sensory involvement with gait ataxia along with a demyelinating neuropathy with prolonged distal latencies and absence of conduction block are characteristic of the myelin-associated glycoprotein (MAG) and sulfatide (SGPG) antibody-mediated neuropathies. This patient has an IgM-κ paraprotein on immunofixation and serum anti-MAG titer of 1:51,200 (normal, <1:800) and anti-SGPG titer of 1:819,200 (normal, <1:800). These neuropathies are generally mild clinically and very impressively abnormal electrodiagnostically; they generally do not require treatment (which is less than satisfactory when attempted) and have a favorable prognosis, although there are exceptions.

Clinical Pearls

1. Anti-MAG and anti-sulfatide neuropathy syndromes typically appear to clinically have sensory loss typical of a distal axonal neuropathy but more gait ataxia than would be expected from such.

2. Electrodiagnostically, the findings are relatively unique, with distal demyelination predominant.

3. Unlike in other acquired demyelinating neuropathies, conduction block is not seen in MAG and sulfatide neuropathies.

REFERENCES

1. Braun, P.E., Frail, D.E., Latov, N., Myelin-associated glycoprotein is the antigen for a monoclonal IgM in polyneuropathy, *J. Neurochem.* 1982; 39(5):1261–1265.
2. Capasso, M., Torrieri, F., Di Muzio, A., De Angelis, M.V., Lugaresi, A., Uncini, A., Can electrophysiology differentiate polyneuropathy with anti-MAG/SGPG antibodies from chronic inflammatory demyelinating polyneuropathy?, *Clin. Neurophysiol.* 2002; 113(3):346–353.
3. Dalakas, M.C., Quarles, R.H., Farrer, R.G., Dambrosia, J., Soueidan, S., Stein, D.P., Cupler, E., Sekul, E.A., Otero, C., A controlled study of intravenous immunoglobulin in demyelinating neuropathy with IgM gammopathy, *Ann. Neurol.* 1996; 40(5):792–795.
4. Eurelings, M., Moons, K.G., Notermans, N.C., Sasker, L.D., De Jager, A.E., Wintzen, A.R., Wokke, J.H., Van den Berg, L.H., Neuropathy and IgM M-proteins: prognostic value of antibodies to MAG, SGPG, and sulfatide, *Neurology* 2001; 56(2):228–233.
5. Gorson, K.C., Ropper, A.H., Weinberg, D.H., Weinstein, R., Treatment experience in patients with anti-myelin-associated glycoprotein neuropathy, *Muscle Nerve* 2001; 24(6):778–786.
6. Kaku, D.A., England, J.D., Sumner, A.J., Distal accentuation of conduction slowing in polyneuropathy associated with antibodies to myelin-associated glycoprotein and sulphated glucuronyl paragloboside, *Brain* 1994; 117:941–947.
7. Katz, J.S., Saperstein, D.S., Gronseth, G., Amato, A.A., Barohn, R.J., Distal acquired demyelinating symmetric neuropathy, *Neurology* 2000; 54(3):615–620.
8. Kelly, J.J., Jr., The electrodiagnostic findings in polyneuropathies associated with IgM monoclonal gammopathies, *Muscle Nerve* 1990; 13(12):1113–1117.

9. Nobile-Orazio, E., Meucci, N., Baldini, L., Di Troia, A., Scarlato, G., Long-term prognosis of neuropathy associated with anti-MAG IgM M-proteins and its relationship to immune therapies, *Brain* 2000; 123(pt. 4):710–717.

10. Trojaborg, W., Hays, A.P., van den Berg, L., Younger, D.S., Latov, N., Motor conduction parameters in neuropathies associated with anti-MAG antibodies and other types of demyelinating and axonal neuropathies, *Muscle Nerve* 1995; 18(7):730–735.

PATIENT 42

**A 43-year-old woman with acute generalized weakness developing
1 month into her intensive care unit stay for sepsis and
multi-organ failure**

This 43-year-old woman developed acute ischemic bowel complicated by multi-organ failure and prolonged intensive care unit hospitalization. One month into her stay, she was noted to be nearly quadriplegic. Volitional movements were limited to incomplete lateral and vertical eye movements, partial eye closure, and slight movement of finger flexion.

Electrodiagnostic Study:

Sensory NCS

Nerve	Sites	Recording Site	Onset (ms)	Peak (ms)	Amplitude (μV)	Distance (cm)	Velocity (m/s)
R. median–dig II	1. Wrist	Dig II	2.45	3.30	3.8	13	53.1
R. ulnar–dig V	1. Wrist	Dig V	1.65	2.40	5.3	11	66.7
R. radial–sn box	1. Forearm	Sn box	1.85	2.25	10.8	10	54.1
R. sural–lat mall	1. Mid-calf	Ankle	2.90	3.80	2.4	14	48.3

Motor NCS

Nerve	Sites	Recording Site	Latency (ms)	Amplitude (mV)	Distance (cm)	Velocity (m/s)
R. peroneal–EDB	1. Ankle	EDB	Absent	—	8	—
R. peroneal–tib ant	1. Fib head	Tib ant	Absent	—	—	—
R. tibial–AH	1. Ankle	AH	4.00	0.8	8	—
	2. Pop fossa	AH	—	Absent	40	0
R. median APB	1. Wrist	APB	Absent	—	—	—
R. ulnar–ADM	1. Wrist	ADM	3.00	0.3	7	—
	2. B. elbow	ADM	6.20	0.2	16.5	51.6
	3. A. elbow	ADM	7.75	0.3	14	90.3

Needle EMG Summary Table

	IA	SA Fib	SA Fasc	SA Other	Amplitude (MUs)	Duration (MUs)	PolyP (MUs)	Activation	Recruitment Pattern
R. biceps	Nl	0	0	0	—	—	—	—	No activity
R. triceps	Incr	1+	0	0	—	—	—	—	No activity
R. deltoid	Incr	1+	0	CRD	—	—	—	—	No activity
R. first dors int	Incr	2+	0	0	—	—	—	—	No activity
R. ext dig comm	Incr	3+	0	0	—	—	—	—	No activity
R. tib ant	Incr	2+	0	0	—	—	—	—	No activity
R. vast med	Incr	3+	0	0	—	—	—	—	No activity
R. abd poll br	Incr	3+	0	0	—	—	—	—	No activity

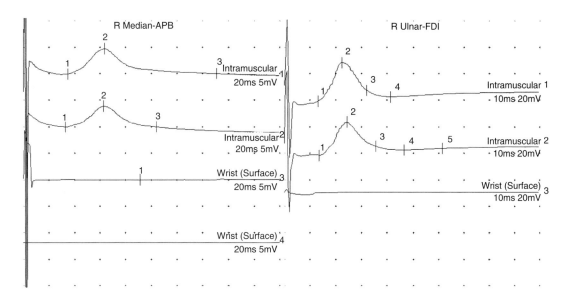

Questions:

1. What are the two most common neuromuscular causes of generalized weakness that develops *after* admission to an intensive care unit?

2. Needle EMG of the right ADM was not performed. Assuming it showed the same findings as that of the right first dorsal interosseous muscle, how would you interpret this together with the right ulnar–ADM motor nerve conduction study?

3. The distinction between a severe myopathy resulting in inexcitable muscle and a severe neuropathy resulting in inexcitable motor nerve can be made using additional studies, the results of which are demonstrated in the figure and the accompanying tabular results. What studies are these? What do the results imply?

Answers:

1. Critical illness myopathy and critical illness neuropathy
2. Indicative of distal conduction block or ongoing Wallerian degeneration
3. Surface and intramuscular needle stimulation, with needle recording in both, suggests inexcitable nerve but excitable muscles, which indicates a neuropathy is the cause of weakness.

Discussion: The nerve conduction studies are remarkable for moderate reduction in the SNAP amplitudes and severely reduced amplitudes of the CMAP amplitudes. These findings provide evidence for a peripheral neuropathy, with motor involvement being much greater than sensory nerve involvement. The process is likely not length dependent, given that the sural SNAP is still recordable despite moderate reduction in the median and ulnar SNAP amplitudes and the EMG shows no recruitment of motor units in both proximal and distal arm and leg muscles. These features suggest a possible demyelinating neuropathy, although no specific evidence of such is available in the electrodiagnostic study.

A more significant problem is the nature of the patient's profound paralysis. Although the sensory nerve abnormalities do imply the existence of a peripheral neuropathy, one wonders whether there could be a mild axonal sensory neuropathy together with a separate cause for the profound motor abnormalities. In particular, a myopathy or neuromuscular junction disorder could account for generalized paralysis with absent or severely reduced CMAP amplitudes and fibrillation potentials. Definitive localization of weakness by electrodiagnostic studies requires observation of the pattern of motor unit recruitment, and in this case there is no recruitment to observe. This makes it impossible to be definitive as to the localization of the weakness. For example, lack of effort could result in no recruited units (but would not result in distal CMAP amplitude reduction or diffuse fibrillation potentials). If a single muscle would have shown a severely reduced pattern of recruitment, localization of the weakness to the motor neuron could have been made.

Hypothetically, by assuming that the right ADM had been studied by needle EMG and showed fibrillation potentials and no recruitment of motor units, together with the small but obtainable ulnar–ADM CMAP, one would be able to say there was electrophysiological evidence of a demyelinating neuropathy or acute Wallerian degeneration of the motor axons supplying ADM proximal to the wrist. This is because the inability to voluntarily recruit units in the setting of being able to electrically excite the distal motor portion of the nerve is due to either conduction block proximal to the stimulation site or acute axonal injury that has not yet resulted in complete distal neuromuscular transmission failure or axonal degeneration.

The important differential diagnostic consideration here is between *critical illness myopathy* (CIM) and *critical illness polyneuropathy* (CIP). CIM, also known as acute quadriplegic myopathy, generally occurs in the setting of treatment with high-dose steroids and neuromuscular blocking agents, or sepsis with multi-organ failure. Some but not all patients have elevated serum CK, and electromyography usually shows fibrillation potentials but abundant motor units recruited early and with full interference patterns despite profound weakness of the muscle. However, the process may be severe enough that no motor units are recruited at all. CIP is a poorly understood entity that, in our opinion, has not been adequately defined. Certainly many ICU patients develop mild distal axonal predominantly or exclusively sensory neuropathies, with a variety of causes stemming directly from multi-organ failure or infection or the treatment of these disorders. Severe acute generalized weakness of neurogenic origin has another specific diagnosis, namely the Guillain–Barré syndrome and its clinical variants. The relationship of CIP to Guillain–Barré syndrome variants is uncertain.

The figure shows the results of both surface stimulation of nerve and needle stimulation of muscle, both with needle recording in muscle. The left panel is that of the median nerve and APB, and the right shows the ulnar nerve and FDI. The top two tracings in each panel show a large reproducible needle-recorded compound muscle action potential with direct needle stimulation of the muscle, while the bottom tracings show no electrical muscle response to surface stimulation of the nerve. Thus, the motor nerve is inexcitable, but the muscle membrane is excitable and muscle stimulation can result in a large potential (29 mV in the case of the FDI). This study provides definite evidence that this patient has a neuropathy, not a myopathy, with nerve membrane inexcitablity accounting for her weakness.

Nerve	Sites	Recording Site	Latency (ms)	Amplitude (mV)
R. median–APB	1. Intramuscular	Intramuscular APB	3.45	4.8
	2. Intramuscular	Intramuscular APB	3.25	3.8
	3. Wrist (surface)	Intramuscular APB	Absent	—
	4. Wrist (surface)	Intramuscular APB	Absent	—
R. ulnar–FDI	1. Intramuscular	Intramuscular FDI	1.30	29.3
	2. Intramuscular	Intramuscular FDI	1.35	25.5
	3. Wrist (surface)	Intramuscular FDI	Absent	—

Clinical Pearls

1. Definitive localization of weakness by electrodiagnostic studies requires observation of the pattern of motor unit recruitment.

2. Direct intramuscular stimulation may sometimes distinguish a neuropathy from myopathy in patients with critical care neuromuscular weakness.

REFERENCES

1. Lacomis, D., Petrella, J.T., Causes of neuromuscular weakness in the intensive care unit: a study of ninety-two patients, *Muscle Nerve* 1998; 21:610–617.
2. Rich, M.M., Bird, S.J., Raps, E.C., McCluskey, L.F., Teener, J.W., Direct muscle stimulation in acute quadriplegic myopathy, *Muscle Nerve* 1997; 20:665–673.

PATIENT 43

A 41-year-old woman with an 11-year history of progressive numbness in her limbs

At the age of 30, this woman became aware of decreased sensation in her right hand. One or two years later similar numbness in the right foot developed, both with gradual progression in intensity since then. At the age of 35, she became aware of left foot and intermittent left hand numbness. Symptoms have gradually increased though remained confined to the right leg up to the middle shin, the left foot up to the ankle, the right hand (particularly D2 and D1), and only intermittently in the left hand. She notes reduction in the ability to feel heat in her hands. She has had several painless burns in her right hand. She notes difficulty walking in a dark room.

Neurological exam was notable for normal strength and the findings shown in the figure. The patient was asked to close her eyes and keep her arms steady in the same position and was reminded of these instructions several times during performance.

On sensory examination, there was severe loss of joint position sense in the right foot to the ankle and right hand to the wrist, with moderate left toe and mild left ankle and finger loss. Vibration sense was nearly absent in the right foot, moderately diminished in the left foot and right hand, and mildly diminished in the left hand. Light touch was nearly absent in her hand in the tip of right D2. Pin sensation was reduced moderately bilaterally and distally. Reflexes were absent at the biceps, triceps, knees, and ankles, and the plantar responses were flexor. Gait and station were wide based, and she had difficulty standing with her feet together. Romberg's sign was present.

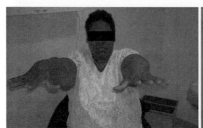 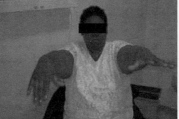 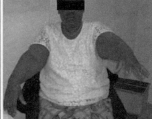

| Eyes Open | 15 sec after eyes closed | 1 minute after eyes closed |

Electrodiagnostic Study:

Sensory NCS

Nerve	Sites	Recording Site	Response	Onset (ms)	Peak (ms)	BP Amplitude (μV)	Distance (cm)	Velocity (m/s)
L. ulnar–dig V	1. Wrist	Dig V	No	Absent	—	—	11	—
L. radial–sn box	1. Forearm	Sn box	No	Absent	—	—	10	—
L. med AB cut	1. Elbow	Forearm	No	Absent	—	—	12	—
L. lat AB cut	1. Elbow	Forearm	No	Absent	—	—	12	—
L. sural–lat mall	1. Mid-calf	Ankle	No	Absent	—	—	14	—
L. median–dig II	1. Wrist	Dig II	No	Absent	—	—	13	—
R. median–dig II	1. Wrist	Dig II	No	Absent	—	—	13	—
R. ulnar–dig V	1. Wrist	Dig V	No	Absent	—	—	11	—
R. radial–sn box	1. Forearm	Sn box	No	Absent	—	—	10	—
R. lat AB cut	1. Elbow	Forearm	No	Absent	—	—	12	—
R. sural–lat mall	1. Mid-calf	Ankle	No	Absent	—	—	14	—

Motor NCS

Nerve	Sites	Recording Site	Latency (ms)	Amplitude (μV)	Distance (cm)	Velocity (m/s)
R. median–APB	1. Wrist	APB	4.10	8.8	7	
	2. Elbow	APB	9.45	6.7	25	46.7
R. ulnar–ADM	1. Wrist	ADM	2.90	8.3	7	—
	2. B. elbow	ADM	7.30	8.4	26	59.1
	3. A. elbow	ADM	9.55	7.1	13	57.8
R. peroneal–EDB	1. Ankle	EDB	4.20	4.6	8	—
	2. Fib head	EDB	11.00	4.0	33	48.5
	3. Pop fossa	EDB	12.90	3.9	9	47.4
R. tibial–AH	1. Ankle	AH	4.85	15.8	8	—
	2. Pop fossa	AH	14.30	5.5	40	42.3

EMG Summary Table

	IA		SA		Amplitude (MUs)	Duration (MUs)	PolyP (MUs)	Activation	Recruitment Pattern
		Fib	Fasc	Other					
R. biceps	Nl	0	0	0	Nl	Nl	Nl	Full	Nl
R. triceps	Nl	0	0	0	Nl	Nl	Nl	Full	Nl
R. vast med	Nl	0	0	0	Nl	Nl	Nl	Full	Nl
R. tib ant	Nl	0	0	0	Nl	Nl	Nl	Full	Nl

Blink Reflex

Nerve	Sites	Muscle	R1 (ms)	R2 (ms)
Supraorbital	1. Right	L.oculi	—	30.00
	2. Right	R.oculi	12.25	30.00
Supraorbital	1. Left	L.oculi	12.05	37.40
	2. Left	R.oculi	—	37.30

Questions:
1. What finding is demonstrated in the figure?
2. What is the electrodiagnostic interpretation?
3. Considering the clinical and electrodiagnostic features together, is this process symmetric or asymmetric? Is it length dependent or non-length dependent?
4. What is the differential diagnosis for this patient?
5. What is the value of a blink reflex in this setting?

Answers:

1. Asymmetric proprioceptive impairment
2. Sensory neuronopathy
3. Asymmetric, non-length dependent
4. Sjögren's syndrome, paraneoplastic
5. Abnormalities in blink reflexes are said to favor a non-paraneoplastic cause.

Discussion: The finding demonstrated in the figure is that of a proprioceptive disturbance in the right greater than left arm. A symmetric posture is easily maintained by the patient with her eyes open (left panel), but closing the eyes results in a droop in her right fingers and wrist (right panel) that she is unaware of. This progresses to a downward drift in her entire right arm and in the left hand after a minute. This finding is a consequence of substantial, asymmetric proprioceptive loss.

The electrodiagnostic study demonstrates complete absence of all sensory nerve action potentials with normal motor and needle EMG studies. The loss of sensory axons is non-length dependent and is electrodiagnostically, though not clinically, symmetric. This apparent electrodiagnostic symmetry is due to sufficient bilateral, though asymmetric, severity to surpass the limits of detection by nerve conduction studies. The interpretation of the electrodiagnostic study is that of a sensory neuronopathy, also known as a dorsal root ganglionopathy.

A chronic progressive dorsal root ganglionopathy has no other well-established cause than Sjögren's syndrome. A subacute more rapidly progressive similar clinical syndrome may be seen in the setting of an anti-Hu or anti-CV2 antibody-associated paraneoplastic syndrome. There are other scattered reports of asymmetric progressive sensory neuronopathies with HTLV-I infection and with *cis*-platinum toxicity (complicating treatment of an underlying cancer). Nevertheless, the syndrome present in this patient should result in a very high index of suspicion of Sjögren's syndrome. Recognition of her distinct neuropathy led to serological testing showing negative ANA, anti-Ro, anti-La, and anti-Hu and anti-CV2 antibody studies. Minor sicca syndromes of dry mouth and eyes were present for 2 years prior, and minor salivary gland biopsy was normal. The potential value of a blink reflex is in demonstrating trigeminal sensory neuropathy evident through an absent afferent response, not present in this case. Abnormalities in the blink reflex favor non-paraneoplastic causes.

Clinical Pearls

1. Sensory neuronopathies are distinct clinical syndromes with a very limited differential diagnosis. Sensory loss is not length dependent and is typically asymmetric.

2. Electrodiagnostic findings are limited to reduction in amplitude or absence of sensory nerve action potentials that may be markedly asymmetric.

REFERENCES

1. Auger, R.G., Windebank, A.J., Lucchinetti, C.F., Chalk, C.H., Role of the blink reflex in the evaluation of sensory neuronopathy, *Neurology* 1999; 53:407–408.
2. Caroyer, J.M., Manto, M.U., Steinfeld, S.D., Severe sensory neuronopathy responsive to infliximab in primary Sjögren's syndrome, *Neurology* 2002; 59(7):1113–1114.
3. Graus, F., Pou, A., Kanterewicz, E., Anderson, N.E., Sensory neuronopathy and Sjögren's syndrome: clinical and immunologic study of two patients, *Neurology* 1988; 38:1637–1639.
4. Kaplan, J.G., Schaumburg, H.H., Predominantly unilateral sensory neuronopathy in Sjögren's syndrome, *Neurology* 1991; 41:948–949.
5. Kaplan, J.G., Rosenberg, R., Reinitz, E., Buchbinder, S., Schaumburg, H.H., Invited review: peripheral neuropathy in Sjögren's syndrome, *Muscle Nerve* 1990; 13:570–579.
6. Laloux, P., Brucher, J.M., Guerit, J.M., Sindic, C.J., Laterre, E.C., Subacute sensory neuronopathy associated with Sjögren's sicca syndrome, *J. Neurol.* 1988; 235:352–354.
7. Lauria, G., Pareyson, D., Grisoli, M., Sghirlanzoni, A., Clinical and magnetic resonance imaging findings in chronic sensory ganglionopathies, *Ann. Neurol.* 2000; 47:104–109.
8. Malinow, K., Yannakakis, G.D., Glusman, S.M., Edlow, D.W., Griffin, J., Pestronk, A., Powell, D.L., Ramsey-Goldman, R., Eidelman, B.H., Medsger, T.A., Jr. *et al.*, Subacute sensory neuronopathy secondary to dorsal root ganglionitis in primary Sjögren's syndrome, *Ann. Neurol.* 1986; 20:535–537.
9. Valls-Sole, J., Graus, F., Font, J., Pou, A., Tolosa, E.S., Normal proprioceptive trigeminal afferents in patients with Sjögren's syndrome and sensory neuronopathy, *Ann. Neurol.* 1990; 28(6):786–790.

SECTION III. NEUROMUSCULAR JUNCTION DISEASE

The electrodiagnostic assessment of disorders of the neuromuscular junction (NMJ) is frequently challenging. The techniques used are often not performed frequently enough to ensure the ideal degree of practical and technical experience. The principle disorder of the NMJ is myasthenia gravis (MG). Others, including the Lambert–Eaton myasthenic syndrome (LEMS), the congenital myasthenic syndromes (CMSs), botulism, and effects of various toxins, are either extremely rare or quite uncommon. It is important to recognize that neuromuscular junctions may be abnormal in a number of disorders that do not primarily involve the NMJ. In acute axonal nerve lesions, neuromuscular transmission fails before Wallerian degeneration. In chronic disorders of lower motor neurons, such as amyotrophic lateral sclerosis, the immature neuromuscular junctions present during reinnervation may demonstrate blocking and abnormal degrees of decrement on repetitive stimulation. Accordingly, both repetitive nerve stimulation and single-fiber EMG may be abnormal in many neuromuscular disorders.

The various elements of the electrodiagnostic study in patients with suspected NMJ disorders are:
- Routine sensory and motor nerve conduction studies, and routine needle EMG
- Repetitive nerve stimulation (RNS)
  - Low frequency (2 to 5 Hz)
  - High frequency (25 to 50 Hz)
  - Post-exercise facilitation
  - Post-exercise exhaustion
  - Special procedures
- Single-fiber electromyography (SFEMG)
  - Voluntary
  - Axonal-stimulated SFEMG

The purpose of routine studies in the NMJ evaluation is to exclude other diagnoses, such as a neuropathy or myopathy, and to exclude other technically confounding disorders, such as an ulnar neuropathy that produces abnormal decrement in a repetitive nerve stimulation ulnar-ADM study. Very occasionally, routine studies will provide direct evidence of a NMJ disorder, such as the occurrence of repetitive CMAPs after a single motor nerve stimulus in patients with organophosphate toxicity or some of the congenital myasthenic syndromes (AChE deficiency and slow channel syndrome).

It is worthwhile to briefly review the history of repetitive nerve stimulation. Repetitive nerve stimulation was described in 1941 by Harvey and Masland,[9] who reported findings in the ulnar-ADM CMAP in various neurological disorders and 3 patients with MG. In 1952 Botelho et al.[4] reported on 21 patients with MG and noted that the greatest decrement occurred at around the 5th potential. In 1968, Slomic et al.[18] studied 23 patients with MG and reported that the degree of decrement increased several minutes after exercise. In 1971, Odzemir and Young[12] studied 30 patients with MG and 30 normals, recording CMAPs from ADM, FCR, and deltoid at baseline and post exercise every 30 seconds for 5 minutes. Using a cutoff of 10% decrement as abnormal, their approach had a sensitivity of 87%. In 1974, Borenstein and Desmedt[3] noted the effects of temperature on RNS in 30 patients with MG: warming increases and cooling decreases decrement. In 1982 Oh et al.[11] recommended avoiding anticholinesterase medication for 12 hours prior to RNS and emphasized distinct RNS sensitivities in ocular (17%) and generalized MG (85%).

The range of sensitivities reported for RNS in MG has been 10% to 50% in ocular myasthenia, and 75% in generalized untreated myasthenia when one distal and one proximal muscle are examined. The specificity has not been rigorously studied. It is quite clear that focal neuropathy or anterior horn cell disease may result in abnormal decrement. Accordingly, *normal RNS does not argue appreciably against MG as a diagnosis (RNS is relatively insensitive). Abnormal RNS strongly suggests an NMJ disorder, though motor neuron disease should also be considered (RNS is relatively specific).*

Single fiber EMG (SFEMG) was first described by Ekstedt in 1964.[8] The concept of "jitter" was reported by Stalberg in 1971[19] and Sanders et al.[15] reported findings in 127 patients with myasthenia gravis in 1979. Stimulated single fiber EMG, as opposed to the voluntary SFEMG previously reported, was first described by Trontelj et al.[20] in 1986. In that year, Sanders and Howard[16] reported that studying 1 muscle demonstrated an abnormality in 85% of patients with MG and 2 muscles demonstrated an abnormality in 99% of patients with MG. The reported range of sensitivity of SFEMG in MG is 82% to 99% among 3 different studies meeting evidenced based medicine criteria as reviewed by an AAEM subcommittee in 2001.

This technique may be over-rated as a clinical diagnostic tool. The technical demands of the study both for patients and examiners are substantial. The test is highly sensitive but likely highly non-specific (its specificity has never been adequately studied and reported in the literature). Many disorders of motor nerves or muscle result in increased jitter, including neuropathy, some myopathies, and anterior horn cell diseases. Accordingly, *an abnormal SFEMG study has limited diagnostic value*. The value of this test is that *a normal SFEMG study makes generalized MG highly unlikely*. These straightforward conclusions suggest the following approach. If the patient clearly has a neuromuscular disorder clinically, SFEMG is likely of no added value. If the goal instead is to exclude a neuromuscular disorder as the cause of symptoms in a patient with a normal neurological examination, the test is quite likely to do that.

The various technical elements of SFEMG are briefly summarized below:
- SFEMG Technique
  - 50 discharges for each pair
  - 20 pairs
  - 3-4 different skin insertions
- Technical Considerations
  - Amplitude of AP > 200 mV
  - Rise time < 300 msec
  - IPI may be influenced by preceding interdischarge interval
  - Effect of variable firing rates on IPI taken into account with MSD
  - Temperature: Stalberg et al. 1971: "Lowering of temperature caused an increase of the jitter and increasing the temperature resulted in a decrease of the jitter"
- SFEMG Criteria For Abnormality
  - A study is abnormal if either:
    - The mean jitter is increased; OR
    - More than 10% of pairs have increased jitter

REFERENCES

1. AAEM. Literature review of the usefulness of repetitive nerve stimulation and single fiber EMG in the electrodiagnostic evaluation of patients with suspected myasthenia gravis or Lambert-Eaton myasthenic syndrome. Muscle Nerve. 2001; 24:1239-1247.
2. AAEM. Practice parameter for repetitive nerve stimulation and single fiber EMG evaluation of adults with suspected myasthenia gravis or Lambert-Eaton myasthenic syndrome: summary statement. Muscle Nerve. 2001; 24:1236-1238.
3. Borenstein S, Desmedt JE. Temperature and weather correlates of myasthenic fatigue. Lancet 1974; 63-66.
4. Botelho SY, Deaterly CF, Austin S, Comroe JH Jr. Evaluation of the electromyogram of patients with myasthenia gravis. Arch Neurol Psychiatry 1952; 67:441-450.
5. Bril V, Werb MR, Greene DA, Sima AA. Single-fiber electromyography in diabetic peripheral polyneuropathy. Muscle Nerve. 1996 Jan; 19(1):2-9.
6. Chaudhry V, Crawford TO. Stimulation single-fiber EMG in infant botulism. Muscle Nerve. 1999 Dec; 22(12):1698-703.
7. Chaudhry V, Watson DF, Bird SJ, Cornblath DR. Stimulated single-fiber electromyography in Lambert-Eaton myasthenic syndrome. Muscle Nerve. 1991 Dec; 14(12):1227-30.
8. Ekstedt J. Human single muscle fiber action potential. Acta Physiol Scand 1964; 61(suppl):226:1-96.
9. Harvey AM, Masland RL. A method for the study of neuromuscular transmission in human subjects. Bull Johns Hopkins Hosp 1941; 68:81-93.
10. Lange DJ, Rubin M, Greene PE, Kang UJ, Moskowitz CB, Brin MF, Lovelace RE, Fahn S. Distant effects of locally injected botulinum toxin: a double-blind study of single fiber EMG changes. Muscle Nerve. 1991 Jul; 14(7):672-5.
11. Oh SJ, Eslami N, Nishihara T, Sarala PK, Kuba T, Elmore RS, Sunwoo IN, Ro YI. Electrophysiological and clinical correlation in myasthenia gravis. Ann Neurol 1982; 12:348-354.
12. Ozdemir C, Young RR. Electrical testing in myasthenia gravis. Ann NY Acad Sci 1971; 183: 287-302.
13. Padua L, Aprile I, Monaco ML, Fenicia L, Anniballi F, Pauri F, Tonali P. Neurophysiological assessment in the diagnosis of botulism: usefulness of single-fiber EMG. Muscle Nerve. 1999 Oct; 22(10):1388-92.
14. Padua L, Stalberg E, LoMonaco M, Evoli A, Batocchi A, Tonali P. SFEMG in ocular myasthenia gravis diagnosis. Clin Neurophysiol. 2000 Jul; 111(7):1203-7.
15. Sanders DB, Howard JF Jr, Johns TR. Single-fiber electromyography in myasthenia gravis. Neurology. 1979 Jan; 29(1): 68-76
16. Sanders DB, Howard JF Jr. AAEE minimonograph #25: Single-fiber electromyography in myasthenia gravis. Muscle Nerve. 1986 Nov-Dec; 9(9):809-19.

17. Single fiber EMG reference values: a collaborative effort. Ad Hoc Committee of the AAEM Special Interest Group on Single Fiber EMG. Muscle Nerve. 1992 Feb; 15(2):151-61.
18. Slomic A, Rosenfalck A, Buchthal F. Electrical and mechanical responses of normal and myasthenic muscle. Brain Res 1968; 10:1-78.
19. Stålberg E, Ekstedt J, Broman A. The electromyographic jitter in normal human muscles. Electroencephalogr Clin Neurophysiol 1971; 31:429-438.
20. Trontelj JV, Mihelin M, Fernandez J, Stålberg E. Axonal stimulation for end-plate jitter studies. J Neurol Neurosurg Psychiatry 1986; 49:677-685.
21. Trontelj JV. Stimulation SFEMG in myasthcnia gravis. Muscle Nerve. 1990 May; 13(5):458-9.
22. Wiechers D. Single fiber EMG evaluation in denervation and reinnervation. Muscle Nerve. 1990 Sep; 13(9):829-32.
23. Weinberg DH, Rizzo JF 3rd, Hayes MT, Kneeland MD, Kelly JJ Jr. Ocular myasthenia gravis: predictive value of single-fiber electromyography. Muscle Nerve. 1999 Sep; 22(9):1222-7.

PATIENT 44

**A 17-year-old woman with progressive dysarthria and dysphagia
for 4 months**

This 17-year-old woman noted progressive nasal and slurred speech and difficulty with both chewing and swallowing initially only present later in the day. Examination showed bilateral varying ptosis and facial and palatal weakness.

Electrodiagnostic Study:

Muscle	Train	Rate (pps)	Amplitude (mV)	4–1 (%)
L. abd dig min	Baseline	3	14.1	−7.4
	Post 1 min exercise	3	14.0	−9.1
	After 1 min	3	13.4	−1.6
	After 2 min	3	14.8	−10.2
	After 3 min	3	13.9	−4.4
	After 4 min	3	13.7	−5
L. trapezius (u)	Baseline	3	5.2	−2.1
	Post 1 min exercise	3	6.0	−8.5
	After 1 min	3	5.8	0.3
	After 2 min	3	5.5	−10.6
	After 3 min	3	5.5	−14.5
	After 4 min	3	5.3	−15.1
	After 5 min	3	5.3	−20.9
L. nasalis	Baseline	3	2.5	−28.1
	Post 1 min exercise	3	2.5	−25.2
	After 1 min	3	1.3	−18.1
	After 2 min	3	1.2	−21.7
	After 3 min	3	1.4	−29.6
	After 4 min	3	0.7	−25.1

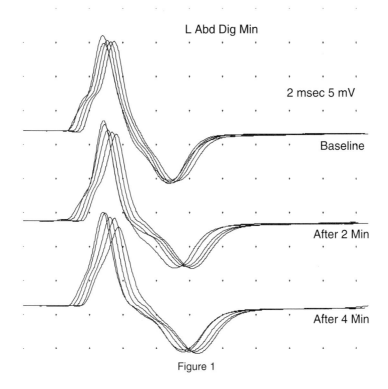

L Abd Dig Min

2 msec 5 mV

Baseline

After 2 Min

After 4 Min

Figure 1

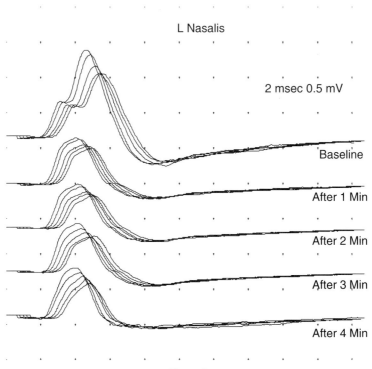

L Nasalis

2 msec 0.5 mV

Baseline

After 1 Min

After 2 Min

After 3 Min

After 4 Min

Figure 2

179

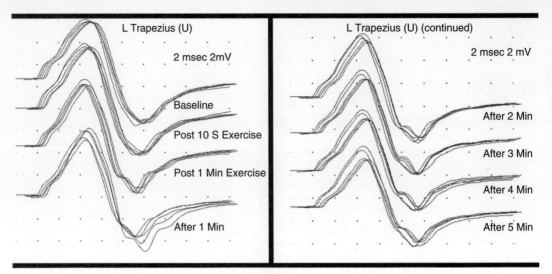

Figure 3

Questions:
1. What are the main clinical diagnoses to consider in this patient?
2. The table lists results of repetitive nerve stimulation studies. What procedure is being used and what abnormalities are being sought?
3. What is the rationale for performing studies of trapezius or nasalis if the ADM study appears normal?
4. What is the most likely explanation for the waveforms for nasalis in the second figure?
5. For the nasalis study in figure 2, was it strictly necessary to perform the exercise and post-exercise recordings for this muscle?
6. For the trapezius study shown in figure 3, again, was it necessary to perform exercise and post-exercise recordings?

Answers:

1. Myasthenia gravis; congenital myasthenic syndrome; oculopharyngeal muscular dystrophy; brain-stem mass
2. Repetitive nerve stimulation after exercise to look for post-exercise exhaustion
3. Proximal muscles may be more likely to be abnormal.
4. Electrode movement occurred during exercise.
5. No
6. Yes

Discussion: The chief clinical consideration given the history is myasthenia gravis. When this diagnosis is considered in children and adolescents, congenital myasthenic syndromes should always be considered as well. The repetitive nerve stimulation studies above were performed as follows:

- Baseline stimulation at 3 Hz for five impulses. This study aims at detecting abnormalities in the *baseline decrement to low frequency stimulation.*
- The patient performed brief exercise for 10 seconds and immediately afterwards, stimulation at 3 Hz for five impulses was performed. This study aims at detecting abnormalities in *post-exercise facilitation.* Such abnormalities are diagnostic of presynaptic neuromuscular transmission disorders.
- The patient then performed sustained exercise for 1 minute; subsequent trains of five impulses were recorded immediately afterwards and then every minute for 5 minutes. This study aims at detecting abnormalities in *post-exercise exhaustion.*

An abnormal decrement to low-frequency stimulation (2 or 3 Hz) is usually defined as a greater than 10% decrement in the baseline-to-peak or peak-to-peak amplitude of the fourth or fifth potential compared to the first. Meticulous attention to technical factors is required to achieve this low of a cutoff for abnormality; slight movement of the recording electrodes, muscle position, or stimulating electrodes can easily produce larger apparent decrements in normal muscles. The measured decrement can also vary significantly depending on which measure of amplitude and which waveform (*i.e.,* fourth or fifth) is used. Unfortunately, there is no published consensus as to which of these measures should be used or a body of literature that supports one approach over another. Accordingly, and for other reasons as well, we recommend caution in interpreting borderline values around 10%.

The abnormal baseline decrement to low-frequency stimulation is the hallmark of neuromuscular transmission defects and occurs in both pre- and postsynaptic disorders; however, the test is relatively insensitive, and many patients with myasthenia gravis will have normal baseline decrement studies. Several approaches to increasing the sensitivity of repetitive nerve stimulation for the diagnosis of MG have been devised. The two commonly used ones are (1) performing more muscle studies (*e.g.,* distal and proximal), and (2) performing exercise to look for post-exercise exhaustion. Studies suggest that the addition of a single proximal muscle study to that of a distal muscle already performed results in a sensitivity of 76% in patients with untreated generalized MG and 48% in patients with purely ocular MG. Commonly both approaches are used.

The phenomenon of post-exercise exhaustion is poorly understood but quite helpful diagnostically. It may be a consequence of depletion of acetylcholine reserves. After 1 minute of voluntary exercise, a train of 5 impulses is delivered each minute for 5 minutes. A typical abnormality consists of the appearance of a decrementing response (fourth or fifth impulse compared to first impulse within a single given train) between 2 and 4 minutes and recovery of the decrement at the fifth minute. However, the appearance of a >10% decrement at any of the time points is taken to be abnormal. This study is very useful in that a significant number of patients with MG will have abnormalities limited to post-exercise exhaustion.

In the current study, we see from the table that the maximal ADM decrement was 10.2% at minute 2—a borderline value—so the results of this nerve were initially taken as normal, and the electromyographer proceeded with a more proximal study. However, review of the waveforms in the figure shows a more impressive drop in the decrement when measured to the fifth potential, particularly at minute 4. Here, the EMG software-computed drop from the first to fourth potential was only 5%. For the fifth potential, estimating from the figure, there is about half of a vertical box drop, which translates to 2.5 mV from a 13.7-mV first potential, or an 18% decrement, which is clearly abnormal. This emphasizes one of the cardinal rules of interpreting repetitive nerve stimulation results: *Always review the waveforms.* The waveforms must be reproducible and free from technical problems, and computer software cannot always be relied upon for proper computation of decrement.

Inspection of the nasalis waveforms in the second figure are notable for the change in morphology of the CMAP waveform that is present in all of the post-exercise tracings compared to the baseline. This likely reflects movement of one of the recording electrodes during forced exercise of the muscle. If the waveform morphology changes within a train of 5, the train needs to be discarded and cannot be interpreted. In this case, the change between trains and the subsequent consistency of the waveform morphologies afterward indicate that the movement of the electrode does not affect the demonstration of decrement within a train of impulses, and the study remains interpretable.

As the nasalis baseline study demonstrated a 28% decrement in amplitude, it was not necessary to perform exercise to demonstrate post-exercise exhaustion as well. For the trapezius, however, the situation is different, and it was necessary to perform exercise to demonstrate an abnormality in this muscle, as can be seen in the third figure. The decrements at baseline, immediately after exercise, and 1 minute post-exercise are not impressive, but at 2, 3, 4, and 5 minutes are quite impressive.

Clinical Pearls

1. Look for post-exercise exhaustion in the evaluation of patients with suspected myasthenia gravis.

2. Always review the waveforms yourself; automated software will calculate decrements but will not detect technical problems with the recordings.

REFERENCES

1. AAEM, Literature review of the usefulness of repetitive nerve stimulation and single fiber EMG in the electrodiagnostic evaluation of patients with suspected myasthenia gravis or Lambert–Eaton myasthenic syndrome, *Muscle Nerve* 2001; 24:1239–1247.
2. AAEM, Practice parameter for repetitive nerve stimulation and single fiber EMG evaluation of adults with suspected myasthenia gravis or Lambert–Eaton myasthenic syndrome: summary statement, *Muscle Nerve* 2001; 24:1236–1238.
3. Gilchrist, J.M., Massey, J.M., Sanders, D.B., Single fiber EMG and repetitive stimulation of the same muscle in myasthenia gravis, *Muscle Nerve* 1994; 17(2):171–175.
4. Keesey, J.C., AAEE Minimonograph 33: electrodiagnostic approach to defects of neuromuscular transmission, *Muscle Nerve* 1989; 12(8):613–626.
5. Killian, J.M., Wilfong, A.A., Burnett, L., Appel, S.H., Boland, D., Decremental motor responses to repetitive nerve stimulation in ALS, *Muscle Nerve* 1994; 17(7):747–754.
6. Morita, H., Shindo, M., Yanagawa, S., Yanagisawa, N., Neuromuscular response in man to repetitive nerve stimulation, *Muscle Nerve* 1993; 16(6):648–654.
7. Rutkove, S.B., Shefner, J.M., Wang, A.K., Ronthal, M., Raynor, E.M., High-temperature repetitive nerve stimulation in myasthenia gravis, *Muscle Nerve* 1998; 21(11):1414–1418.
8. Sanders, D.B., Andrews, P.I., Howard, J.F., Massey, J.M., Seronegative myasthenia gravis, *Neurology* 1997; 48:S40–S45.
9. Schumm, F., Stohr, M., Accessory nerve stimulation in the assessment of myasthenia gravis, *Muscle Nerve* 1984; 7(2):147–151.
10. Sonoo, M., Uesugi, H., Mochizuki, A., Hatanaka, Y., Shimizu, T., Single fiber EMG and repetitive nerve stimulation of the same extensor digitorum communis muscle in myasthenia gravis, *Clin. Neurophysiol.* 2001; 112(2):300–303.
11. Tim, R.W., Sanders, D.B., Repetitive nerve stimulation studies in the Lambert–Eaton myasthenic syndrome, *Muscle Nerve* 1994; 17(9):995–1001.

PATIENT 45

A 71-year-old man with subacute symmetrical proximal weakness

This 71-year-old man developed symptoms of symmetric proximal arm and leg weakness 1 year prior, which remitted spontaneously over 3 months and then again recurred 2 to 3 months ago. Brief neurological examination demonstrated mild symmetric weakness of neck flexion, deltoids, and biceps and mild-moderate weakness of first dorsal interosseous (FDI) bilaterally. The left biceps reflex was initially absent, but after 10 seconds of exercise was a normal 2+. Right biceps reflex was trace to 1+. The patient was referred for a question of motor neuron disease.

Electrodiagnostic Study:

Sensory NCS

Nerve	Sites	Recording Site	Onset (ms)	Peak (ms)	Amplitude (µV)	Distance (cm)	Velocity (m/s)
L. median–dig II	1. Wrist	Dig II	3.10	4.00	30.3	13	41.9
L. ulnar–dig V	1. Wrist	Dig V	2.45	3.35	19.7	11	44.9
L. radial–snbox	1. Forearm	Sn box	1.70	2.40	38.0	10	58.8
L. sural–lat mall	1. Mid-calf	Ankle	3.05	3.85	7.0	14	45.9

Motor NCS

Nerve	Sites	Recording Site	Latency (ms)	Amplitude (mV)	Distance (cm)	Velocity (m/s)
L. median–APB	1. Wrist	APB	4.45	10.3	7	—
	2. Elbow	APB	8.80	9.6	21	48.3
	3. Axilla	APB	12.55	9.1	18	48.0
L. ulnar–ADM	1. Wrist	ADM	3.60	3.3	7	—
	2. B. elbow	ADM	8.90	2.3	24	45.3
	3. A. elbow	ADM	12.00	2.0	13	41.9
	4. Axilla	ADM	13.85	1.6	10	54.1
L. ulnar–FDI	1. Wrist	FDI	6.15	2.3	—	—
	2. B. elbow	FDI	9.70	1.6	20	56.3
	3. A. elbow	FDI	12.10	1.4	13	54.2
	4. Axilla	FDI	13.80	1.2	10	58.8
R. ulnar–ADM	1. Wrist	ADM	3.90	6.1	7	—
	2. B. elbow	ADM	8.50	5.3	22	47.8
L. peroneal–EDB	1. Ankle	EDB	5.25	1.4	8	—
	2. Fib head	EDB	13.75	0.9	32	37.6
	3. Pop fossa	EDB	15.70	0.9	10	51.3
L. tibial–AH	1. Ankle	AH	3.85	4.1	8	—
	2. Pop fossa	AH	14.85	4.0	36	32.7

Although the reduced CMAP amplitudes are compatible with motor neuron disease, the history of symmetric proximal weakness that remits and then relapses again is not particularly suggestive of a motor neuron disorder. Reduced amplitudes of CMAPs should raise the possibility of Lambert–Eaton myasthenic syndrome and prompt the electromyographer to have the patient exercise the appropriate muscle for 10 seconds and then repeat the CMAP measurement. High-frequency repetitive stimulation at 50 Hz for 1 second can be performed as an alternative in patients who cannot cooperate. Low-frequency stimulation at 2 or 3 Hz should also be performed. Observe the following figures and tables.

Pre- and Post-Exercise CMAPs

Nerve	Sites	Recording Site	Latency (ms)	Amplitude (mV)	Relative Amplitude (%)	Distance (cm)
L. ulnar–ADM	At rest	ADM	4.40	3.1	100	7
Immediately post 10 s exercise	ADM	4.25	6.8	221	—	
L. median–APB	At rest	APB	4.05	9.3	100	7
Immediately post 10 s exercise	APB	4.10	12.3	132	—	
R. median–APB	At rest	APB	4.00	6.1	100	7
Immediately post 10 s exercise	APB	3.90	10.3	168	—	
R. ulnar–ADM	At rest	ADM	3.50	2.5	100	7
Immediately post 10 s exercise	ADM	3.50	4.6	182	—	

Repetitive Nerve Stimulation

Muscle	Train	Time	Rate (pps)	Amplitude (mV)	4–1 (%)	5–1 (%)	Fac Amplitude (%)
L. abd dig min	Baseline	0:01:21	3	2.6	−39.9	−30.2	103

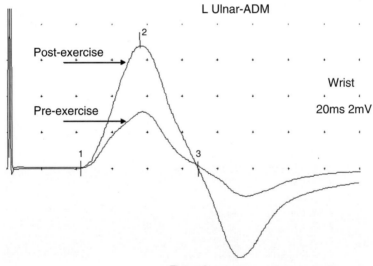

Figure 1

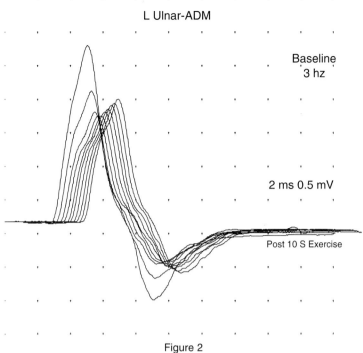

L Ulnar-ADM

Baseline
3 hz

2 ms 0.5 mV

Post 10 S Exercise

Figure 2

Questions:
1. What are the relevant abnormalities?
2. The bilateral ulnar–ADM and left peroneal–EDB CMAPs are reduced in amplitude. Are these findings compatible with motor neuron disease? What other electrodiagnostic procedures should be done when multiple CMAPs have reduced amplitude?
3. What finding is shown in figure 1?
4. What is the generally accepted upper limit of normal (ULN, as percent of baseline) for physiological post-exercise increment of a CMAP amplitude?
5. What finding is shown in figure 2?
6. What additional non-electrophysiological diagnostic evaluation is indicated for this patient?

Answers:

1. Low amplitude bilateral ulnar-ADM CMAPs; post-exercise facilitations, low frequency decrement
2. Yes; post-exercise nerve stimulation
3. Abnormal post-exercise CMAP facilitation
4. 100% increment
5. Abnormal decrement to low frequency stimulation
6. Measurement of serum P/Q voltage-gated calcium channels

Discussion: The first figure shows abnormal post-exercise facilitation of the left ulnar–ADM CMAP. A 100% increment is generally accepted as the upper limit of normal; this CMAP shows a 121% increment. As seen in the table, several other nerves have large increments, particularly the right ulnar (82%). The 100% cutoff is likely a very conservative estimate; in clinical practice, post-exercise increments of even 25% or more are quite uncommon, except in myasthenia gravis. The second figure shows a decrement at low-frequency stimulation, maximal at the fourth potential, that then repairs partially by the tenth potential.

These findings are diagnostic of a presynaptic disorder of neuromuscular transmission, and in this clinical setting are diagnostic of Lambert–Eaton myasthenic syndrome. Additional studies of value include measurement of serum voltage-gated P/Q calcium channel antibodies and chest CT scan for evidence of small-cell lung cancer. In this patient, the calcium channel antibody titer was highly abnormal at 51 U (normal, <19 U). CT scan did not show chest abnormalities but did show liver lesions, and biopsy revealed small-cell cancer. The patient's weakness progressed, and he became nonambulatory. The patient was treated with chemotherapy and 3,4-diaminopyridine, and his strength improved to independent ambulation.

The Lambert-Eaton myasthenic syndrome is the second most common disorder of neuromuscular transmission but is nevertheless rare. Its prevalence is unknown but has been estimated to be as low as a total of 400 cases in the entire United States. Approximately two-thirds of patients have a paraneoplastic disorder, primarily associated with small-cell lung cancer, and the other third have an otherwise uncharacterized autoimmune disorder.

The clinical features are muscular weakness (proximal legs greater than arms; diplopia uncommon), hyporeflexia, and cholinergic autonomic dysfunction (dry mouth, sluggish pupillary reflexes, urinary retention, and erectile dysfunction in males). Rapid progression over weeks or months favors the paraneoplastic form as a cause.

Antibodies directed against the P/Q type voltage-gated calcium channels (VGCCs) of the motor nerve terminals are present in over 90% of patients with LEMS, resulting in destruction and loss of these presynaptic calcium channels. Arriving action potentials consequently do not generate sufficient calcium influx for release of acetylcholine. Electrodiagnostic studies typically demonstrate low-amplitude CMAP amplitudes that show a greater than 100% increment with high-frequency repetitive stimulation (50 Hz). At low-frequency stimulation, a decrement may occur in LEMS as in MG. Treatment with 3,4-diaminopyridine, requiring an investigational new drug approval from the Food and Drug Administration in the United States, is the treatment of choice. Immunosuppressive or immunomodulatory treatments similar to those for MG are effective, although less so than with MG. Treatment of underlying malignancy when present is also important and may improve strength.

As a rule, both pre-synaptic and post-synaptic neuromuscular junction disorders typically have abnormal decrements with low-frequency stimulation; presynaptic disorders have abnormal increments with high-frequency stimulation.

Clinical Pearls

1. Consider performing 10 seconds of exercise followed by a repeat CMAP recording in patients with low CMAP amplitudes.

2. In Lambert-Eaton myasthenic syndrome, the increment does not necessarily exceed 100% in all motor nerves.

3. Low-frequency stimulation may produce an abnormal decrement in pre-synaptic disorders also; abnormalities are not specific to myasthenia gravis.

REFERENCES

1. Tim, R.W., Massey, J.M., Sanders, D.B., Lambert–Eaton myasthenic syndrome: electrodiagnostic findings and response to treatment, *Neurology* 2000; 54(11):2176–2178.
2. AAEM Quality Assurance Committee, Literature review of the usefulness of repetitive nerve stimulation and single fiber EMG in the electrodiagnostic evaluation of patients with suspected myasthenia gravis or Lambert–Eaton myasthenic syndrome, *Muscle Nerve* 2001; 24:1239–1247.

PATIENT 46

A 34-year-old woman with generalized weakness since infancy

This 34-year-old woman was a floppy baby and has had longstanding generalized weakness leading to use of a wheelchair for most activities. She carried a diagnosis of spinal muscular atrophy and was referred for electrodiagnostic studies. Exam was notable for bilateral fatigable ptosis, and bilateral proximal greater than distal weakness of the upper and lower extremities.

Electrodiagnostic Study: Routine sensory and motor studies were normal.

Repetitive Nerve Stimulation

Muscle	Train	Time	Rate (pps)	Amplitude (mV)	4–1 (%)
R. abd dig min	Baseline	0:00:00	3	7.6	−10.2
	Post 1 min exercise	0:02:22	3	8.0	−2.3
	After 1 min	0:03:15	3	8.4	−6.3
	After 2 min	0:04:14	3	8.5	−6.8
	After 3 min	0:05:19	3	8.1	−7.9
	After 4 min	0:06:14	3	8.5	−9.9
	After 5 min	0:07:18	3	8.5	−11.8
R. trapezius (u)	Baseline	0:00:00	3	4.8	−33
	Post 10 s exercise	0:00:33	3	5.3	−8.6
	Post 1 min exercise	0:01:42	3	5.4	−11.1
	After 1 min	0:02:49	3	5.4	−27.6
	After 2 min	0:03:56	3	5.2	−38.4
	After 3 min	0:05:07	3	4.9	−37.8
	After 4 min	0:06:13	3	5.3	−41.3
	After 5 min	0:07:14	3	5.4	−41.7

Needle EMG Summary Table

		SA			Amplitude (MUs)	Duration (MUs)	PolyP (MUs)	Activation	Recruitment Pattern
	IA	Fib	Fasc	Other					
R. biceps	Nl	0	0	0	Small	Brief	Few	Full	Early
R. deltoid	Nl	0	0	0	Small	Brief	Few	Full	Early

SFEMG Stimulation

Muscle		N	Jitter (μs)	Block	MIPI (μs)	MCD (μs)	MSD (μs)	FR (pps)
R. ext dig comm	1.1	15	46.26	—	2999	46.26	46.26	3
	2.1	99	45.89	—	2925	45.89	45.89	3
	5.1	99	53.07	—	3171	53.07	53.07	3
	6.1	40	56.59	—	2896	56.59	56.59	3
	7.1	98	58.62	—	2464	58.62	58.62	3
	7.2	100	118.44	5	5629	118.44	118.44	3

MIPI = mean interpotential interval, MCD = mean consecutive difference, MSD = mean sorted difference, FR = firing rate

Continued

187

Muscle	N	Jitter (μs)	Block	MIPI (μs)	MCD (μs)	MSD (μs)	FR (pps)
8.1	100	139.56	60	11003	139.56	139.56	3
10.1	95	45.25	—	3809	45.25	45.25	3
11.1	100	68.17	0	3728	68.17	68.17	3
11.2	100	74.12	0	6563	74.12	74.12	3
11.3	100	117.78	20	10748	117.78	117.78	3
11.4	100	133.37	73	14705	133.37	133.37	3
Mean	—	79.76	—	—	—	—	—
% Blocked	—	—	46	—	—	—	—

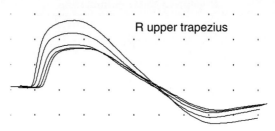

R upper trapezius

Figure 1

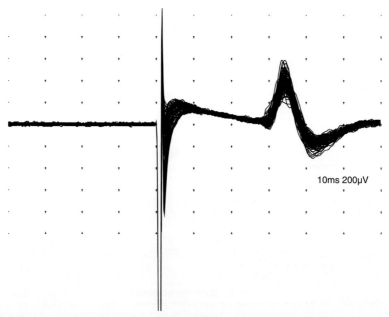

10ms 200μV

Figure 2

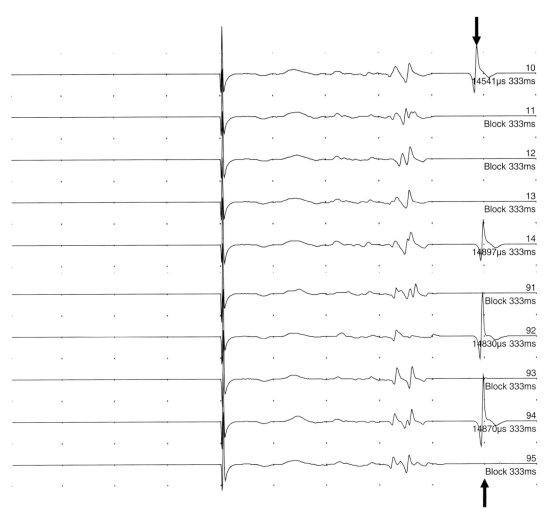

Figure 3

Questions:

1. What do the needle EMG studies suggest?
2. What is the overall interpretation of the electrodiagnostic study?
3. Can you identify what is being demonstrated in each of the figures?
4. What do you think is the most likely diagnosis for this patient?

Answers:
1. A myopathy or neuromuscular junction disorder
2. A neuromuscular junction disorder
3. Abnormal decrement; abnormal jitter; intermittent blocking
4. A congenital myasthenic syndrome

Discussion: The electrodiagnostic study shows an abnormal decrement in the trapezius muscle at low-frequency stimulation: 33% at baseline and 42% 5 minutes after exercise. There was no abnormal increment after 10 seconds of exercise, and the baseline CMAP amplitudes were normal. There were also no after-discharges seen on single motor stimuli during routine motor studies. The first figure shows intermittent blocking of a single fiber potential (arrows) in a series of 10 consecutive recordings.

The most likely diagnosis for this patient is a congenital myasthenic syndrome. The history of weakness since infancy, fatigable ptosis on examination, and demonstration of a postsynaptic disorder of neuromuscular transmission are all suggestive of such. Laboratory studies showed repeatedly absent acetylcholine receptor antibodies over 2 decades of testing.

The congenital myasthenic syndromes (CMSs) are a diverse group of molecular genetic defects affecting the neuromuscular junction. The classification and molecular basis for these are still evolving. A review by Engel *et al.*[4] covers this topic in depth. The table below highlights the main disorders. The diagnosis of a CMS should be suspected from a history of fluctuating weakness involving ocular, bulbar, and limb muscles since infancy or early childhood, a history of similarly affected relatives, a decremental EMG response to low-frequency stimulation, and negative tests for acetylcholine receptor (AChR) antibodies. In some CMSs, however, the onset is delayed, and patients may present with an apparent myopathy in adulthood.

- *CMS with defect in resynthesis/packing:* This disorder is also known as CMS with episodic apnea and as familial infantile myasthenia. The presentation is in infancy or early childhood with a range of myasthenic symptoms, including apnea provoked by fever or excitement. The molecular basis is choline acetyltransferase mutations. This enzyme catalyzes the reversible synthesis of ACh from acetyl CoA and choline, resulting in stimulus-dependent depletion of ACh.

- *Paucity of synaptic vesicles:* The clinical features are similar to myasthenia gravis, the molecular basis is unknown, and diagnosis requires specialized techniques (quantitative electron microscopy of the endplate).

- *Lambert-Eaton–like CMS:* Only two patients have been described with this syndrome. The defect lies in a subunit of the presynaptic voltage-gated P/Q-type calcium channel or in a component of the synaptic vesicle release complex. Patients have marked facilitation of CMAPs with high-frequency repetitive stimulation.

Congenital Myasthenic Syndromes

Defects	Inheritance	Molecular Genetics
Presynaptic defects		
Defect in ACh resynthesis/packaging	AR	ChAT
Paucity of synaptic vesicles (1 patient to date)	?	Unknown
Lambert–Eaton syndrome like	AR	Unknown
Reduced quantal release (3 patients to date)	?	Unknown
Synaptic defect		
Endplate AChE deficiency	AR	ColQ gene
Postsynaptic defects		
Primary kinetic abnormality	AR	—
Slow channel syndromes	AD	α, β, or ε AChR subunit
Fast channel syndromes	AR	α, δ, or ε AChR subunit
Primary AChR deficiency	AR	AChR ε-subunit null mutation
Rapsyn deficiency	AR	Rapsyn
Myasthenic syndrome with plectin deficiency	AR	—
No identified defect		

AR = autosomal recessive; AD = autosomal dominant

- *Endplate acetylcholinesterase deficiency:* Patients born with a congenital deficiency of acetylcholinesterase present soon after birth or in early childhood with fluctuating ptosis, extraocular muscle weakness, generalized delay in motor development, weakness exacerbated by exertion, poor cry and suck, and respiratory muscle weakness. The disorder is due to mutations in the gene encoding for ColQ, the collagen tail of AChE anchoring it to the basement membrane. A single electrical stimulus produces repetitive compound muscle action potentials during routine nerve conduction studies.
- *Slow channel syndromes:* These disorders result from mutations in various subunits of the AChR. Individuals with the slow channel syndrome may present at essentially any time (*i.e.*, infancy, childhood, or adulthood). Most patients show selective and severe involvement of cervical, scapular, wrist, and finger extensor muscles. In effect, these patients have a myopathy due to prolonged opening episodes of the AChR channel in the presence of ACh (the channel is slow to close). Even choline in its normal serum concentration opens the channel and renders it leaky in the resting state. The result is cationic overloading of the junctional sarcoplasm resulting in degeneration of the junctional folds with loss of AChR, widening of the synaptic space, and subsynaptic cellular degeneration. This disorder is the only CMS that is autosomal dominant. Repetitive CMAPs evoked from a single supramaximal nerve impulse is a common finding, as in AChE deficiency.
- *Fast channel syndromes:* This disorder is rare. The clinical features are generally severe weakness at birth with poor suck and weak cry. The AChR channel opens and closes too quickly, resulting in the ineffectiveness of acetylcholine to effect muscle depolarization. Mutations in AChR subunits, as in slow channel syndromes, appear to be the cause. A mutation of the fetal δ-subunit may result in arthrogryposis multiplex congenita due to absence of fetal movement *in utero*.
- *Primary AChR deficiency:* Several patients have been described with a presentation during the neonatal period characterized by feeding difficulties, nasal regurgitation, ptosis, impaired eye movements, and reduced overall tone. These disorders mainly result from AChR ε-subunit null or low expression mutations resulting in severe loss of function of the subunit. In these patients, the few AChR present include the γ-subunit (a fetal subunit typically found replacing the ε-subunit during AChR development) instead of the ε-subunit. It may be that null mutations of the other AChR subunits are lethal.

Clinical Pearl

The diagnosis of a CMS should be suspected from a history of fluctuating weakness involving ocular, bulbar, and limb muscles since infancy or early childhood, a history of similarly affected relatives, a decremental EMG response to low-frequency stimulation, and negative tests for acetylcholine receptor (AChR) antibodies.

REFERENCES

1. Brownlow, S., Webster, R., Croxen, R., Brydson, M., Neville, B., Lin, J.P., Vincent, A., Newsom-Davis, J., Beeson, D., Acetylcholine receptor delta subunit mutations underlie a fast-channel myasthenic syndrome and arthrogryposis multiplex congenita, *J. Clin. Invest.* 2001; 108(1):125–130.
2. Croxen, R., Young, C., Slater, C., Haslam, S., Brydson, M., Vincent, A., Beeson, D., End-plate gamma- and epsilon-subunit mRNA levels in AChR deficiency syndrome due to epsilon-subunit null mutations, *Brain* 2001; 124(pt. 7):1362–1372.
3. Engel, A.G., 73rd ENMC International Workshop: congenital myasthenic syndromes, 22–23 October, 1999, Naarden, The Netherlands, *Neuromuscul. Disord.* 2001; 11(3):315–321.
4. Engel, A.G., Ohno, K., Sine, S.M., Congenital myasthenic syndromes: progress over the past decade, *Muscle Nerve* 2003; 27:4–25.
5. Ohno, K., Tsujino, A., Brengman, J.M., Harper, C.M., Bajzer, Z., Udd, B., Beyring, R., Robb, S., Kirkham, F.J., Engel, A.G., Choline acetyltransferase mutations cause myasthenic syndrome associated with episodic apnea in humans, *Proc. Natl. Acad. Sci. USA* 2001; 98(4):2017–2022.
6. Zhou, M., Engel, A.G., Auerbach, A., Serum choline activates mutant acetylcholine receptors that cause slow channel congenital myasthenic syndromes, *Proc. Natl. Acad. Sci. USA* 1999; 96:10466–10471.

SECTION IV.   MOTOR NEURON DISEASE AND MOTOR NEUROPATHIES

The electrodiagnosis of motor neuron diseases and of motor neuropathies are intricately associated. As the principal motor neuron disease, amyotrophic lateral sclerosis (ALS) is universally fatal, while motor neuropathies are effectively treatable, the physician must thoroughly explore the possibility that a motor neuropathy is present in patients with suspected motor neuron diseases.

In a patient with a suspected motor neuron disease, the broad goals of the study include:

- *Demonstration of a "generalized" disorder of lower motor neurons.* "Generalized" can be variously defined, and the electromyographer should state the definition in the study's report. Because many clinical trials have adopted the Revised World Federation of Neurology's El Escorial criteria for patient enrollment,[7] this is one commonly used definition. These criteria require needle EMG abnormalities in two of four regions: bulbar, cervical, thoracic (paraspinals at or below T6, or abdominal muscles), and lumbar. For the bulbar or thoracic region, one abnormal muscle is required, while for the cervical or lumbosacral, two abnormal muscles innervated by different roots and peripheral nerves are required. Another commonly used definition is the presence of abnormalities in at least two distinct nerve distributions (including root, plexus, or peripheral nerve) in each of three limbs. Specific abnormalities indicating lower motor neuron (LMN) disease include signs of acute denervation (fibrillation potentials and positive sharp waves), reinnervation (increased amplitude or duration of motor unit action potentials or the presence of satellite potentials), and reduced interference patterns. Some advocate that the presence of varying motor unit morphology should also be considered an abnormality. Fasciculation potentials should be sought, although they do not provide evidence of definite abnormalities by themselves.

- *Demonstration of a lack of focal motor demyelination to exclude a treatable motor neuropathy.* An extensive search for a segment of focal motor demyelination should include at least bilateral median–APB and ulnar–ADM motor studies with multiple stimulation sites, including axillary stimulation, and, if possible, bilateral peroneal–EDB and tibial–AH studies as well. A careful F-wave study should also be performed on all motor nerves studied.

- *Demonstration of normal sensory nerve studies, particularly in anatomic territories overlapping with those of severe motor involvement.* The demonstration of normal sensory nerve action potential (SNAP) amplitudes helps exclude focal neuropathies (such as a median and ulnar neuropathy) and X-linked bulbospinal neuronopathy, a lower motor neuron disorder that frequently has reduced SNAP amplitudes in the absence of sensory symptoms or signs. A very strong case for a motor neuron disorder is often made by the demonstration of normal SNAP amplitudes in distributions with severe motor axonal loss. For example, an absent median–APB compound muscle action potential (CMAP) along with normal median–D2 and ulnar–D5 SNAPs would be difficult to attribute to a focal peripheral lesion, such as a median neuropathy or medial cord plexus lesion.

- *Note the presence of suprasegmental recruitment patterns, possibly indicative of upper motor neuron weakness.* ALS is a disorder of upper and lower motor neurons. Upper motor neuron weakness is evidenced on needle EMG studies as a suprasegmental interference pattern: a small number of motor units firing at low frequency in a weak muscle, despite the patient's stated full effort not limited by pain. One should not be definitive about concluding the presence of a disorder of upper motor neurons by needle EMG interference patterns, but such a pattern is highly suggestive of such.

- *Note the presence and distribution of fasciculation potentials.* Fasciculation potentials by themselves are not generally considered abnormal. In the setting of a probably generalized disorder of lower motor neurons, however, they often indicate a diseased motor unit and may be a prelude to denervation. As such, they indicate muscles that might be valuable in demonstrating future abnormalities should a subsequent electrodiagnostic study be required.

A number of specialized electrodiagnostic techniques, including motor unit number estimation (MUNE) and the use of transcranial magnetic stimulation for calculation of central motor conduction time, are currently primarily of research value and are not routine in clinical practice.

REFERENCES

1. Brooks, B.R., El Escorial World Federation of Neurology: criteria for the diagnosis of amyotrophic lateral sclerosis, *J. Neurol. Sci.* 1994; 124(suppl.):96–107.
2. Cornblath, D.R., Kuncl, R.W., Mellits, E.D., Quaskey, S.A., Nerve conduction studies in amyotrophic lateral sclerosis, *Muscle Nerve* 1992; 15:1111–1115.
3. Daube, J.R., Electrodiagnostic studies in amyotrophic lateral sclerosis and other motor neuron disorders. *Muscle Nerve* 2000; 23:1488–1502.
4. Layzer, R.B., The origin of fasciculations and cramps. *Muscle Nerve* 1994; 17:1243–1249.
5. Olney, R.K., American Association of Electrodiagnostic Medicine. Consensus criteria for the diagnosis of partial conduction block, *Muscle Nerve* 1999; 22:(suppl. 8):225–229.
6. Olney, R.K., Aminoff, M.J., So, Y.T., Clinical and electrodiagnostic features of X-linked recessive bulbospinal neuronopathy, *Neurology* 1991; 41:823–828.
7. Ross, M.A., Miller, R.G., Berchert, L., Parry, G., Barohn, R.J., Armon, C., Bryan, W.W., Petajan, J., Stromatt, S., Goodpasture, J., McGuire, D., Toward earlier diagnosis of amyotrophic lateral sclerosis: revised criteria, *Neurology* 1998; 50:768–772.
8. Yuen, E.C., Olney, R.K., Longitudinal study of fiber density and motor unit number estimate in patients with amyotrophic lateral sclerosis, *Neurology* 1997; 49:573–578.

PATIENT 47

A 55-year-old man with progressive left hand weakness for 6 months

Over the previous 6 months, this man has noted difficulty writing, buttoning a shirt, and turning a key. He has noted frequent left hand finger extensor cramps and infrequent similar cramps in the right hand. Neurological exam showed atrophy and frequent fasciculations diffusely in left arm muscles, particularly in ventral forearm flexors, thenar, and hypothenar muscles, but also deltoid, biceps, and triceps. Reflexes were brisker in the left arm than the right; for example, the left biceps was MRC grade 3 strength with a 3+ reflex.

Electrodiagnostic Study:

Sensory NCS

Nerve	Sites	Recording Site	Onset (ms)	Peak (ms)	Amplitude (µV)	Distance (cm)	Velocity (m/s)
L. median–dig II	1. Wrist	Dig II	2.80	3.55	13.2	13	46.4
R. median–dig II	1. Wrist	Dig II	2.65	3.35	21.6	13	49.1
L. ulnar–dig V	1. Wrist	Dig V	2.25	3.05	13.8	11	48.9
R. ulnar–dig V	1. Wrist	Dig V	2.65	3.35	6.4	11	41.5
L. radial–sn box	1. Forearm	Sn box	1.60	2.15	18.8	10	62.5
L. med AB cut	1. Elbow	Forearm	2.10	2.50	3.8	12	57.1
R. med AB cut	1. Elbow	Forearm	1.80	2.30	6.4	12	66.7
L. lat AB cut	1. Elbow	Forearm	2.00	2.50	8.9	12	60.0

Motor NCS

Nerve	Sites	Recording Site	Latency (ms)	Amplitude (mV)	Distance (cm)	Velocity (m/s)
L. median–APB	1. Wrist	APB	5.30	0.6	7	—
	2. Elbow	APB	10.25	0.4	24	48.5
R. median–APB	1. Wrist	APB	3.80	6.5	7	—
	2. Elbow	APB	7.95	6.3	24.5	59.0
	3. Axilla	APB	11.45	6.5	20	57.1
L. ulnar–ADM	1. Wrist	ADM	4.65	0.8	7	—
	2. B. elbow	ADM	9.80	0.7	23	44.7
	3. A. elbow	ADM	12.90	0.6	14	45.2
R. ulnar–ADM	1. Wrist	ADM	3.35	9.3	7	—
	2. B. elbow	ADM	7.25	8.2	23.5	60.3
	3. A. elbow	ADM	9.20	7.6	11	56.4
	4. Axilla	ADM	11.65	7.3	15	61.2
L. ulnar–FDI	1. Wrist	FDI	5.55	1.1	—	—
	2. B. elbow	FDI	9.75	1.0	23	54.8
	3. A. elbow	FDI	13.55	0.9	14	36.8

F-Wave

Nerve	F_{min} (ms)	F_{max} (ms)	Max − Min (ms)	%F
L. ulnar	Absent	—	—	—
R. median	29.60	31.65	2.05	80
R. ulnar	28.30	30.95	2.65	80

Needle EMG Summary Table

		SA			Amplitude (MUs)	Duration (MUs)	PolyP (MUs)	Activation	Recruitment Pattern
	IA	Fib	Fasc	Other					
Left arm									
L. deltoid	Incr	2+	2+	0	Nl	Nl	Nl	Full	Nl
L. biceps	Incr	2+	4+	0	Nl	Nl	Nl	Full	Nl
L. triceps	Incr	3+	3+	0	Nl	Nl	Few	Full	Mod red
L. ext Indicis	Nl	0	0	0	Nl	Nl	Nl	Full	Nl
L. ext dig comm	Incr	3+	2+	0	Nl	Nl	Nl	Central	Sev red
L. first dors int	Incr	3+	Rare	0	Nl	Nl	Nl	Central	Sev red
Left leg									
L. tib ant	Nl	0	Rare	0	Nl	Nl	Nl	Full	Nl
L. gastroc med	Nl	0	Rare	0	Nl	Nl	Nl	Full	Nl
L. vast med	Nl	0	0	0	Nl	Nl	Nl	Full	Nl
L. glut med	Nl	0	0	0	Nl	Nl	Nl	Full	Nl
L. bic fem SH	Nl	0	0	0	Nl	Nl	Nl	Full	Nl
Thoracic paraspinals									
L. thoracic PSP lower	Nl	0	0	0	—	—	—	—	—
L. thoracic PSP mid	Nl	1+	1+	0	—	—	—	—	—
L. thoracic PSP upper	Nl	1+	1+	0	—	—	—	—	—
Right arm									
R. deltoid	Nl	0	Rare	0	Nl	Nl	Nl	Full	Nl
R. biceps	Nl	0	0	0	Nl	Nl	Nl	Full	Nl
R. triceps	Nl	0	0	0	Nl	Nl	Nl	Full	Nl
R. pron teres	Nl	0	Rare	0	Nl	Nl	Nl	Full	Nl
R. abd poll br	Nl	0	0	0	Nl	Nl	Nl	Full	Nl
R. first dors int	Incr	1+	0	0	Nl	Nl	Nl	Full	Nl
Right leg									
R. tib ant	Nl	0	0	0	Nl	Nl	Nl	Full	Nl
R. vast med	Nl	0	0	0	Nl	Nl	Nl	Full	Nl

Questions:
1. Does this study provide evidence of a generalized disorder of motor neurons?
2. Is there electrophysiological evidence of a potentially treatable motor neuropathy?
3. Is the prolonged left median–APB distal motor latency likely due to carpal tunnel syndrome?
4. Are the sensory amplitudes normal?
5. What muscles might be valuable to study in a follow-up EMG examination should one be needed for diagnosis?

Answers:

1. Yes
2. No
3. Possibly
4. All except the right ulnar-D5
5. Right deltoid, pronator teres, left tibialis anterior, gastrocnemius

Discussion: We analyze this case from the perspective put forth in the introduction to this section:

- *Is there electrophysiological evidence of a generalized disorder of motor neurons?* We look for reduction in CMAP amplitudes and for the presence of fibrillation potentials or reduced recruitment of motor units. The left median–APB, ulnar–ADM, and ulnar–FDI CMAPs are all reduced, and fibrillation potentials are present in at least two myotomes in the left arm, C5/6 (deltoid) and C8/T1 (FDI). Fibrillation potentials are also present in thoracic paraspinal muscles and in right FDI. Accordingly, the World Federation of Neurology revised El Escorial criteria for "generalized" are met, but not the criteria of at least two distinct nerve distributions in each of three different limbs.

- *Is there electrophysiological evidence of conduction block of motor axons?* We have looked at multiple motor segments including bilateral median and ulnar nerves and including axillary stimulation and F-wave responses. There is mild prolongation of left median–APB and ulnar–ADM distal motor latencies, and all other motor segments, including F-waves, are normal (no conduction block or focal slowing). Can this be accounted for by the degree of axonal loss? The answer is probably, but there are no definite data that establish this. If we apply the conservative research criteria for focal demyelination commonly used in the diagnosis of acute inflammatory demyelinating polyneuropathies (AIDP) or chronic inflammatory demyelinating polyneuropathy (CIDP) (see case 32), requiring a distal motor latency (DML) of greater than 150% the upper limit of normal (ULN), a median DML of greater than 6.8 or ulnar DML of greater than 6.0 would be required. In answer to question 3, it is possible that the mild prolongation in the left median–APB DML is due to carpal tunnel syndrome, and we note a mild but not clearly abnormal reduction in the left median–D2 SNAP amplitude compared to the right (13 µV vs. 21 µV). However, the across-wrist sensory velocity is normal (46 m/s). Ideally, a more sensitive test (see case 2) such as the median–ulnar palm–wrist interlatency difference would best answer this question.

- *Is the neuronal degeneration selective (i.e., are the SNAP amplitudes normal)?* Seven of eight SNAP amplitudes are normal. The right ulnar–D5 SNAP amplitude is reduced in isolation, a likely incidental finding or suggestive of a separate nonlocalizing right ulnar neuropathy. As evidence of selectivity of the neuronal degeneration, we note the reduced amplitudes of the left median–APB and ulnar–ADM CMAPs, but preserved left median–D2 and ulnar–D5 SNAP amplitudes.

- *Which muscles normal in the current study should particularly be studied if a follow-up needle EMG exam is performed in the future?* These are the muscles with fasciculations present: the right deltoid and pronator teres and the left tibialis anterior and gastrocnemius. The appearance of fibrillation potentials in these muscles in a follow-up exam would allow the study to meet the "generalized" criteria of two distinct nerve distributions in each of three limbs.

This patient has ALS. Six months after the initial study, his left arm weakness had progressed, and right hand and left leg weakness had developed.

Clinical Pearls

The following questions should be addressed in the electrophysiological evaluation of possible motor neuron disorders:

1. Is there electrophysiological evidence of a generalized disorder of motor neurons?
2. Is there electrophysiological evidence of conduction block of motor axons?
3. Is the neuronal degeneration selective (i.e., are the SNAP amplitudes normal)?
4. Which muscles normal in the current study should particularly be studied if a follow-up needle EMG exam is performed in the future?

REFERENCES

See the references listed in the introduction to this section.

PATIENT 48

A 3-month-old boy with congenital hypotonia and weakness

A 3-month-old boy was referred for evaluation of congenital hypotonia and weakness since birth. The mother noted reduced fetal movements during this pregnancy compared to when she was pregnant with her other healthy 2-year-old son. On exam, the child was lying in a frog-leg posture. There was little spontaneous movement of the extremities. He was floppy and muscle bulk was diminished. There was decreased suck and quivering movements of the tongue. Muscle stretch reflexes were absent.

Electrodiagnostic Study:

Sensory NCS

Nerve	Sites	Recording Site	BP Amplitude (µV)	Velocity (m/s)
L. median–dig II	1. Wrist	Dig II	16	35
L. sural–lat mall	1. Mid-calf	Ankle	15	38

Motor NCS

Nerve	Sites	Recording Site	Latency (ms)	Amplitude (mV)	Velocity (m/s)
L. median–APB	1. Wrist	APB	3.0	0.1	—
	2. Elbow	APB	—	Absent	—
L. peroneal–EDB	1. Ankle	EDB	3.3	0.1	—
	2. Fib head	EDB	—	Absent	—

Needle EMG Summary

	IA	SA Fib	SA Fasc	SA Other	Amplitude (MUs)	Duration (MUs)	PolyP (MUs)	Recruitment Pattern
L. vast lat	Incr	3+	2+	0	Many small, few large	Many short, few long	Nl	Marked red
L. tib ant	Incr	3+	2+	0	Many small, few large	Many short, few long	Nl	Marked red

Questions:
1. What is the differential diagnosis of a floppy infant?
2. How would you proceed in evaluating this child?

1. Congenital myopathy, congenital myasthenic syndrome, spinal muscular atrophy, others
2. Genetic testing for SMN gene mutations

Discussion: The nerve conduction studies were remarkable for low-amplitude CMAPs with normal distal latencies. The sensory studies were normal. Needle EMG demonstrated fibrillation potentials, positive sharp waves, and fasciculation potentials at rest. Motor units had a mixed morphology, and recruitment was markedly reduced. The overall clinical picture and electrodiagnostic findings were suggestive of a lower motor neuron syndrome (e.g., spinal muscular atrophy).

Spinal muscular atrophy (SMA) type 1 or Werdnig–Hoffmann disease manifests within the first 6 months of life. About 30% of patients manifest *in utero* with decreased fetal movements. The incidence is approximately 1 in 25,000 live births, with males and females being equally affected. Infants manifest with severe generalized weakness and hypotonia. Most infants are never able to sit without support when placed. Infants have weak sucking motions, and difficulty swallowing and poor clearing of secretions are quite common. Fasciculations are evident in the tongue. A fine tremor of the fingers may be seen secondary to hand intrinsic fasciculations.

Sensory nerve conduction studies are normal in SMA. Motor nerve conduction studies may be normal during the early course of the disease process; however, as the disease progresses and there is considerable loss of anterior horn cells, a resultant drop in CMAP amplitudes is observed. Mild slowing of conduction velocities proportional to the loss of large myelinated axons (usually not more than 25% below the lower limit of normal) may be observed. The needle electromyographic examination is abnormal. Fibrillation potentials, positive sharp waves, and fasciculation potentials are commonly appreciated. Motor unit action potentials (MUAPs) may be decreased in amplitude and short in duration due to the diffuse atrophy and lack of reinnervation, although a few larger units may be appreciated. The MUAPs numbers are decreased and fire at rapid rates (*i.e.*, demonstrate reduced recruitment).

Muscle biopsy reveals severe groups of atrophic, rounded, type 1 and 2 fibers intermixed with scattered large rounded fibers (usually type I fibers). With DNA testing now available, there is little indication for performing muscle biopsies on these patients.

Spinal muscular atrophy types 1 to 3 are due to mutations in the spinal motor neuron gene (SMN) located on chromosome 5q13. Two almost identical SMN genes—telomeric SMN (SMN_t) and centromeric SMN (SMN_c)—differ by five nucleotides. Normal individuals contain two copies of SMN_t and several copies of SMN_c. SMA is caused by mutations in both SMN_t alleles. Approximately 98% of the causes are associated with deletions, usually involving exons 7 and 8, while the other 2% are the result of conversion of the SMN_t genes to the SMN_c sequence. The age of onset and severity of SMA may be modified by the number of intact copies of SMN_c and other neighboring genes.

The SMN protein is present in the cytoplasm of all cells and in nuclear structures called *gems* that associate with nuclear coiled bodies. These gems and coiled bodies are believed to serve as storage sites for spliceosomes that excise introns from newly synthesized small nuclear RNA (snRNA) to produce messenger RNA (mRNA). However, prior to this splicing of the snRNA into mRNA, SMN protein binds to and shuttles snRNA out of the nucleus and into the cytoplasm, where they undergo methylation to form mature small nuclear ribonucelic protein (snRNP), or "snurps." SMN protein then shuttles the mature snRNP back into the nucleus, where splicing to mRNA occurs. Thus, the fundamental defect in SMA appears to involve abnormal trafficking and splicing of RNA species. How this leads to destruction of motor neurons is unclear.

Clinical Pearl

In the evaluation of generalized weakness in an infant, focus on sensory studies (for possible neuropathy) and needle EMG to distinguish lower motor neuron from muscle or neuromuscular junction disease.

REFERENCES

1. Dumitru, D., Amato, A.A., Disorders of motor neurons, in Dumitru, D., Amato, A.A., Swartz, M.J., Eds., *Electrodiagnostic Medicine*, 2nd ed., Hanley & Belfus, Philadelphia, PA, 2002, pp. 581–651.
2. Iannaccone, S.T., Russman, B.S., Brown, R.H. *et al.*, Prospective analysis of strength in spinal muscular atrophy, *J. Child Neurol.* 2000; 15:97–101.
3. Morris, G.E., Nuclear proteins and cell death in inherited neuromuscular disease, *Neuromusc. Dis.* 2000; 10:217–227.

PATIENT 49

A 66-year-old man with a 5-year history of progressive weakness and wasting of his distal right leg

At the age of 61, this man noted the onset of right ankle weakness that gradually increased in a slow, stepwise fashion with prolonged periods of relatively little change. His right foot became essentially flail, with very poor plantar flexion and almost no dorsiflexion. There was no pain, numbness, tingling or any sensory disturbance. Neurological examination at age 66 was remarkable for extensive atrophy of the right leg below the knee, affecting all muscle groups. Eversion and dorsiflexion of foot and toes were trace at best, and plantarflexion and inversion were 2/5. The hamstrings and the buttocks were normal in bulk and strength, and there was no sensory deficit. The knee reflex was normal, the ankle reflex absent, and the plantar response silent. There was no spasticity. There were no symptoms in the other three limbs.

Electrodiagnostic Study:

Sensory NCS

Nerve	Sites	Recording Site	Onset (ms)	Peak (ms)	Amplitude (μV)	Distance (cm)	Velocity (m/s)
R. median–dig II	1. Wrist	Dig II	Absent	—	—	13	—
L. median–dig II	1. Wrist	Dig II	3.75	4.65	17.2	13	34.7
R. ulnar–dig V	1. Wrist	Dig V	2.65	3.55	23.4	11	41.5
L. ulnar–dig V	1. Wrist	Dig V	2.80	3.70	26.0	11	39.3
R. sural–lat mall	1. Mid-calf	Ankle	2.60	3.40	11.6	14	53.8
L. sural–lat mall	1. Mid-calf	Ankle	3.55	4.40	13.3	14	39.4
R. sup peroneal	1. Lat leg	Ankle	3.60	4.30	6.8	14	38.9
L. sup peroneal	1. Lat leg	Ankle	2.55	3.35	5.7	12	47.1

Motor NCS

Nerve	Sites	Recording Site	Latency (ms)	Amplitude (mV)	Relative Amplitude (%)	Distance (cm)	Velocity (m/s)
R. median–APB	1. Wrist	APB	10.8	5.7	100	7	—
	2. Elbow	APB	18.4	0.8	14	25.5	26.8
	3. Axilla	APB	20.8	0.8	14	12	50
L. median–APB	1. Wrist	APB	5.35	8.5	100	7	—
	2. Elbow	APB	9.05	8.8	103	23	62.2
R. ulnar–ADM	1. Wrist	ADM	3.95	8.8	100	7	—
	2. B. elbow	ADM	7.65	7.1	80.9	21	56.8
	3. A. elbow	ADM	9.25	7.0	80	10	62.5
	4. Axilla	ADM	11.15	6.3	71.3	10	52.6
L. ulnar–ADM	1. Wrist	ADM	3.50	10.5	100	7	—
	2. B. elbow	ADM	7.55	6.0	57.2	20.5	50.6
	3. A. elbow	ADM	9.65	6.1	57.8	11.5	54.8
L. median–ADM	1. Elbow	ADM	No Martin–Gruber		—	—	—
R. peroneal–EDB	1. Ankle	EDB	7.25	0.4	100	8	—
	2. Fib head	EDB	15.65	0.4	97.9	32	38.1
	3. Pop fossa	EDB	18.30	0.4	96.2	8	30.2
L. peroneal–EDB	1. Ankle	EDB	7.45	2.7	100	8	—
	2. Fib head	EDB	15.90	2.5	90.3	33	39.1

Continued

Motor NCS—cont'd

Nerve	Sites	Recording Site	Latency (ms)	Amplitude (mV)	Relative Amplitude (%)	Distance (cm)	Velocity (m/s)
	3. Pop fossa	EDB	18.70	2.6	94.8	10	35.7
R. peroneal–tib ant	1. Fib head	tib ant	3.10	1.0	100	10	—
	2. Pop fossa	tib ant	6.95	0.9	87.7	8.5	22.1
R. tibial–AH	1. Ankle	AH	Absent	—	—	8	—
L. tibial–AH	1. Ankle	AH	6.55	6.0	100	8	—
	2. Pop fossa	AH	17.40	4.1	68	40	36.9

F-Wave

Nerve	F_{min} (ms)	F_{max} (ms)	Persistence
L. tibial	70.05	74.35	8/10
L. peroneal	66.15	71.35	6/10
R. median	42.35	48.45	9/10
R. ulnar	31.65	34.15	9/10
L. median	32.65	34.95	7/10
L. ulnar	31.90	33.30	7/10

H-Reflex

Nerve	H Latency (ms)
L. tibial–soleus	Absent
R. tibial–soleus	50.35

EMG Summary Table

		SA			Amplitude (MUs)	Duration (MUs)	PolyP (MUs)	Activation	Recruitment Pattern
	IA	Fib	Fasc	Other					
R. vast lat	Nl	0	0	0	Nl	Nl	Nl	Full	Nl
R. tib ant	Incr	2+	0	0	Nl	Nl	Nl	Full	SevRed
R. gastrocmed	Incr	3+	0	CRD	Nl	Nl	Nl	Full	SevRed
R. peron ln	Incr	3+	0	0	Nl	Nl	Nl	Full	SevRed
R. bic fem SH	Nl	0	0	0	Nl	Nl	Nl	Full	Nl
R. glut med	Nl	0	0	0	Nl	Nl	Nl	Full	Nl
R. L5 para-spinals	Incr	1+	0	0	Nl	Nl	Nl	Full	Nl
R. S1 para-spinal	Nl	0	0	0	Nl	Nl	Nl	Full	Nl
L. L5 para-spinals	Nl	0	0	0	Nl	Nl	Nl	Full	Nl

Motor NCS: R Median - APB

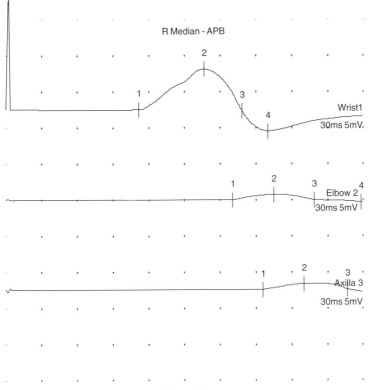

Figure 1

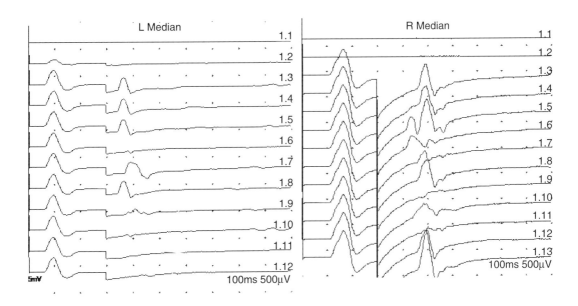

F Wave: L Median   F Wave: R Median

Figure 2

Questions: This patient was initially diagnosed with ALS. How would you classify this syndrome? What would be the potential value and rationale for performing extensive motor conduction studies in all four limbs?

Discussion: The patient's clinical syndrome, prior to electrophysiological characterization, is that of a progressive unilateral distal lower motor neuron degeneration. There is marked motor axonal loss in the distal right leg without sensory or upper motor neuron findings. This syndrome always raises the possibility of ALS but is also indicative of multifocal motor neuropathy (MMN) and rarely structural disorders.

The nerve conduction study abnormalities are:

- Absent right median–D2 SNAP and prolonged left median–D2 distal sensory latency
- Reduced amplitude of the right peroneal–EDB, peroneal–TA, and tibial–AH CMAPs
- Asymmetric prolongation of bilateral median–APB distal motor latencies
- Conduction block (86% amplitude drop) and focal slowing of the right median forearm motor segment (figure 1)
- Probable conduction block (43% amplitude drop) of the left ulnar forearm segment (note that the amplitude drop was not due to the presence of a Martin–Gruber anastomosis)
- Focal slowing of the right peroneal–EDB and right peroneal–TA across-fibular-head motor segments
- Prolongation of the right median, left peroneal, and left tibial minimum F-wave latencies
- Prolongation of the right and absent left tibial–soleus H-reflex

These findings provide evidence of multifocal demyelination of motor nerves and support a diagnosis of multifocal motor neuropathy. In addition, there is evidence of sensory involvement for the median nerves at the wrist, which might reflect the coexistence of bilateral carpal tunnel syndromes. In this case, motor axonal degeneration dominates the clinical and electrodiagnostic picture, but unequivocal evidence of demyelination is crucial for diagnosis and management. This patient was subsequently treated with intravenous immunoglobulin (IVIG) monthly; after 8 months, strength in ankle dorsiflexion and toe extension and flexion had improved. Electrodiagnostic studies (see below and figure 3) showed resolution of the median nerve conduction block and forearm slowing and improvement in peroneal and tibial distal evoked CMAP amplitudes.

Multifocal motor neuropathy has a spectrum of presentations, including a purely demyelinating form, an asymmetric lower motor neuron degeneration (as in this case), and a motor unit hyperactivity disorder (see case 50). The diagnosis of the asymmetric lower motor neuron degeneration form of MMN is one of the most significant contributions the electromyographer can make to the clinical care of a patient. Accordingly, the electrodiagnostic evaluation of patients with suspected ALS and a purely lower motor neuron syndrome should include extensive search for demyelination, including motor conduction studies of as many nerve segments as can be accomplished and F-wave studies. Bilateral median and ulnar studies, including axillary stimulation, and bilateral peroneal and tibial studies including F-waves should almost always be performed in this evaluation. When appropriate, radial motor studies might also be considered. Erb's point and root stimulation to demonstrate conduction block have the disadvantage that a significant number of patients cannot be supramaximally stimulated at these sites, making it impossible to confidently demonstrate conduction block. American Association of Electrodiagnostic Medicine (AAEM) consensus criteria do not recognize Erb's point stimulation for the demonstration of definite partial conduction block, although they do allow it for the demonstration of "probable" partial conduction block. The criteria do not allow for root stimulation at all. Subtle evidence of demyelination is sometimes limited only to F-wave minimum latency prolongation, which should be interpreted attentively but cautiously.

Electrodiagnostic Studies 8 Months After Monthly IVIG Treatment:

Motor NCS

Nerve	Sites	Recording Site	Latency (ms)	Amplitude (mV)	Relative Amplitude (%)	Distance (cm)	Velocity (m/s)
R. median–APB	1. Wrist	APB	11.40	6.0	100	7	—
	2. Elbow	APB	14.60	4.8	79.5	22	68.7
	3. Axilla	APB	16.85	5.4	89.2	10	44.4

Continued

Nerve	Sites	Recording Site	Latency (ms)	Amplitude (mV)	Relative Amplitude (%)	Distance (cm)	Velocity (m/s)
R. peroneal– EDB	1. Ankle	EDB	9.35	1.6	100	8	—
	2. Fib head	EDB	20.25	1.3	82.6	32	29.4
	3. Pop fossa	EDB	25.10	1.3	85.4	10	20.6
R. tibial–AH	1. Ankle	AH	10.70	0.1	100	8	—
	2. Pop fossa	AH	27.15	0.1	79.5	38	23.1

F-Wave

Nerve	F_{min} (ms)	F_{max} (ms)	Max – Min (ms)	%F
R. median	44.70	46.95	2.25	7/10
R. peroneal	Absent	—	—	—
R. tibial	Absent	—	—	—

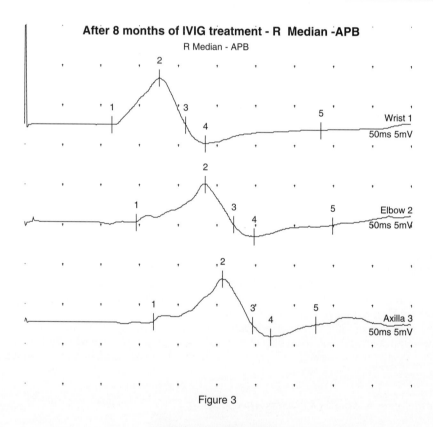

Figure 3

Clinical Pearls

1. The electrodiagnostic evaluation of suspected motor neuron disorders should include a thorough search for conduction block in motor segments, even in asymptomatic distributions. If possible, bilateral median–APB, ulnar–ADM, peroneal–EDB, and tibial–AH motor studies, including F-waves and axillary segments, should be performed.

2. Multifocal motor neuropathy (MMN) is a potentially treatable disorder that can be mistaken for ALS.

REFERENCES

1. Federico, P., Zochodne, D.W., Hahn, A.F., Brown, W.F., Feasby, T.E., Multifocal motor neuropathy improved by IVIg: randomized, double-blind, placebo-controlled study, *Neurology* 2000; 55(9):1256–1262.
2. Katz, J.S., Barohn, R.J., Kojan, S., Wolfe, G.I., Nations, S.P., Saperstein, D.S., Amato, A.A., Axonal multifocal motor neuropathy without conduction block or other features of demyelination, *Neurology* 2002; 58(4):615–620.
3. Katz, J.S., Wolfe, G.I., Bryan, W.W., Jackson, C.E., Amato, A.A., Barohn, R.J., Electrophysiological findings in multifocal motor neuropathy, *Neurology* 1997; 48:700–707.
4. Leger, J.M. *et al.*, Intravenous immunoglobulin therapy in multifocal motor neuropathy: a double-blind, placebo-controlled study, *Brain* 2001; 124:145–153.
5. Lewis, R.A., Sumner, A.J., Brown, M.J., Asbury, A.K., Multifocal demyelinating neuropathy with persistent conduction block, *Neurology* 1982; 32:958–964.
6. Olney, R.K., Consensus criteria for the diagnosis of partial conduction block, *Muscle Nerve* 1999; 22(suppl. 8): S225–S229.
7. Pakiam, A., Parry, G.J., Multifocal motor neuropathy without overt conduction block, *Muscle Nerve* 1998; 21:243–245.
8. Pestronk, A. Chaudhry, V., Feldman, E.L., Griffin, J.W., Cornblath, D.R., Denys, E.H., Glasbery, M., Kuncl, R.W., Olney, R.K., Yee, W.C. Lower motor neuron syndromes defined by patterns of weakness, nerve conduction abnormalities, and high titers of antiglycolipid antibodies, *Ann. Neurol.* 1990; 27:316–326.
9. Taylor, B.V., Wright, R.A., Harper, C.M., Dyck, P.J., Natural history of 46 patients with multifocal motor neuropathy with conduction block. *Muscle Nerve* 23: 900–908, 2000.
10. Van Doorn, P.A., Van der Meche, F.G., IVIg treatment improves multifocal motor neuropathy: easy to start but difficult to stop, *Neurology* 2000; 55:1246–1247.

PATIENT 50

A 45-year-old woman with a 5-year history of cramps and twitching and 2-year history of weakness in her left forearm

This 45-year-old woman complained of frequent cramping of her left hand for the previous 5 years, often precipitated by wrist extension or changes in temperature. In addition, she was aware of nearly continuous left forearm extensor muscle twitching for several years. Over the last year, she noticed weakness of finger extension, particularly for the thumb and digit 3. Examination was most remarkable for continuous twitching, best described as clinical myokymia, in left forearm finger extensor muscles and MRC grade 2 strength in the thumb and third digit extensors, with grade 4+ strength in the other finger extensors. There has been no numbness or paresthesias or neurological symptoms in her other limbs.

Electrodiagnostic Study:

Sensory NCS

Nerve	Sites	Recording Site	Onset (ms)	Peak (ms)	Amplitude (µV)	Distance (cm)	Velocity (m/s)
L. radial–sn box	1. Forearm	Sn box	1.70	2.25	32	10	58.8
R. radial–sn box	1. Forearm	Sn box	1.50	2.00	48	10	66.7
L. median	1. Wrist	D2	2.20	3.00	64	13	59.0
L. ulnar	1. Wrist	D5	2.00	2.6	58	11	65.0

Motor NCS

Nerve	Sites	Recording Site	Area (mVms)	Latency (ms)	Amplitude (mV)	Distance (cm)	Velocity (m/s)
R. radial–EIP	1. Forearm	EIP	48.1	1.80	10.1	—	—
	2. B. spiral gr	EIP	39.6	3.20	8.4	9	64.3
	3. A. spiral gr	EIP	42.4	4.65	8.6	10	69.0
L. radial–EIP	1. Forearm	EIP	64.1	2.00	10.3	—	—
	2. B. spiral gr	EIP	57.3	2.50	9.3	3	60.0
	3. A. spiral gr	EIP	15.7	7.80	2.5	18	34.0
L. median–APB	1. Wrist	APB	—	3.0	16.9	7	
	2. Elbow	APB	—	6.9	16.5	21.5	55.1
	3. Axilla	APB	—	10.0	15.8	19.5	62.9
R. median–APB	1. Wrist	APB	—	3.6	14.6	7	—
	2. Elbow	APB	—	7.7	14.3	23	56
L. ulnar–ADM	1. Wrist	ADM	—	2.9	10.1	7	—
	2. B. elbow	ADM	—	6.1	10.7	21	65.6
	3. A. elbow	ADM	—	8.4	10.7	12	52.6
R. ulnar–ADM	1. Wrist	ADM	—	3.0	10.5	7	—
	2. B. elbow	ADM	—	5.9	9.7	19.5	67
	3. A. elbow	ADM	—	7.9	9.1	10	50
	4. Axilla	ADM	—	9.5	8.8	10	62.5

F-Wave

Nerve	F_min (ms)	Persistence
R. median	28.9	10/10
R. ulnar	27.9	10/10
L. median	27.5	10/10
L. ulnar	27.9	10/10

	SA								
	IA	Fib	Fasc	High-Frequency Discharges	Amplitude (MUs)	Duration (MUs)	PolyP (MUs)	Activation	Recruitment Pattern
L. biceps	Nl	0	0	0	Nl	Nl	Nl	Full	Nl
L. triceps	Nl	0	0	0	Nl	Nl	Nl	Full	Nl
L. ECR	Nl	0	3+	Continuous	Nl	Nl	Nl	Full	Mild red
L. brachiorad	Nl	0	0	0	Nl	Nl	Nl	Full	Nl
L. EDC	Nl	0	3+	0	Nl	Nl	Nl	Full	Mod red
L. FDI	Nl	0	0	0	Nl	Nl	Nl	Full	Nl

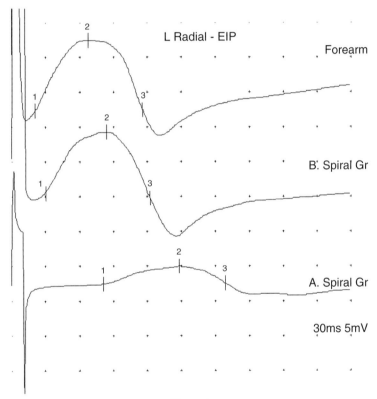

Figure 1

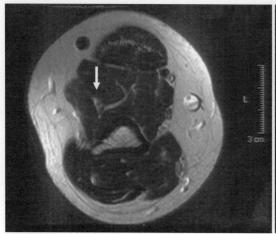 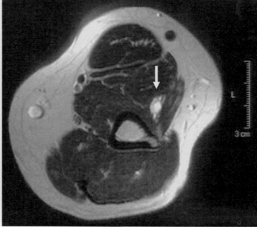

Right radial nerve   Left radial nerve

Figure 2

Questions:
1. What findings are shown in the figures?
2. What is the physiological implication of the needle EMG findings for the left extensor digitorum communis (EDC)?
3. What is the significance of the high-frequency discharges in the left extensor carpi radialis (ECR)?

Answers:

1. Conduction block of left radial-EIP motor nerves; enlargement and increased T2 signal
2. Decreased recruitment without fibrillation potentials suggests focal demyelination
3. Continuous motor unit activity

Discussion: Figure 1 shows conduction block of the left radial–EIP across the spiral groove motor segment. As can be seen from the numerical tabular results, there is a 73% reduction in the CMAP area. In addition, there is focal slowing (34 m/s) of this nerve segment. The needle EMG studies of left EDC show no fibrillation potentials, normal motor unit morphology, and moderately reduced recruitment of motor units. This combination implies demyelination of motor axons (although chronic denervation with partial reinnervation, despite normal motor unit amplitude and duration, is a conceivable possible interpretation). Furthermore, the left ECR continuous, high-frequency discharges indicate a motor unit hyperactivity disorder and can be called *continuous motor unit activity* (CMUA).

An MRI of the forearm (figure 2) demonstrated enlargement and increased T2 signal of the left radial nerve in the across fibular head segment, corresponding to the electrodiagnostic abnormality. The clinical presentation of a motor unit hyperactivity disorder, with cramps, fasciculations, and continuous motor unit activity, argued strongly for a diagnosis of multifocal motor neuropathy (MNN), and the patient was treated with intravenous immunoglobulin (IVIg). The patient described her response to the first infusion as "miraculous" in that it allowed for the first night of sleep without forearm extensor cramps in over a year. Continued periodic treatment resulted in marked improvement in strength and reduced, but did not eliminate, cramps and fasciculations.

The spectrum of MMN and its relationship to several other disorders is outlined in figure 3. Typical chronic inflammatory demyelinating neuropathy (CIDP) has symmetric sensory and motor involvement not confined to individual named nerves. There is generally elevated cerebrospinal fluid (CSF) protein and an excellent treatment response to prednisone. Multifocal CIDP, also called *multifocal inflammatory demyelinating neuropathy* and *multifocal acquired demyelinating sensory and motor neuropathy* (MADSAM), is characterized by multifocal (symmetric or asymmetric) sensory and motor with individual named nerve involvement, variable CSF protein, and excellent but variable response to prednisone. Multifocal motor neuropathy is characterized by multifocal (symmetric or asymmetric) purely motor with individual named nerve involvement, normal CSF protein, and poor response to prednisone but excellent response to IVIg. As indicated in the figure, MMN has several distinct presentations, in decreasing order of incidence: (1) pure, or classic, MMN with prolonged and marked multifocal purely demyelination without axonal loss, often dramatically improved by IVIG; (2) an asymmetric lower motor neuron degeneration with subtle evidence of demyelination (see case 49); and (3) a rarer motor unit hyperactivity syndrome (this case).

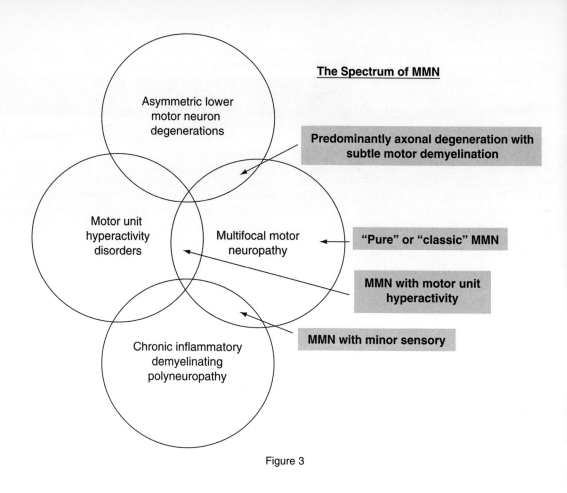

Figure 3

Clinical Pearl

Multifocal motor neuropathy has a spectrum of presentations, including that of a motor unit hyperactivity disorder, dominated by cramps and fasciculations rather than weakness.

REFERENCES

1. Chaudhry, V., Multifocal motor neuropathy, *Semin. Neurol.* 1998; 18(1):73–81.
2. Federico, P., Zochodne, D.W., Hahn, A.F., Brown, W.F., Feasby, T.E., Multifocal motor neuropathy improved by IVIg: randomized, double-blind, placebo-controlled study, *Neurology* 2000; 55:1256–1262.
3. Felice, K.J., Goldstein, J.M., Monofocal motor neuropathy: Improvement with intravenous immunoglobulin, *Muscle Nerve* 2002; 25:674–678.
4. Layzer, R.B., The origin of fasciculations and cramps. *Muscle Nerve* 1994; 17:1243–1249.
5. Lewis, R.A., Sumner, A.J., Brown, M.J., Asbury, A.K., Multifocal demyelinating neuropathy with persistent conduction block, *Neurology* 1982; 32:958–964.
6. Meriggioli, M.N., Sanders, D.B., Conduction block and continuous motor unit activity in chronic acquired demyelinating polyneuropathy, *Muscle Nerve* 1999; 22:532–537.
7. O'Leary, C.P., Mann, A.C., Lough, J., Willison, H.J., Muscle hypertrophy in multifocal motor neuropathy is associated with continuous motor unit activity, *Muscle Nerve* 1997; 20:479–485.
8. Thomas, P.K., Claus, D., Jaspert, A., Workman, J.M., King, R.H., Larner, A.J., Anderson, M., Emerson, J.A., Ferguson, I.T., Focal upper limb demyelinating neuropathy, *Brain* 1996; 119:765–774.
9. Van Doorn, P.A., van der Meche, F.G., IVIg treatment improves multifocal motor neuropathy: easy to start but difficult to stop, *Neurology* 2000; 55:1246–1247.
10. Van Es, H.W., Van den Berg, L.H., Franssen, H., Witkamp, T.D., Ramos, L.M., Notermans, N.C., Feldberg, M.A., Wokke, J.H., Magnetic resonance imaging of the brachial plexus in patients with multifocal motor neuropathy, *Neurology* 1997; 48:1218–1224.

Electrodiagnostic studies are valuable in patients with weakness for distinguishing among nerve, muscle, or other causes. For patients with suspected myopathies, the nerve conduction studies are often normal, and the needle EMG studies are the most informative part of the electrodiagnostic study. There are some exceptions worth noting. Myopathies may result in reduced compound muscle action potential amplitudes in affected muscles. Because routine motor nerve compound muscle action potentials (CMAPs) are recorded from distal muscles (*e.g.*, abductor pollicis brevis, abductor digiti minimi, extensor digitorum brevis, abductor hallucis), reductions in amplitudes occur only in myopathies with involvement of hand or foot muscles (such as myotonic dystrophy or critical illness myopathy).

The needle EMG study in myopathies generally follows the following principles:

- Studies are often limited to one side of the body. Many patients with suspected myopathies ultimately undergo muscle biopsy in the course of their initial diagnostic evaluation, often shortly after referral for an EMG study. It is imperative to avoid the possibility of the biopsy sample including muscle traumatized by a needle EMG study because of the resulting inflammation. The electrodiagnostic practitioner should clearly state what side was studied.

- Both proximal and distal muscles in an arm and a leg should generally be studied. Most myopathies have a proximal predominance, and it is helpful to demonstrate a proximal-to-distal gradient of abnormalities. Muscles that are typically biopsied, such as the biceps and vastus lateralis, should be studied so that, if abnormal, the electromyographer can suggest biopsy of the corresponding muscle on the contralateral study.

- Fibrillation potentials and positive waves may be seen in myopathies. These electrical potentials should never be referred to as "denervation potentials" as one is misled into viewing their presence as indicative of nerve disease. When present in myopathies, fibrillation potentials and positive sharp waves have diagnostic implications, and such myopathies are often reported as myopathies associated with "membrane irritability" or "membrane instability."

- The electrodiagnostic hallmarks of myopathies are small-amplitude, short-duration motor unit action potentials (MUAPs), and early recruitment of MUAPs with full interference patterns in weak muscles. A number of small-amplitude and short-duration motor units are often present in normal muscles, however, and this criterion is only a reliable indicator when abundant sampling of motor units has been performed in a given muscle. Early recruitment is a pattern of motor unit firing in which abundant units are recruited and generate a relatively weak force. Thus, slight movement is associated with many units, rather than the normal pattern of one or a few MUAPs at weak effort.

- Often, the only electrodiagnostic abnormality in patients with myopathies is a full interference pattern in a weak muscle. When there is substantial weakness of a muscle (MRC grade 3 or less) and the examiner is able to overcome the muscle while recording a full interference pattern, a myopathy (or disorder of neuromuscular transmission) is highly likely. Weakness from neurogenic or suprasegmental causes have very different interference patterns in this situation.

- Neuromuscular junction disease may demonstrate myopathic needle EMG abnormalities and should not be neglected as considerations.

REFERENCES

1. Daube, J.R., AAEM minimonograph 11: needle examination in clinical electromyography, *Muscle Nerve* 1991; 14:685–700.
2. Petajan, J.H., AAEM minimonograph 3: motor unit recruitment, *Muscle Nerve* 1991; 14:489–502.

PATIENT 51

A 49-year-old woman with progressive proximal leg weakness for 3 years

A 49-year-old woman developed difficulty getting out of a chair and climbing stairs 3 years ago. She now typically climbs stairs on her hands and knees. She also has difficulty lifting her arms over her head to shampoo her hair and has noticed some protrusion of her shoulder blades. Family history is remarkable for her mother, who had difficulty walking in her late 50s. She had prominent scapulae and some speech and swallowing disturbances, as well, and made a slapping sound with her feet when walking. The patient has four daughters, ages 25, 18, 14, and 13, and two sons, ages 23 and 20, who are alive and well.

Neurological exam was remarkable for bilateral scapular winging and overriding scapulae. Manual muscle testing revealed the following MRC scores: orbicularis oculi, 5; neck flexion, 5–; neck extension, 5; shoulder flexion, 4; and infraspinatus, 4. Shoulder abduction was 4; elbow extension, 5; elbow extension, 4+; wrist extension, 4+ on the left and 5 on the right; wrist flexion, 5; and hand intrinsics, 5. In the lower extremities, hip flexion, abduction, and extension were 4; knee extension and knee flexion were 5; ankle dorsiflexion was 4+; and plantar flexion was 5. On gait testing, she had marked hyperlordotic posture. Her gait was wide based and waddling. Significant paraspinal atrophy, in addition to the hyperlordosis and scapular winging, was evident.

Electrodiagnostic Study:

Sensory NCS

Nerve	Sites	Recording Site	Onset (ms)	Peak (ms)	BP Amplitude (μV)	Distance (cm)	Velocity (m/s)	Temperature (°C)
L. median–dig II	1. Wrist	Dig II	3.00	3.90	25.8	13	43.3	34.9
L. sup peroneal	1. Lat leg	Ankle	2.55	3.15	17.9	12	47.1	—

Motor NCS

Nerve	Sites	Recording Site	Latency (ms)	Amplitude (mV)	Distance (cm)	Velocity (m/s)
L. median–APB	1. Wrist	APB	3.65	12.0	7	—
	2. Elbow	APB	7.45	11.4	22	57.9
L. peroneal–EDB	1. Ankle	EDB	4.10	6.2	8	—
	2. Fib head	EDB	10.05	5.5	29	48.7
	3. Pop fossa	EDB	11.70	5.4	9	54.5

Needle EMG Summary Table

	IA	SA Fib	Fasc	Other	Amplitude (MUs)	Duration (MUs)	PolyP (MUs)	Activation	Recruitment Pattern
R. deltoid	Nl	0	0	0	Few	Short	Few	Full	Early
R. biceps	Nl	0	0	0	Many	Short	Many	Full	Early

	IA	SA Fib	Fasc	Other	Amplitude (MUs)	Duration (MUs)	PolyP (MUs)	Activation	Recruitment Pattern
R. FDI	Nl	0	0	0	Nl	Nl	Nl	Full	Nl
R. glut med	Nl	0	0	0	Small	Short	Few	Full	Early
R. vast lat	Nl	0	0	0	Small	Short	Few	Full	Early
R. tib ant	Nl	0	0	0	Small	Short	Few	Full	Early
R. mid-thoracic paraspinals	Incr	1+	0	0	—	—	—	—	—

Question: What is your differential diagnosis and how would you proceed?

Answer: Limb girdle muscular dystrophy, fascioscapulohumeral muscular dystrophy

Discussion: There was electrophysiological evidence of a myopathic process affecting proximal muscles more than distal and in which there was little evidence of muscle membrane instability. Clinically, the patient has a limb-girdle pattern of weakness associated with marked winging of the scapulae, hyperlordotic posture, and paraspinal muscle atrophy. There was also a family history, which is most likely autosomal dominant in nature, but we cannot exclude a mitochondrial inheritance pattern, as the disorder was passed down only from her mother and there were no other affected family members. The most common disorder or form of disorders that would cause this pattern of weakness would be a limb-girdle muscular dystrophy (LGMD). There are at least five genetically distinct forms of autosomal dominant LGMD; three causative mutated genes have been identified (see table below). These include mutations directed against myotilin, lamin A/C, and caveolin-3. In addition, fascioscapulohumeral dystrophy can rarely present with a limb-girdle pattern of weakness. Some congenital myopathies can have a limb-girdle pattern of weakness, but most do not present this late in life. One that can is myofibrillar or desmin myopathy.

The patient had a mildly increased serum CPK of 1010 IU/L (normal, <200 IU/L). Left biceps muscle biopsy demonstrated variability in muscle fiber size, scattered necrotic and regenerating fibers, and increased endomysial connective tissue suggestive of a dystrophy. In addition, many fibers had rimmed vacuoles, a finding typical of autosomal dominant LGMD type 1A, which has an age of onset ranging from late teens to the late 60s (mean, 24.8 years). Affected individuals have proximal greater than distal weakness, with the legs more affected than the arms. Distal weakness is evident in a few patients. Rare patients develop dysarthria secondary to palatal muscle involvement and mild facial weakness. Serum creatine kinase (CK) levels are normal or elevated up to 9 times normal. Muscle biopsies are notable for the frequent occurrence of rimmed vacuoles. LGMD 1A 1 is caused by mutations in the gene that encodes for myotilin located on chromosome 5q22.3–31.3. Myotilin is a sarcomeric protein that colocalizes with α-actinin on the Z-disk. Mutations in myotilin do not appear to affect its binding with α-actinin but may perturb the normal structure of the Z-disk.

Limb-Girdle Muscular Dystrophies

Disease	Inheritance	Gene Locus	Gene Product
LGMD1A	AD	5q22–q34	Myotilin
LGMD1B	AD	1q11–q21	Lamin A/C
LGMD1C	AD	3p25	Caveolin-3
LGMD1D	AD	6q22	—
LGMD1E	AD	7	—
LGMD2A	AR	15q15	Calpain
LGMD2B	AR	2p13	Dysferlin
LGMD2C	AR	13q12	γ-Sarcoglycan
LGMD2D	AR	17q12–21	α-Sarcoglycan
LGMD2E	AR	4q12	β-Sarcoglycan
LGMD2F	AR	5q33–q34	δ-Sarcoglycan
LGMD2G	AR	17q11–q12	Telethionin
LGMD2H	AR	9q3–q34	—

AD = autosomal dominant; AR = autosomal recessive

Clinical Pearl

Limb-girdle muscular dystrophies are a heteorgenous group of genetically determined diseases; type I diseases are autosomal dominant, and type II diseases are autosomal recessive.

REFERENCES

1. Cohn, R.D., Campbell, K.P., Molecular basis of muscular dystrophies, *Muscle Nerve* 2000; 23:1456–1471.
2. Gilchrist, J.M., Pericak-Vance, M., Silverman, L., Clinical and genetic investigation in autosomal dominant limb-girdle muscular dystrophy, *Neurology* 1988; 38:5–9.
3. Hauser, M.A., Horrigan, S.K., Salmikangas, P. *et al.*, Myotilin is mutated in limb-girdle dystrophy 1A, *Hum. Mol. Genet.* 2000; 9:2141–2147.

PATIENT 52

A 6-month-old girl with generalized weakness since birth

A 6-month-old infant girl was referred for generalized weakness that was noted at birth and for recent respiratory failure requiring a mechanical ventilator. Her exam revealed generalized hypotonia and weakness, no ptosis, and full extraocular movements. Muscle stretch reflexes were absent.

Electrodiagnostic Study:

Sensory NCS

Nerve	Sites	Recording Site	BP Amplitude (μV)	Velocity (m/s)
L. median–dig II	1. Wrist	Dig II	15	22
L. sural–lat mall	1. Mid-calf	Ankle	8	24

Motor NCS

Nerve	Sites	Recording Site	Latency (ms)	Amplitude (mV)	Velocity (m/s)
L. median–APB	1. Wrist	APB	3.2	7	—
	2. Elbow	APB	—	7	22
L. peroneal–EDB	1. Ankle	EDB	3.3	5	—
	2. Fib head	EDB	—	5	23

Needle EMG Summary Table

		SA			Amplitude (MUs)	Duration (MUs)	PolyP (MUs)	Recruitment Pattern
	IA	Fib	Fasc	Other				
L. deltoid	Incr	2+	0	0	Many small	Many short	Many	Early
L. biceps	Incr	2+	0	0	Many small	Many short	Many	Early
L. vast lat	Incr	2+	0	0	Many small	Many short	Many	Early
L. tib ant	Incr	2+	0	0	Many small	Many short	Many	Early

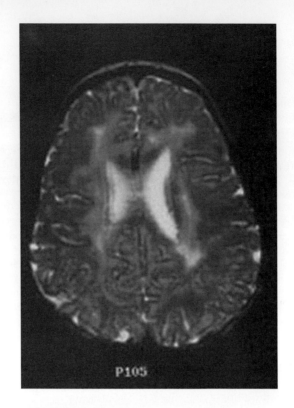

Questions:
1. What is your differential diagnosis and how would you proceed?
2. What other tests would be helpful?
3. What other tests might you consider?

Answers:

1. Mitochondrial disorders, merosin deficiency
2. Serum CK, muscle biopsy
3. Immunostaining of the muscle biopsy for merosin

Discussion: The motor and sensory nerve conduction studies were remarkable for normal amplitudes but mildly slow conduction velocities for age. The EMG demonstrated abnormalities suggestive of a myopathy with muscle membrane instability. Myopathies associated with peripheral nerve abnormalities in children include mitochondrial disorders and the congenital muscular dystrophy associated with merosin deficiency (CMD 1). The serum creatine kinase level was elevated over 2000 IU/L. An MRI scan of the brain revealed hypomyelination. A muscle biopsy subsequently demonstrated features of a dystrophy. Immunostaining for merosin demonstrated absence on the sarcolemma.

The congenital muscular dystrophies (CMDs) are a heterogeneous group of autosomal recessive inherited disorders characterized by perinatal onset of hypotonia with proximal weakness; joint contractures affecting the elbows, hips, knees, and ankles (arthrogryposis); dystrophic appearing muscle biopsies; and exclusion of other recognizable causes of myopathy of the newborn. The CMDs are classified according to clinical, ophthalmological, radiological, and pathological features. The major categories of CMDs are (1) the classic or Occidental/Western type; (2) the Fukuyama type, characterized by defects in neuronal migration (*i.e.*, polymicrogyria) with severe mental retardation, seizures, and a progressively deteriorating course; (3) the Walker-Warburg or cerebral-ocular-dysplasia syndrome; and (4) Santivouri type, or muscle-eye-brain disease.

The classical type of CMD is divided into the merosin-negative and merosin-positive subgroups. Merosin, or α-2 laminin, is connected to the dystrophin–glycoprotein complex. At least 40 to 50% of patients with CMD have absent or decreased merosin. Infants with classical CMD are characteristically hypotonic and weak at birth. Weakness is generalized with a predilection for proximal shoulder and hip girdle muscles. Sensation appears normal. Deep tendon reflexes are diminished or absent. Arthrogryposis may or may not be present. Patients with partial merosin deficiency have been identified. These patients have a milder course and can present in childhood with a Duchenne muscular dystrophy (DMD) phenotype or in early adulthood similar to Becker muscular dystrophy (BMD) or limb-girdle muscular dystrophy (LGMD).

Serum CK levels are elevated, usually over 2000 IU/L, in merosin-negative infants. In contrast, most infants with merosin-positive CMD have normal or mildly elevated serum CKs, typically less than 1000 IU/L. Interestingly, magnetic resonance images (MRIs) demonstrate diffuse white matter abnormalities suggestive of dysmyelination in most infants with merosin-negative CMD. MRI in merosin-positive patients is typically normal. Patients with partial merosin deficiency may or may not have cerebral hypomyelination on MRI.

The classical-type CMD with cerebral hypomyelination is associated with mutations in the α-2 subchain of merosin. Merosin binds to α-dystroglycan of the dystrophin glycoprotein complex and α7β1D integrin. Merosinopathies may result in a disruption and loss of integrity of the muscle membrane. Merosin is also present in the basal lamina of myelinated nerves. Abnormal expression of merosin may interfere with myelinogenesis and may account for the hypomyelination evident in the central and peripheral nervous system.

Clinical Pearl

The combination of a demyelinating neuropathy and a myopathy in a child suggests a mitochondrial disorder or congenital muscular dystrophy with merosin deficiency.

REFERENCES

1. Amato, A.A., Dumitru, D., Hereditary myopathies, in: Dumitru, D., Amato, A.A., Swartz, M.J., Eds., *Electrodiagnostic Medicine*, 2nd ed., Hanley & Belfus, Philadelphia, PA, 2002, pp. 1265–1370.
2. Pegoraro, E., Marks, H., Garcia, C.A., Crawford, T., Mancias, P., Connolly, A.M., Fanin, M., Martinello, F., Trevisan, C.P., Angelini, C., Stella, A., Scavina, M., Munk, R.L., Servidei, S., Bonnermann, C.C, Bertorini, T., Acsadi, G., Thompson, E.C., Gagnon, D., Goganson, G., Carver, V., Zimmerman, R.A., Hoffman, E.P., Laminin α2 muscular dystrophy: genotype/phenotype studies of 22 patients, *Neurology* 1998; 50:101–110.

PATIENT 53

A 29-year-old man with a cardiomyopathy

A 29-year-old white man complained of progressive dyspnea related to a dilated cardiomyopathy since the age of 22. About a year ago, he noted difficulty swallowing. Of note, over the past 7 or 8 years, he had noticed progressive hearing loss. Recent pulmonary function tests showed a forced vital capacity (FVC) of 80%. He had decreased mean inspiratory and expiratory pressures of 52 and 40%, respectively, of predicted. Family history was remarkable as follows. He has a 32-year-old sister who is healthy. Of note, his mother, who is in her mid-50s, has been deaf for over 10 years and had a cochlear implant 2 years ago. She also has had a history of diabetes for a long period of time. The patient's father is healthy. The patient has no known medical allergies. General physical examination was remarkable for his short stature: 5 foot, 3 inches in height.

On neurological examination, there was evidence of pigmentary retinopathy in the macula of both eyes and mild bilateral ptosis. He had marked limitations of all upward and lateral eye movements with normal down-gaze. Orbicularis oculi and oris strength was 5/5. Jaw, palate, and tongue strength likewise was 5/5. Motor exam revealed thin muscle bulk proximally and distally in the arms and legs. On manual muscle testing, he had the following MRC scores: neck flexion, 4+; neck extension, 5; shoulder abduction, 5; elbow flexion, 5–; and elbow extension, 5. Wrist extension and flexion and hand intrinsics were grade 5. Hip flexion, abduction, and extension were grade 4; knee extension and flexion, 5; and ankle dorsiflexion and plantar flexion, 5. Complex motor skills revealed normal coordination. Deep tendon reflexes were 1 at the biceps and at the ankles, but 0 at the triceps, brachioradialis, and knees. Plantar responses were flexor.

Electrodiagnostic Study:

Sensory NCS

Nerve	Sites	Recording Site	Onset (ms)	Peak (ms)	BP Amplitude (µV)	Distance (cm)	Velocity (m/s)
L. median–dig II	1. Wrist	Dig II	2.50	3.30	111.1	13	52.0
L. radial–sn box	1. Forearm	Sn box	1.90	2.45	42.2	10	52.6
L. sural–lat mall	1. Mid-calf	Ankle	3.00	3.70	28.0	14	46.7

Motor NCS

Nerve	Sites	Recording Site	Latency (ms)	Amplitude (mV)	Distance (cm)	Velocity (m/s)
L. median–APB	1. Wrist	APB	3.25	12.7	7	—
	2. Elbow	APB	6.95	12.6	19	51.4
L. ulnar–ADM	1. Wrist	ADM	2.85	13.8	7	—
	2. B. elbow	ADM	5.75	13.5	16.5	56.9
	3. A. elbow	ADM	7.50	13.4	10	57.1
L. peroneal–EDB	1. Ankle	EDB	4.00	6.1	8	—
	2. Fib head	EDB	9.35	5.8	26	48.6
	3. Pop fossa	EDB	11.20	5.7	9	48.6
L. tibial–AH	1. Ankle	AH	4.10	20.0	8	—
	2. Pop fossa	AH	11.45	16.9	37	50.3

Needle EMG Summary Table

| | IA | SA | | | Amplitude (MUs) | Duration (MUs) | PolyP (MUs) | Activation | Recruitment Pattern |
		Fib	Fasc	Other					
L. deltoid	Nl	0	0	0	Nl	Nl	Nl	Full	Nl
L. biceps	Nl	0	0	0	Nl	Nl	Nl	Full	Nl
L. vast lat	Nl	0	0	0	Nl	Nl	Nl	Full	Nl
L. tib ant	Nl	0	0	0	Nl	Nl	Nl	Full	Nl

Questions:
1. How would you interpret these studies?
2. Would normal EMG/NCS exclude an underlying neuromuscular disorder in the patient?

Answers:
1. Normal
2. No

Discussion: The patient has normal EMG/NCS. Based on his clinical features (ptosis, ophthalmoparesis, deafness, short stature, mild extremity weakness, and cardiomyopathy), a mitochondrial myopathy was suspected. This would also explain his mother's deafness. The patient had a mildly elevated serum CK and lactic acid. He underwent a biopsy of the right biceps brachii muscle, which demonstrated numerous ragged red fibers and abnormal mitochondria on electron microscopy. Importantly, EMG is often normal in patients with a mitochondrial myopathy. Some syndromes are associated with peripheral neuropathies, which are typical axonal in nature. His electrophysiological studies were completely normal.

This patient falls into the category of progressive external ophthalmoplegia (PEO), which is a heterogeneous group of mitochondrial disorders. There are autosomal dominant and maternally inherited forms of PEO. Some sporadic patients with PEO have single large mtDNA deletions indistinguishable from those seen in Kearns–Sayre syndrome (KSS). These patients could represent partial expressions of KSS. Importantly, these deletions are felt to be sporadic in occurrence and not inheritable. Point mutations have been demonstrated within various mitochondrial tRNA (Leu, Ile, Asn, Trp) genes in several kinships with maternal inheritance of PEO. In addition, multiple mtDNA deletions have been described in a few kinships with autosomal dominant inheritance.

The molecular defects are suspected to lie in nuclear genes involved in regulating the mitochondrial genome. Autosomal dominant PEO appears to be genetically heterogeneous, because the disorder has been localized to mutations in the genes encoding for adenine nucleotide translocator 1 (ANT1) on chromosome 4q34–q35, the twinkle gene on chromosome 10q23.3–q24.3, and polymerase-γ on 15q22–q26. ANT1 is responsible for transporting adenosine triphosphate across the inner mitochondrial membrane, while twinkle and polymerase-γ are involved in mitochondrial DNA replication.

Clinical Pearl

Many patients with myopathies have normal electrodiagnostic studies. Although it may be diagnostically useful to perform them in suspected myopathy, normal EMG studies provide little evidence against a myopathy.

REFERENCES

1. Hirano, M., DiMauro, S., ANT1, Twinkle, POLG, and TP: new genes open our eyes to ophthalmoplegia, *Neurology* 2001; 57:2163–2165.
2. Kawai, H., Akaike, M., Yokoi, K., Nishida, Y., Kunishige, M., Mine, H., Saito, S., Mitochondrial encephalomyopathy with autosomal dominant inheritance: a clinical and genetic entity of mitochondrial diseases, *Muscle Nerve* 1995; 18:753–760.
3. Li, F.Y., Tariq, M., Croxen, R., Morten, K., Squier, W., Newsom-Davis, J., Beeson, D., Larsson, C., Mapping of autosomal dominant progressive external ophthalmoplegia to a 7-cM critical region on 10q24, *Neurology* 1999; 53:1265–1271.

PATIENT 54

A 62-year-old man with slowly progressive weakness

A 62-year-old right-handed man noted insidious onset of weakness in his neck flexors, hands, and hips about 3 years ago. He also has a feeling occasionally of food getting stuck in his throat. He denies dysarthria, dyspnea, ptosis, diplopia, or sensory loss. There is no significant past medical history or family history of neuromuscular disease. Neurological examination was notable for 4–/5 strength of neck flexors and 5/5 strength of neck extensors. In the upper extremities strength was 5–/5 in the deltoids, 4+/5 in the biceps, 4/5 in the triceps, 4+ in wrist extensors, 4 on left wrist flexion, 4– in right wrist flexion, 4+/5 in the finger extensors, 4 on left finger flexors, and 4– on right finger flexors. In the lower extremities, strength was 4/5 in the hip flexors, abductors, and extensors; 3– in knee extension (quadriceps), 4 in ankle dorsiflexors, and 5 in plantar flexors. On gait testing there was noticeable hyperextension of the knees. Serum creatine kinase level was 200 IU/L (upper limit of normal).

Electrodiagnostic Study:

Sensory NCS

Nerve	Sites	Recording Site	Onset (ms)	Peak (ms)	BP Amplitude (μV)	Distance (cm)	Velocity (m/s)
L. median–dig II	1. Wrist	Dig II	2.30	3.15	80.1	13	56.5
L. ulnar–dig V	1. Wrist	Dig V	2.25	3.20	76.5	11	48.9
L. sural–lat mall	1. Mid-calf	Ankle	3.15	4.05	12.2	14	44.4

Motor NCS

Nerve	Sites	Recording Site	Latency (ms)	Amplitude (mV)	Distance (cm)	Velocity (m/s)
L. median–APB	1. Wrist	APB	3.65	5.4	7	—
	2. Elbow	APB	7.55	4.5	21.5	55.1
L. ulnar–ADM	1. Wrist	ADM	3.15	10.5	7	—
	2. B. elbow	ADM	5.80	9.2	16	60.4
	3. A. elbow	ADM	7.40	9.4	12.5	78.1
L. peroneal–EDB	1. Ankle	EDB	5.30	4.5	8	—
	2. Fib head	EDB	11.90	3.7	28	42.4
	3. Pop fossa	EDB	13.75	4.2	9	48.6

Needle EMG Summary Table

	IA	SA			Amplitude (MUs)	Duration (MUs)	PolyP (MUs)	Activation	Recruitment Pattern
		Fib	Fasc	Other					
L. deltoid	Incr	1+	0	0	Nl	Nl	Nl	Full	Nl
L. biceps	Incr	2+	0	0	Small	Brief	Few	Full	Early
L. triceps	Incr	2+	0	0	Small	Brief	Many	Full	Early
L. FCU	Incr	3+	0	CRD	Small	Brief and long	Many	Full	Early
L. first dors int	Incr	1+	0	0	Nl	Nl	Nl	Full	Nl
L. glut med	Incr	2+	0	0	Small	Brief	Few	Full	Early
L. vast lat	Incr	3+	0	0	Small	Brief and long	Many	Full	Early
L. iliopsoas	Incr	2+	0	0	Small	Brief and long	Many	Full	Early
L. tib ant	Incr	2+	0	0	Small	Brief and long	Many	Full	Early
L. thoracic PSP upper	Incr	1+	0	0	—	—	—	—	—

Questions:
1. What is your differential diagnosis?
2. How would you interpret this study?
3. What is the most common myopathy in this age group?
4. How would you proceed with the diagnostic evaluation?
5. What does the muscle biopsy show?

Answers:
1. Inflammatory myopathy, myasthenia gravis, sarcoid myopathy
2. Myopathy with muscle membrane irritability
3. Inclusion body myositis
4. Muscle biopsy
5. Vacuolated muscle fibers

Discussion: The early recruitment of motor units and the presence of short-duration and small-amplitude motor unit action potentials is characteristic of a myopathy, and the fibrillation potentials provide evidence of associated muscle membrane irritability. The most common myopathy with age of onset over the age of 50 is inclusion body myositis (IBM). A muscle biopsy would be indicated to pursue the diagnosis, and this was done (see figure).

On the basis of the exam findings, a diagnosis of IBM was suspected. Muscle biopsy confirmed the diagnosis, showing vacuolated muscle fibers (see figure) and invasion of non-necrotic muscle fibers (not shown). IBM is characterized clinically by the insidious onset of slowly progressive proximal and distal weakness that generally develops after the age of 50 years. The slow evolution of the disease process probably accounts in part for the delay in diagnosis, averaging approximately 6 years from the onset of symptoms. Men are much more commonly affected than women, in contrast to the female predominance seen in dermatomyositis (DM) and polymyositis (PM). The clinical hallmark of IBM is early weakness and atrophy of the quadriceps, volar forearm muscles (*i.e.*, wrist and finger flexors), and ankle dorsiflexors. We have invariably found that the manual muscle scores of the finger and wrist flexors are lower than those of the shoulder abductors, and the muscle scores of the knee extensors are lower than those of the hip flexors in patients with IBM. The opposite relationship between muscles scores is present in DM and PM. In addition, muscle involvement in IBM is often asymmetric, in contrast to the symmetrical involvement in DM and PM. The presence of slowly progressive, asymmetric quadriceps and wrist/finger flexor weakness in a patient over 50 years of age strongly suggests the diagnosis of IBM.

Serum CK is normal or only mildly elevated (less than tenfold above normal). EMG studies demonstrate increased spontaneous and insertional activity, small polyphasic MUPs, and early recruitment. In addition, large polyphasic MUPs can also be demonstrated in one third of patients; however, large polyphasic MUPs can also be seen in DM, PM, and other muscle disorders (*e.g.*, muscular dystrophies) and probably reflect chronicity of the disease process rather than a neurogenic etiology. Nevertheless, nerve conduction studies reveal evidence of a mild axonal sensory neuropathy in up to 30% of patients.

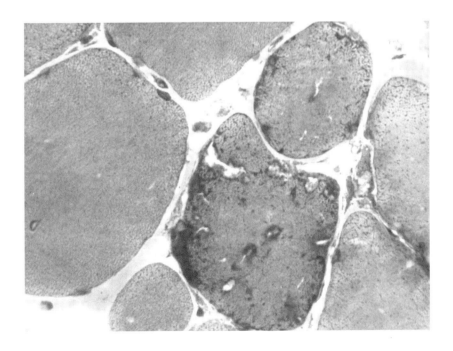

The characteristic light microscopic findings are endomysial inflammation, small groups of atrophic fibers, eosinophilic cytoplasmic inclusions, and muscle fibers with one or more rimmed vacuoles lined with granular material. Amyloid deposition is evident on Congo red staining using polarized light or fluorescence techniques. Increased numbers of ragged red fibers and COX-negative fibers are also evident in IBM compared to DM and PM patients and age-matched controls. Electron microscopy demonstrates 15- to 21-nm cytoplasmic and intranuclear tubulofilaments, although a minimum of three vacuolated fibers may have to be scrutinized to confirm their presence. Vacuolated fibers also contain cytoplasmic clusters of 6- to 10-nm amyloid-like fibrils. Because of sampling error, repeat muscle biopsies may be required to identify the rimmed vacuoles and abnormal tubulofilament or amyloid accumulation in order to histologically confirm the diagnosis of IBM. This sampling error probably accounts for IBM being misdiagnosed as PM.

The pathogenesis of IBM is unknown. Whether IBM is a primary inflammatory myopathy like DM and PM or a myopathy in which the inflammatory response plays a secondary role is the subject of intense research. IBM is slowly progressive and unfortunately does not respond well to immunosuppressive medications.

Clinical Pearls

1. The most common myopathy with onset after age 50 is inclusion body myositis.
2. EMG studies typically show muscle membrane irritability with fibrillation potentials and positive sharp waves in the inflammatory myopathies.

REFERENCES

1. Barohn, R.J., Amato, A.A., Kissel, J.T., Sahenk, Z., Mendell, J.R., Inclusion body myositis: response to immunosuppressive therapy, *Neurology* 1995; 45:1302–1304.
2. Amato, A.A., Gronseth, G.S., Jackson, C.E., Wolfe, G.I., Katz, J.S., Bryan, W.W., Barohn, R.J., Inclusion body myositis: clinical and pathological boundaries, *Ann. Neurol.* 1996; 40:581–586.
3. Greenberg, S.A., Sanoudou, D., Haslett, J.N., Kohane, I.S., Kunkel, L.M., Beggs, A.H., Amato, A.A., Molecular profiles of inflammatory myopathies, *Neurology* 2002; 59:1170–1182.

PATIENT 55

A 46-year-old woman with a 2-year history of proximal leg and arm weakness

This 46-year-old woman noted that approximately 2 years ago she began having difficulty walking down steps and getting up out of a chair. Additionally, she began having difficulty swallowing approximately 15 months ago. She has difficulty swallowing solid foods and feels that they get caught at the back of her throat. She has had no numbness or tingling. She has not had any rashes on the face, neck, or shawl area. Neurological examination was notable for normal muscle bulk and tone. No action or percussion myotonia, paramyotonia, or fasciculations were noted. Muscle strength was as follows: neck flexion, 4–; extension, 5; deltoids, 4; biceps, 4; triceps, 4; wrist extension, 5–; wrist flexion, 5; and finger extension and flexion, 5 bilaterally. No winging of the scapula was seen. In the lower extremities, hip flexion, extension and abduction were 4–/5; knee extension, 5–; knee flexion, 4+; and ankle dorsiflexion and plantar flexion, 5.

Electrodiagnostic Study:

Sensory NCS

Nerve	Sites	Recording Site	Onset (ms)	Peak (ms)	BP Amplitude (µV)	Distance (cm)	Velocity (m/s)
R. median–dig II	1. Wrist	Dig II	2.35	3.05	32.7	13	55.3
R. ulnar–dig V	1. Wrist	Dig V	1.95	2.65	29.5	11	56.4
R. sural–lat mall	1. Mid-calf	Ankle	2.90	3.90	16.4	14	48.3

Motor NCS

Nerve	Sites	Recording Site	Latency (ms)	Amplitude (mV)	Distance (cm)	Velocity (m/s)
R. peroneal–EDB	1. Ankle	EDB	4.45	5.4	8	—
	2. Fib head	EDB	10.75	4.9	33.5	53.2
	3. Pop fossa	EDB	12.70	4.7	10	51.3
R. tibial–AH	1. Ankle	AH	4.00	10.8	8	—
	2. Pop fossa	AH	13.30	8.5	43	46.2
R. median–APB	1. Wrist	APB	3.65	5.4	7	—
	2. Elbow	APB	7.45	5.4	22.5	59.2
R. ulnar–ADM	1. Wrist	ADM	2.95	11.1	7	—
	2. B. elbow	ADM	6.55	9.6	21.5	59.7
	3. A. elbow	ADM	8.85	9.0	12	52.2

Needle EMG Summary Table

		SA							
	IA	Fib	Fasc	Other	Amplitude (MUs)	Duration (MUs)	PolyP (MUs)	Activation	Recruitment Pattern
R. deltoid	Incr	Nl	0	0	Nl	Nl	Nl	Full	Nl
R. biceps	Nl	Nl	0	0	Nl	Nl	Nl	Full	Nl
R. FDI	Nl	Nl	0	0	Nl	Nl	Nl	Full	Nl

Continued

		SA		Amplitude	Duration	PolyP		Recruitment
	IA	Fib	Fasc	Other	(MUs)	(MUs)	(MUs)	Activation	Pattern
R. low thoracic paraspinals	Incr	2+	0	0	—	—	—	—	—
R. glu medius	Incr	2+	0	0	Small	Short	Many	Full	Early
R. vastus lateralis	Incr	2+	0	0	Small	Short	Many	Full	Early
R. FHL	Nl	Nl	0	0	Nl	Nl	Nl	Full	Nl

Questions:
1. How would you interpret the EMG/NCS findings?
2. Does this help narrow the differential diagnosis?
3. What further tests and work-up would be helpful?
4. What does the muscle biopsy demonstrate?

Answers:
1. Myopathy with membrane irritability in proximal muscles
2. Narrows to myopathy
3. Serum CK, muscle biopsy
4. Invasion of non-necrotic fibers by inflammatory cells

Discussion: There is electrophysiological evidence of a myopathy with muscle membrane irritability in proximal muscle groups. This is a nonspecific finding and may be seen in inflammatory myopathies, muscular dystrophies, toxic myopathies, certain congenital myopathies (*e.g.*, myofibrillar myopathy), and some metabolic myopathies (*e.g.*, acid maltase deficiency). The differential diagnosis in a middle-aged adult with an insidious onset of progressive, symmetrical, proximal greater than distal weakness would include a form of motor neuron disease (*e.g.*, adult-onset spinal muscular atrophy, Kennedy's disease), a neuromuscular junction disorder (*e.g.*, myasthenia gravis, Lambert–Eaton syndrome), polyneuropathy (*e.g.*, chronic inflammatory polyradiculoneuropathy), and various myopathies (myositis, limb-girdle muscular dystrophy, and endocrine, metabolic, toxic, and some congenital myopathies). The electrodiagnostic studies in this case were very helpful in pointing toward a myopathic etiology. Further, the muscle membrane irritability excludes many of the endocrine myopathies (*i.e.*, hypothyroid, Cushing's syndrome) and congenital myopathies that have little in the way of abnormal insertional and spontaneous activity. However, the EMG cannot narrow the differential diagnosis any further, and additional tests are required, including a muscle biopsy. Laboratory work-up revealed creatine phosphokinase (CPK) ranging from 684 to 713 IU/L. A muscle biopsy of the left quadriceps was performed (see figure).

The biopsy demonstrated endomysial inflammation with invasion of non-necrotic muscle fibers consistent with the diagnosis of polymyositis. Polymyositis is a major form of idiopathic inflammatory myopathy, along with dermatomyositis and inclusion body myositis (IBM). Although it is often thought to be the most common form of myositis, it is in fact the least common. Many cases of IBM and limb-girdle muscular dystrophy with inflammation have been incorrectly diagnosed as polymyositis. The pattern of muscle weakness with symmetric proximal greater than distal weakness can help distinguish polymyositis from IBM. The clinical examination and special stains on muscle biopsy are useful in differentiating polymyositis from limb-girdle muscular dystrophy, acid maltase deficiency, and congenital myopathies that may have similar clinical presentations and electrodiagnostic findings. Polymyositis is usually responsive to corticosteroids. Intravenous immunoglobulin (IVIg), methotrexate, azathioprine, or mycophenolate mofetil may be used in patients refractory to steroids or as steroid sparing agents.

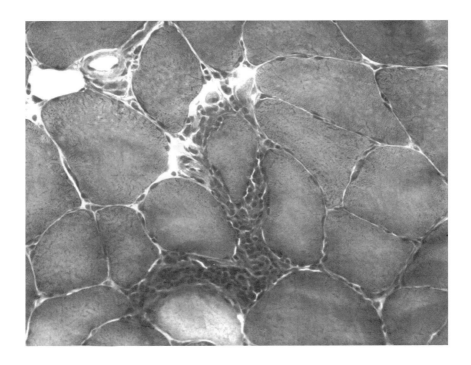

Clinical Pearls

1. Polymyositis is the least common of the inflammatory myopathies.
2. Treatment-resistant polymyositis is usually a mistaken diagnosis—most such patients have inclusion body myositis (IBM) or a muscular dystrophy.

REFERENCES

1. Amato, A.A., Barohn, R.J., Idiopathic inflammatory myopathies, *Neurol. Clin*. 1997; 15:615–648.
2. Briemberg, H.R., Amato, A.A., Dermatomyositis and polymyositis, *Curr. Treat. Options Neurol*. 2003; 5:349–356.
3. Dalakas, M.C., Progress in inflammatory myopathies: good but not good enough, *J. Neurol. Neurosurg. Psychiatry* 2001; 70:569–573.
4. Dalakas, M.C., Hohlfeld, R., Polymyosits and dermatomyositis, *Lancet* 2003; 362: 971–982.
5. Van Der Meulen, M.F., Bronner, I.M., Hoogendijk, J.E., Burger, H., Van Venrooij, W.J., Voskuyl, A.E., Dinant, H.J., Linssen, W.H., Wokke, J.H., De Visser, M., Polymyositis: an overdiagnosed entity, *Neurology* 2003; 61:316–321.

PATIENT 56

A 59-year-old woman with proximal weakness and a rash

This 59-year-old woman noted an erythematous rash on her face, trunk, and extremities 1 year prior to evaluation. Eight months ago she began to develop symmetrical proximal leg weakness followed by proximal arm weakness. She complained of arthralgias but no myalgias. She denies dysphagia, dyspnea, or ocular symptoms. She has had no sensory symptoms, numbness, tingling, or paresthesia. She has had no fevers, night sweats. General physical examination showed an erythematous papular rash present all over the extensor surfaces. This was particularly prominent over the knuckles of her hands (Gottron's papules), and she also had evidence of some telangiectasia of her nail beds. The rash was also present over her anterior neck, face, back, and on her thighs and buttocks.

Motor examination revealed normal muscle bulk and tone. Strength in her neck flexion was 4+/5. Neck extension was 5/5. Strength diffusely in her upper extremities seemed to be 4/5 in her deltoids bilaterally. Biceps and triceps were 4+/5. Wrist flexion and extension were also 4+/5, as was distally finger extension and finger flexion. In her lower extremities, her hip flexion, abduction, and extension were 4/5. Knee flexion was 4+/5 and knee extension was 5–. Ankle dorsiflexion was 4+/5 and plantar flexion was 5. Laboratory investigations showed that her sedimentation rate was normal at 18 mm/hr, and the serum CPK was normal at 80 IU/L.

Electrodiagnostic Study:

Sensory NCS

Nerve	Sites	Recording Site	Onset (ms)	Peak (ms)	BP Amplitude (μV)	Distance (cm)	Velocity (m/s)
R. median–dig II	1. Wrist	Dig II	2.50	3.50	40.8	13	52.0
R. ulnar–dig V	1. Wrist	Dig V	2.20	3.10	24.3	11	50.0
R. sural–lat mall	1. Mid-calf	Ankle	2.85	3.65	24.7	14	49.1
L. sural–lat mall	1. Mid-calf	Ankle	3.10	3.95	9.7	14	45.2

Motor NCS

Nerve	Sites	Recording Site	Latency (ms)	Amplitude (mV)	Distance (cm)	Velocity (m/s)
R. median–APB	1. Wrist	APB	3.50	4.0	7	—
	2. Elbow	APB	7.00	3.8	20.5	58.6
R. median–APB	1. Wrist	APB	3.45	3.8	7	—
10 s post-exercise	2. Wrist	APB	3.45	3.8	—	—
R. ulnar–ADM	1. Wrist	ADM	2.85	8.2	7	—
	2. B. elbow	ADM	5.50	8.0	17	64.2
	3. A. elbow	ADM	7.10	8.1	12	75.0
R. peroneal–EDB	1. Ankle	EDB	4.05	4.7	8	—
	2. Fib head	—	9.40	4.5	27	50.5
	3. Pop fossa	—	10.35	4.5	6	63.2
R. tibial–AH	1. Ankle	AH	5.35	10.6	8	—
	2. Pop fossa	—	11.20	11.3	33.5	57.3

F-Wave

Nerve	F_{min} (ms)	F_{max} (ms)	Max − Min (ms)	%F
R. median	25.50	28.80	3.30	80
R. ulnar	24.40	27.55	3.15	100
R. peroneal	41.10	47.20	6.10	50
R. tibial	44.80	53.65	8.85	100

Needle EMG Summary Table

		SA			Amplitude (MUs)	Duration (MUs)	PolyP (MUs)	Activation	Recruitment Pattern
	IA	Fib	Fasc	Other					
R. deltoid	Incr	0	0	0	Small	Brief	Many	Full	Early
R. biceps	Nl	0	0	0	Small	Brief	Nl	Full	Early
R. first dors int	Nl	0	0	0	Nl	Nl	Nl	Full	Nl
R. glut med	Incr	1+	0	0	Small	Brief	Many	Full	Early
R. iliopsoas	Incr	0	0	0	Small	Brief	Many	Full	Early
R. vast lat	Nl	0	0	0	Small	Brief	Nl	Full	Early
R. flexor hal	Nl	0	0	0	Nl	Nl	Nl	Full	Nl
R. thoracic PSP lower	Incr	2+	0	0	—	—	—	—	—

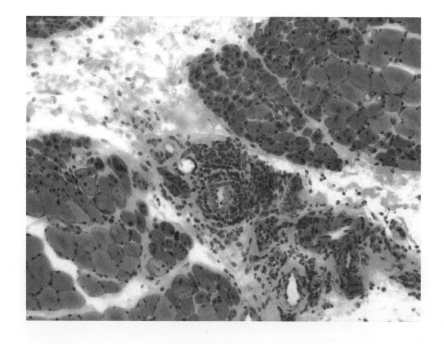

Question: What is your differential diagnosis?

Answer: Dermatomyositis, inflammatory myopathy with systemic lupus erythematosus

Discussion: Nerve conduction studies were normal, but the electromyography revealed evidence of a proximal myopathy with muscle membrane irritability. The history, clinical examination (particularly the characteristic rash), and the electrophysiologic findings are suggestive of a diagnosis of dermatomyositis. The patient underwent a muscle biopsy of her left deltoid muscle, which confirmed the clinical impression of dermatomyositis. Dermatomyositis is a humorally mediated microangiopathy that can present at any age, including childhood. The characteristic histological abnormality is perifascicular atrophy, but this is not always present. Inflammation, when evident, is perivascular and located in the perimysium. This patient's biopsy demonstrated both perivascular inflammation and perifasicular atrophy. As with other autoimmune disorders, women are affected more frequently than men (2:1 ratio). The characteristic rash usually precedes or accompanies muscle weakness. Importantly, serum CK can be normal in dermatomyositis. The severity of muscle weakness does not correlate with the degree of CK elevation. EMG usually demonstrates evidence of increased insertional activity and muscle membrane instability in the form of fibrillation potentials, positive sharp waves, and complex repetitive discharges in proximal more than distal muscles. In early or mild disease, these abnormalities may only be appreciated in the proximal muscles, as they are the most proximal muscle group. We routinely study the thoracic paraspinals, as these muscles do not typically have muscle membrane irritability related to degenerative disease of spine.

There is an increased risk of malignancy in patients with dermatomyositis; therefore, patients should undergo yearly malignancy screening to include complete physical exam, breast, pelvic and rectal exams, mammogram, pelvic ultrasound/CT, and colonoscopy if over 50 years of age or if rectal exams demonstrate blood. Dermatomyositis is typically very responsive to corticosteroids. IVIg, methotrexate, or azathioprine may be used in patients refractory to steroids or as steroid sparing agents.

Clinical Pearls

1. The pathogenesis of dermatomyositis (DM) is distinct from polymyositis; perifascicular atrophy, when present, is specific for DM.
2. The serum CK may be normal in dermatomyositis.

REFERENCES
1. Amato, A.A., Barohn, R.J., Idiopathic inflammatory myopathies, *Neurol. Clin.* 1997; 15:615–648.
2. Briemberg, H.R., Amato, A.A., Dermatomyositis and polymyositis, *Curr. Treat. Options Neurol.* 2003; 5:349–356.
3. Dalakas, M.C., Progress in inflammatory myopathies: good but not good enough, *J. Neurol. Neurosurg. Psychiatry* 2001; 70:569–573.
4. Dalakas, M.C., Therapeutic approaches in patients with inflammatory myopathies, *Semin. Neurol.* 2003; 23:199–206.

PATIENT 57

A 70-year-old man with difficulty climbing stairs for several years

A 70-year-old white man complained of difficulty climbing stairs for about 2 or 3 years. He described stiffness in his leg muscles that was worse in the morning and better with activity. Past medical history was remarkable for excision of cataracts when he was about 37 years of age. Family history is only remarkable for his mother having leg weakness in her 70s. Review of systems was remarkable for hearing loss and impotence. On examination, he was a well-developed male. There was thinning of his quadriceps muscles bilaterally. No action or percussion myotonia, paramyotonia, myoedema, or fasciculations were evident in proximal or distal muscle groups. Manual muscle testing revealed the following MRC scores: orbicularis oculi, 4; neck flexion, 4; extension, 5; shoulder abduction and elbow extension, 4; elbow flexion, 4; wrist flexion and extension, 5–; and hand intrinsics, 5. In the lower extremities, he was 4– in the hip girdle, 5 in knee extension, and 5 in ankle dorsiflexion and plantar flexion. Sensation, coordination, gait, and reflexes were normal.

Electrodiagnostic Study:

Sensory NCS

Nerve	Sites	Recording Site	Onset (ms)	Peak (ms)	BP Amplitude (µV)	Distance (cm)	Velocity (m/s)
L. ulnar–dig V	1. Wrist	Dig V	2.40	3.15	14.9	11	45.8
L. radial–sn box	1. Forearm	Sn box	1.95	2.45	22.0	10	51.3
L. sural–lat mall	1. Mid-calf	Ankle	3.50	4.25	5.3	14	40.0
R. sural–lat mall	1. Mid-calf	Ankle	3.45	4.55	5.5	14	40.6

Motor NCS

Nerve	Sites	Recording Site	Latency (ms)	Amplitude (mV)	Distance (cm)	Velocity (m/s)
L. median–APB	1. Wrist	APB	3.85	4.7	7	—
	2. Elbow	APB	8.35	4.4	23.5	52.2
L. ulnar–ADM	1. Wrist	ADM	2.80	9.6	7	—
	2. B. elbow	ADM	6.55	9.0	21	56.0
	3. A. elbow	ADM	8.50	8.9	12	61.5
L. peroneal–EDB	1. Ankle	EDB	4.85	2.6	8	—
	2. Fib head	EDB	13.30	2.4	32.5	38.5
	3. Pop fossa	EDB	16.00	2.4	10	37.0
L. tibial–AH	1. Ankle	AH	5.15	3.4	8	—
	2. Pop fossa	AH	15.50	2.9	42	40.6

F-Wave

Nerve	F_{min} (ms)	F_{max} (ms)	Max – Min (ms)	%F
L. peroneal	61	64	3.30	60
L. tibial	59.95	64.80	4.85	60
L. median	29.40	33.25	3.85	50
L. ulnar	29.35	32.35	3.00	100

		SA			Amplitude (MUs)	Duration (MUs)	PolyP (MUs)	Activation	Recruitment Pattern
	IA	Fib	Fasc	Other					
R. deltoid	Incr	2+	0	Myot	Nl	Nl	Few	Full	Nl
R. biceps	Incr	2+	0	Myot	Small	Small	Few	Full	Early
R. FDI	Incr	1+	0	Myot	Nl	Nl	Nl	Full	Nl
R. glut med	Incr	2+	0	Myot	Small	Small	Few	Full	Early
R. vast lat	Incr	2+	0	Myot	Nl	Nl	Few	Full	Nl
R. FHL	Incr	1+	0	Myot	Nl	Nl	Nl	Full	Nl

Questions:
1. What is your differential diagnosis?
2. Were there any clues from the history?
3. What other work-up would you recommend?

Answers:

1. Myotonic dystrophy type 1 and 2, myotonia congenita, paramyotonia congenita, toxic myopathy
2. Positive family history of cataracts and deafness
3. Genetic testing for PROMM

Discussion: There was electrophysiologic evidence of a generalized myopathy with associated muscle membrane irritability and myotonic discharges. Myopathies that can present with proximal weakness, clinical myotonia, and myotonic discharges on needle EMG include myotonic dystrophy (types 1 and 2), myotonia congenita, paramyotonia congenita, and potassium-sensitive periodic paralysis. Disorders that present with proximal weakness and myotonic discharges on EMG but no clinical myotonia include acid maltase deficiency, rarely inflammatory myopathies, myofibrillar myopathy, certain vacuolar myopathies, and some toxic myopathies secondary to drugs (*e.g.*, colchicines, chloroquine, statin agents).

The patient's positive family history (mother developing proximal leg weakness in her 70s), history of early cataracts, impotence, deafness and significant proximal weakness along with the electrophysiologic evidence of a myopathy with myotonic discharges raised the possibility of proximal myotonic myopathy (PROMM) or myotonic dystrophy type 2. Usually, but not invariably, these patients also have clinical myotonia, which he did not appear to have. DNA testing was subsequently performed which confirmed a mutation in the zinc finger-9 (*ZNF9*) gene, which is responsible for PROMM. Whereas DM1 has a predilection for the distal muscles, patients with DM2 or PROMM have greater stiffness, pain, and weakness in proximal than distal muscles. Transmission is also by autosomal dominant inheritance. Cataracts are part of the phenotype, but gonadal atrophy and cardiac conduction defects are much less common than in DM1. The initial complaints—muscle stiffness and pain—usually have their onset in adult life. The pain is a sense of discomfort and varies from sharp to a deep visceral ache. The stiffness is a sense of having a tight muscle that causes reluctance to move. It commonly affects the thighs and may be asymmetrical. The severity of myotonia may vary from day to day.

The prognosis is relatively good. Patients with PROMM usually do not have significant cardiac disease as seen in DM1. EMG shows myotonia but may require a careful search of several muscles. Muscle histology shows features similar to DM1. The serum CK concentration may be elevated. The genetic defect has been localized to mutations in the gene that encodes for *ZNF9* on chromosome 3q21. The mutations are expanded CCTG repeats in intron 1. As with DM1, the expanded repeat probably leads to the expression of a toxic pre-mRNA that impairs the splicing of other mRNA species, including those of ion channels.

Clinical Pearl

The differential diagnosis for a myopathy with myotonic discharges is limited, as noted in the text.

REFERENCES

1. Day, J.W., Ricker, K., Jacobsen, J.F., Rasmussen, L.J., Dick, K.A., Kress, W., Schneider, C., Koch, M.C., Beilman, G.J., Harrison, A.R., Dalton, J.C., Ranum, L.P., Myotonic dystrophy type 2: molecular, diagnostic and clinical spectrum, *Neurology* 2003; 60:657–664.
2. Liquori, C.L., Ricker, K., Mosely, M.L. *et al.*, Myotonic dystrophy type 2 caused by a CCTG expansion in intron 1 of *ZNF9*, *Science* 2001; 293:864–867.
3. Mankodi, A., Takahashi, M.P., Jiang, H., Beck, C.L., Bowers, W.J., Moxley, R.T., Cannon, S.C., Thornton, C.A., Expanded CUG repeats trigger aberrant splicing of ClC-1 chloride channel pre-mRNA and hyperexcitability of skeletal muscle in myotonic dystrophy, *Mol. Cell* 2002; 10:35–44.
4. Mankodi, A., Thornton, C.A., Myotonic syndromes, *Curr. Opin. Neurol.* 2002; 15:545–552.
5. Meola, G., Sansone, V., Marinou, K., Cotelli, M., Moxley, R.T., 3rd, Thornton, C.A., De Ambroggi, L., Proximal myotonic myopathy: a syndrome with a favourable prognosis?, *J. Neurol. Sci.* 2002; 193:89–96.
6. Moxley. R.T., 3rd, Proximal myotonic myopathy: mini-review of a recently delineated clinical disorder, *Neuromuscul. Disord.* 1996; 6:87–93.

PATIENT 58

A 50-year-old woman with HIV infection and weakness of her arms and legs for 6 months

A 50-year-old woman with an 11-year history of HIV infection complained of weakness in her arms and legs for at least 6 months. She also had numbness and paresthesia in her feet for several years. She denied myalgias or muscle cramps. She noted some swallowing difficulties for at least 2 years and denied double vision, ptosis, fluctuation of her weakness in her extremities, and back or neck pain.

Laboratory studies showed serum CK persistently elevated, as high as 1900 IU/L. Thyroid function tests were normal and antinuclear antibody (ANA) was negative. Her HIV viral load was high, while the CD-4 count was low. Her medications were antiretroviral medications, including nevirapine. Of note, she was off these medications for 1 month without any change in her symptoms. Examination was notable for no rash. Motor exam revealed normal muscle bulk and tone. There was no evidence of atrophy or fasciculations. Muscle strength testing revealed symmetric, proximal greater than distal weakness in the arms and legs. Sensory testing demonstrated decreased vibratory perception in the toes. The patient had a normal gait. She did have difficulty arising from a squat. Deep tendon reflexes were 2+ at the biceps, triceps, brachioradialis, and knees but 0 at the ankles. Plantar responses were flexor bilaterally.

Electrodiagnostic Study:

Sensory NCS

Nerve	Sites	Recording Site	Onset (ms)	Peak (ms)	BP Amplitude (μV)	Distance (cm)	Velocity (m/s)
R. median–dig II	1. Wrist	Dig II	2.70	3.45	38.5	13	48.1
R. ulnar–dig V	1. Wrist	Dig V	1.95	2.75	28.6	11	56.4
R. radial–sn box	1. Forearm	Sn box	1.55	2.05	26.6	10	64.5
R. sural–lat mall	1. Mid-calf	Ankle	3.80	4.55	2.7	14	36.8
L. sural–lat mall	1. Mid-calf	Ankle	3.60	4.25	1.6	14	38.9

Motor NCS

Nerve	Sites	Recording Site	Latency (ms)	Amplitude (mV)	Distance (cm)	Velocity (m/s)
R. median–APB	1. Wrist	APB	3.50	6.7	7	—
	2. Elbow	APB	7.45	6.3	21.5	54.4
R. ulnar–ADM	1. Wrist	ADM	2.55	8.9	7	—
	2. B. elbow	ADM	5.85	8.1	18.5	56.1
	3. A. elbow	ADM	8.05	8.1	12	54.5
R. peroneal–EDB	1. Ankle	EDB	3.55	3.5	8	—
	2. Fib head	EDB	11.00	3.3	32.5	43.6
	3. Pop fossa	EDB	12.35	2.9	8	59.3
R tibial–AH	1. Ankle	AH	5.95	6.2	8	—
	2. Pop fossa	AH	12.90	4.5	38.5	55.4

F-Wave

Nerve	F_{min} (ms)	F_{max} (ms)	Max – Min (ms)	%F
R. median	28.10	29.55	1.45	70
R. tibial	61.45	64.80	3.35	40

Needle EMG Summary Table

		SA			Amplitude (MUs)		Duration (MUs)		PolyP (MUs)	Activation	Recruitment Pattern
	IA	Fib	Fasc	Other							
R. deltoid	Incr	2+	0	0	Nl	—	Nl	—	Nl	Full	Nl
R. biceps	Incr	3+	0	0	Few	Small	Few	Brief	Few	Full	Mild early
R. triceps	Incr	2+	0	0	Few	Small	Few	Mixed	Few	Full	Mild early
R. pron teres	Incr	2+	0	0	Few	Mixed	Few	Brief	Few	Full	Early
R. first dors int	Incr	2+	0	0	Few	Mixed	Few	Mixed	Few	Full	Nl

Questions:
1. What is your differential diagnosis?
2. How would you interpret this study? Does it narrow down your differential diagnosis?
3. Would you perform any other tests?
4. How would you treat the patient?

Answers:
1. Toxic myopathy, primary inflammatory myopathy, HIV associated myopathy
2. Myopathy and distal axonal sensory neuropathy
3. Muscle biopsy
4. Corticosteroids

Discussion: The patient's history and examination suggested a long-standing sensory neuropathy that was supported by the nerve conduction studies demonstrating low-amplitude sural sensory nerve action potentials (SNAPs). It is possible that the neuropathy is the HIV-associated distal symmetric polyneuropathy (HIV-DSP) or a toxic neuropathy related to her use of nucleoside analogs. In addition, the EMG demonstrated evidence of a diffuse myopathic process with muscle membrane instability and small, polyphasic motor units that recruited early. She had a muscle biopsy that demonstrated features of HIV myositis. She was treated with IVIg without response. Subsequently, she was started on corticosteroids and had significant improvement in strength and normalization of her serum CK.

Patients with HIV infection can manifest with weakness secondary to central etiologies (*e.g.*, myelopathy), motor neuropathies, peripheral neuropathies, and myopathies. Myopathies associated with HIV infection are uncommon but certainly occur. These include mitochondrial myopathy related to antiretroviral medication (*e.g.*, zidovudine AZT), inflammatory myopathies (HIV myositis, inclusion body myositis, secondary infections of muscle), and type 2 muscle fiber atrophy secondary to HIV-wasting syndrome. Unfortunately, the exact cause of the myopathy is often not clear, as patients may have a combination of myositis, AZT myopathy, and HIV-wasting syndrome, not to mention a peripheral neuropathy related to the infection or medications. Differentiating these conditions requires a detailed history, neurological examination, laboratory studies, neurophysiological testing, and sometimes a muscle biopsy. Inflammatory myopathies are associated with symmetric proximal greater than distal weakness, elevated serum CKs, and EMG demonstrating myopathic MUAPs and abnormal insertional and spontaneous activity (*e.g.*, fibrillation potentials and positive sharp waves). A toxic myopathy related to the antiviral medication AZT is usually associated with impaired mitochondria, which on muscle biopsy is characterized by the presence of ragged red fibers. Usually, patients have symmetric proximal greater than distal weakness and pain. EMG may demonstrate myopathic units, but there is usually no abnormal insertional or spontaneous activity. Wasting disease occurs in 25 to 50% of patients with AIDS and is associated with severe weight loss and easy fatigability. Serum CK and EMG are usually normal.

At least 20% of patients with HIV develop some form of polyneuropathy during the course of their illness. The seven major types of peripheral neuropathy associated with HIV infection are (1) distal symmetric polyneuropathy (DSP), (2) inflammatory demyelinating polyneuropathy (including both AIDP and CIDP), (3) mononeuropathy multiplex (*e.g.*, vasculitis, CMV related), (4) progressive polyradiculopathy (usually CMV related), (5) autonomic neuropathy, (6) sensory ganglionitis, and (7) toxic neuropathy secondary to nucleoside analogs. DSP is the most common form of peripheral neuropathy associated with HIV infection and usually is seen in patients with AIDS. The nucleoside analogs zalcitabine (dideoxycytidine, or ddC), didanosine (dideoxyinosine, or ddI), stavudine (d4T), lamivudine (3TC), and antiretroviral nucleoside reverse transcriptase inhibitor (NRTI) are used in the treatment of HIV infection. One of the major dose-limiting side effects of these medications is a predominantly sensory, length-dependent, symmetric, painful neuropathy. Patients with DSP and toxic neuropathies related to treatment with nucleoside analogs present with numbness and painful paresthesias of the hands and feet. Nerve conduction studies demonstrate features of a length-dependent axonal neuropathy. It is often difficult to distinguish whether a patient's neuropathy is secondary to DSP or is medication induced; discontinuation of medication and observation are usually required for such a determination.

Clinical Pearl

HIV or its treatment may produce a myopathy with fibrillation potentials.

REFERENCES

1. Barohn, R.J., Gronseth, G.S., LeForce, B.R. *et al.*, Peripheral nervous system involvement in a large cohort of human immunodeficiency virus infected individuals, *Arch. Neurol.* 1993; 50:167–171.
2. Dalakas, M.C., Illa, I., Pezeshkpour, G.H., Mitochondrial myopathy caused by long-term zidovudine therapy, *New Engl. J. Med.* 1990; 322:1098–1105.
3. Simpson, D.M., Citak, K.A., Godfrey, E., Godbold, J., Wolfe, D., Myopathies associated with human immunodeficiency virus and zidovudine: can their effects be distinguished?, *Neurology* 1993; 43:971–976.
4. Simpson, D.M., Olney, R.K., Peripheral neuropathies associated with human immunodeficiency virus infection, *Neurol. Clin.* 1992; 10:685–711.

PATIENT 59

An 85-year-old woman with progressive leg weakness and myalgias

An 85-year-old woman reported a 2-month history of progressive leg weakness and myalgias with significant difficulty going up stairs. She has not noted any upper extremity weakness, dysphagia, ocular symptoms, or significant shortness of breath. She denies any history of cramps or fasciculations. There are no sensory symptoms. She does suffer from chronic mild low back pain but denies any radicular symptoms. Past medical history is significant for hypertension and hypercholesterolemia. She was started on atorvastatin 1 year ago, and additional medications include enalapril, nifedipine, atenolol, and aspirin. Neurological examination showed mild weakness in her deltoids and biceps bilaterally at 4+/5. Strength in her triceps, wrist extensors, wrist flexors, finger extensors, finger flexors, and interossei was 5/5 bilaterally. She had moderate weakness in her hip girdle and hamstrings at 4/5 bilaterally. Quadriceps, dorsiflexors, plantar flexors, invertors, and evertors were all 5/5. There was moderate neck flexor weakness at 4–/5. Sensory exam revealed a mild decrease in vibration in her toes bilaterally. Her gait was narrow based but somewhat shuffling. Her reflexes were 2+ and symmetric at the biceps, brachial radialis, triceps, knees, and ankles. Plantar responses were flexor.

Electrodiagnostic Study:

Sensory NCS

Nerve	Sites	Recording Site	Onset (ms)	Peak (ms)	BP Amplitude (µV)	Distance (cm)	Velocity (m/s)
R. median–dig II	1. Wrist	Dig II	2.85	3.90	21.6	13	45.6
R. sural	1. Calf	Ankle	3.45	4.55	5.5	14	41

Motor NCS

Nerve	Sites	Recording Site	Latency (ms)	Amplitude (mV)	Distance (cm)	Velocity (m/s)
R. median–APB	1. Wrist	APB	4.20	5.0	7	—
R. median–APB	2. Elbow	APB	7.70	5.0	17	48.6
R. tibial–AH	1. Ankle	AH	5.15	3.4	8	—
R. tibial–AH	2. Pop fossa	AH	15.50	2.9	42	40.6

Needle EMG Summary Table

		SA			Amplitude (MUs)	Duration (MUs)	PolyP (MUs)	Activation	Recruitment Pattern
	IA	Fib	Fasc	Other					
R. deltoid	Incr	0	0	0	Few small	Few short	Nl	Full	Early
R. biceps	Incr	1+	0	Myotonia	Few small	Few short	Nl	Full	Early
R. FDI	Nl	0	0	0	Nl	Nl	Nl	Full	Nl
R. iliopsoas	Incr	1+	0	Myotonia	Few small	Few short	Nl	Full	Early
R. vast lat	Incr	0	0	0	Few small	Few short	Nl	Full	Early
R. tib ant	Incr	0	0	0	Nl	Nl	Nl	Full	Nl
R. FHL	Nl	0	0	0	Nl	Nl	Nl	Full	Nl
R. thoracic PSP-mid	Incr	2+	0	0	—	—	—	—	—

1. What is your differential diagnosis?
2. What other recommendations and tests would you suggest?

Answers:
1. Myopathy with myotonic discharges
2. Serum CK, muscle biopsy, genetic testing for myotonic dystrophy type 2

Discussion: There was electrophysiologic evidence of a generalized myopathy with associated muscle membrane irritability and myotonic discharges. Myopathies that can present with proximal weakness, clinical myotonia, and myotonic discharges on EMG include myotonic dystrophy (types 1 and 2), myotonia congenita, paramyotonia congenita, and potassium-sensitive periodic paralysis. Disorders that present with proximal weakness and myotonic discharges on EMG but no clinical myotonia include acid maltase deficiency, rarely inflammatory myopathies, myofibrillar myopathy, certain vacuolar myopathy, and some toxic myopathies secondary to drugs (*e.g.*, chloroquine, statin agents).

Initial work-up revealed an elevated CK of between 5300 and 6000 IU/L. In order to exclude a treatable inflammatory myopathy, we opted to perform a biopsy of the left biceps muscle. This muscle was chosen because it was clinically weak and the contralateral muscle had abnormalities on EMG. The muscle biopsy demonstrated scattered necrotic and regenerating muscle fibers with increased internal nuclei. There was no evidence of a primary inflammatory myopathy. The atorvastatin was subsequently stopped, and the patient was closely followed in the clinic. Her serum CKs and muscle strength gradually returned to normal, and the myalgias resolved within a couple of months.

Another option would have been to have stopped the atorvastatin and to follow her before proceeding with a biopsy; however, the duration of the toxic side effects are not well known. We have seen patients who continue to complain of symptoms for several months after stopping the medication. We did not want to delay treatment of a possible inflammatory myopathy in a patient who is clinically weak, thus the biopsy.

Clinical Pearl

The statin agents may be associated with a myopathy in which myotonic discharges are frequently seen. In rare cases, rhabdomyolysis may result.

REFERENCES
1. Meriggioli, M.N., Barboi, A., Rowin, J., Cochran, E.J., HMG-CoA reductase inhibitor myopathy: clinical, electrophysiologic, and pathologic data in five patients. *J. Clin. Neuromusc. Dis.* 2001; 2:129–134.
2. Thompson, P.D., Clarkson, P., Karas, R.H., Statin-associated myopathy, *JAMA* 2003; 289:1681–1690.

PATIENT 60

A 38-year-old man with myasthenia gravis complaining of muscular stiffness and rippling

A 38-year-old man developed bilateral arm flexion weakness, hypophonia, dysphagia, and nasal regurgitation of liquids which progressed over 1 year. Serum CK ranged from 130 to 240 mg/dl (normal, 200 mg/dl). Left deltoid muscle biopsy showed degenerating and regenerating muscle fibers and epimysial and endomysial inflammatory cell infiltrates. He was diagnosed with an inflammatory myopathy and treated with prednisone; within 2 weeks, he noted substantial improvement. He tapered his prednisone over 9 months, and relapsed with proximal arm weakness, diplopia, jaw fatigue, dysphagia, and head drop, and he had a marked response to edrophonium testing. Further evaluation showed a 25% decrement to low-frequency repetitive nerve stimulation of the spinal accessory nerve and normal needle EMG studies of a single deltoid muscle. The acetylcholine receptor antibody level was 65.2 (normal, <0.08), and chest CT showed a 3×3×2-cm anterior mediastinal mass. He was treated with 60 mg/day of prednisone for 6 weeks without benefit, underwent plasmapharesis with improvement, and underwent thymectomy, with pathology revealing a thymoma.

He gradually improved and by the age of 42 was without symptoms on low-dose prednisone for 6 months when he started to note rippling waves of muscle contractions across his chest, back, and limbs that were precipitated by percussion. Rapid extension of his arms became painful with a sensation that a muscle was catching. Serum CK increased over an 18-month period of increasing muscular symptoms from 63 to 788 mg/dl. The acetylcholine receptor antibody level was 5.7. Needle EMG studies did not show fibrillation potentials or myotonic or neuromyotonic discharges. Electrical silence was present during episodes of muscle rippling. Carbamazepine was without significant benefit. He continued to taper his prednisone and went on pyridostigmine alone for 2 years without symptoms of myasthenia gravis but continued to have persistent symptoms of muscle rippling and stiffness with rapid limb movement (see figures).

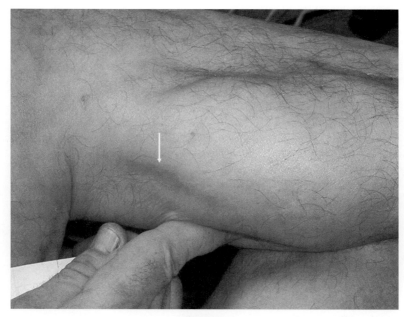

Figure 1

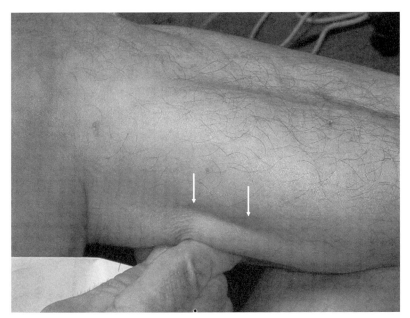

Figure 2

Question: What is the name of this rippling muscle phenomenon?

Answer: Rippling muscle disease

Discussion: Rippling muscle disease has two forms: genetic and acquired. The genetic form may have been commented on in 1974 in the dermatology literature as a transient rippling of the skin in an infant. The syndrome was really identified in 1975 by Torbergsen,[11] who described a family with dominant myotonia. At least two distinct genetic loci exist: a 1q41–q42 locus, for which the gene has not been identified, and a locus at 3p25 at the caveolin 3 gene. Mutations in this gene are also implicated in limb-girdle muscular dystrophy type 1c (LGMD1C) and in some patients with idiopathic elevations of serum CK.

The disorder is a rare, generally benign disorder of muscle stiffness, muscular hypertrophy, and modestly elevated serum CK. It is named for the self-propagating rolling or rippling of muscles induced by passive stretch or percussion, with velocity of ~0.6 m/s (10 times slower than muscle fiber conduction velocity). The muscle contraction is electrically silent and has been hypothesized to be a consequence of intracellular local contraction that induces stretch of mechanosensitive calcium channels in the neighboring sarcomere, initiating a new local contraction and a repetition of the cycle. Additional clinical features are myoedema, a localized mounding of muscle lasting several to 30 seconds and induced by percussion, and percussion contracture, a clinical sign identical to percussion myotonia.

Thymoma is most commonly associated with myasthenia gravis but may be associated with polymyositis or the rare syndromes of rippling muscle disease (RMD) or neuromyotonia. Rippling muscle disease in association with myasthenia gravis had been reported in seven patients as of 2002, the first in 1996. Two of these patients have had thymoma, five have not. Three patients were reported to have electrically active contraction, in stark contrast to all patients with genetic RMD and the other four patients with acquired RMD. Modestly elevated serum CK and very high titers of acetylcholine receptor antibodies have been present in all patients.

Clinical Pearl

Rippling muscle disease is typically familial, although an acquired form reported exclusively in association with myasthenia gravis has been reported in a few patients since 1996.

REFERENCES

1. Ansevin, C.F., Agamanolis, D.P., Rippling muscles and myasthenia gravis with rippling muscles, *Arch. Neurol.* 1996; 53(2):197–199.
2. Ansevin, C.F., Phenotypic variability in rippling muscle disease, *Neurology* 2000; 54(1):273–274.
3. Betz, R.C., Schoser, B.G., Kasper, D., Ricker, K., Ramirez, A., Stein, V., Torbergsen, T., Lee, Y.A., Nothen, M.M., Wienker, T.F., Malin, J.P., Propping, P., Reis, A., Mortier, W., Jentsch, T.J., Vorgerd, M., Kubisch, C., Mutations in CAV3 cause mechanical hyperirritability of skeletal muscle in rippling muscle disease, *Nat. Genet.* 2001; 28(3):218–219.
4. Fine, H.L., Possick, P.A., Myrow, P.F., Transient rippling of the skin (smooth muscle hamartoma?), *Arch. Dermatol.* 1974; 110:141.
5. Greenberg, S.A., Acquired rippling muscle disease with myasthenia gravis, *Muscle Nerve* 2004; 29:143–146.
6. Kosmorsky, G.S., Mehta, N., Mitsumoto, H., Prayson, R., Intermittent esotropia associated with rippling muscle disease, *J. Neuroophthalmol.* 1995; 15(3):147–151.
7. Koul, R.L., Chand, R.P., Chacko, A., Ali, M., Brown, K.M., Bushnarmuth, S.R., Escolar, D.M., Stephan, D.A., Severe autosomal recessive rippling muscle disease, *Muscle Nerve.* 2001; 24(11):1542–1547.
8. Muller-Felber, W., Ansevin, C.F., Ricker, K., Muller-Jenssen, A., Topfer, M., Goebel, H.H., Pongratz, D.E., Immunosuppressive treatment of rippling muscles in patients with myasthenia gravis, *Neuromuscul. Disord.* 1999; 9(8):604–607.
9. So, Y.T., Zu, L., Barraza, C., Figueroa, K.P., Pulst, S.M., Rippling muscle disease: evidence for phenotypic and genetic heterogeneity, *Muscle Nerve* 2001; 24(3):340–344.
10. Stephan, D.A., Hoffman, E.P., Physical mapping of the rippling muscle disease locus, *Genomics* 1999; 55(3):268–274.
11. Torbergsen, T., Rippling muscle disease: a review, *Muscle Nerve* 2002; 11(suppl.):S103–S107.
12. Vernino, S., Auger, R.G., Emslie-Smith, A.M., Harper, C.M., Lennon, V.A., Myasthenia, thymoma, presynaptic antibodies, and a continuum of neuromuscular hyperexcitability, *Neurology* 1999; 53(6):1233–1239.
13. Vorgerd, M., Ricker, K., Ziemssen, F., Kress, W., Goebel, H.H., Nix, W.A., Kubisch, C., Schoser, B.G., Mortier, W., A sporadic case of rippling muscle disease caused by a *de novo* caveolin-3 mutation, *Neurology* 2001; 57(12):2273–2277.
14. Walker, G.R., Watkins, T., Ansevin, C.F., Identification of autoantibodies associated with rippling muscles and myasthenia gravis that recognize skeletal muscle proteins: possible relationship of antigens and stretch-activated ion channels, *Biochem. Biophys. Res. Commun.* 1999; 264(2):430–435.

PATIENT 61

A 75-year-old woman with difficulty holding her head up

This 75-year-old woman noted 2 years of increasing difficulty holding her head up straight, sometimes requiring her to use her arm to support it. There was no fluctuation of the weakness over the course of a day and no weakness in her limbs, swallowing, or other axial muscles. Examination showed severe weakness of neck extensors with normal neck flexion and limb strength (see figure).

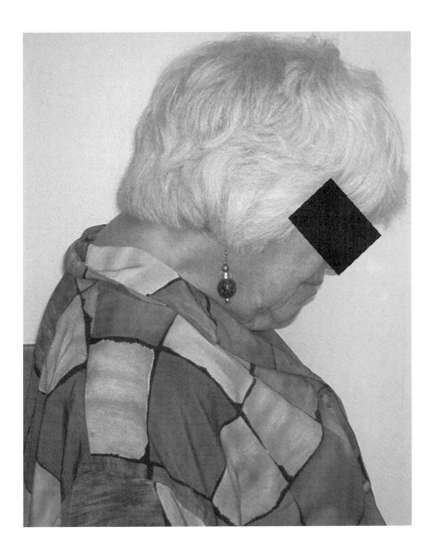

Electrodiagnostic Study:

Sensory NCS

Nerve	Sites	Recording Site	Onset (ms)	Peak (ms)	BP Amplitude (μV)	Distance (cm)	Velocity (m/s)
L. median–dig II	1. Wrist	Dig II	3.45	4.35	12.8	13	37.7
L. ulnar–dig V	1. Wrist	Dig V	2.50	3.55	17.0	11	44.0
L. radial–sn box	1. Forearm	Sn box	1.85	2.50	21.8	10	54.1
L. median–ulnar	1. Median-palm	Wrist	2.20	2.80	20.3	8	36.4
(palmar)	2. Ulnar-palm	Wrist	1.60	2.20	13.9	8	50.0

Motor NCS

Nerve	Sites	Recording Site	Latency (ms)	Amplitude (mV)	Distance (cm)	Velocity (m/s)
L. median–APB	1. Wrist	APB	4.80	5.7	7	—
	2. Elbow	APB	9.35	4.9	21	46.2
L. ulnar–ADM	1. Wrist	ADM	3.00	5.4	7	—
	2. B. elbow	ADM	6.90	5.1	20	51.3
	3. A. elbow	ADM	8.85	4.1	11	56.4
L. tibial–AH	1. Ankle	AH	4.65	5.2	8	—
	2. Pop fossa	—	12.90	3.1	39	47.3

F-Wave

Nerve	F_{min} (ms)	F_{max} (ms)	Max − Min (ms)	%F
L. tibial	59.05	60.90	1.85	80
L. ulnar	31.20	32.05	0.85	80

Needle EMG Summary Table

	IA	SA Fib	SA Fasc	SA Other	Amplitude (MUs)	Duration (MUs)	PolyP (MUs)	Activation	Recruitment Pattern
L. deltoid	Nl	0	0	0	Nl	Nl	Nl	Full	Nl
L. biceps	Nl	0	0	0	Nl	Nl	Nl	Full	Nl
L. pron teres	Nl	0	0	0	Nl	Nl	Nl	Full	Nl
L. ext dig comm	Nl	0	0	0	Nl	Nl	Nl	Full	Nl
L. vast lat	Nl	0	0	0	Nl	Nl	Nl	Full	Nl
L. vast med	Nl	0	0	0	Nl	Nl	Nl	Full	Nl
L. tib ant	Nl	0	0	0	Nl	Nl	Nl	Full	Nl
L. gastroc med	Nl	0	0	0	Nl	Nl	Nl	Full	Nl
L. L5 para-spinals	Nl	0	0	0	Nl	Nl	Nl	Full	Nl
R. vast lat	Nl	0	0	0	Nl	Nl	Nl	Full	Nl
R. vast med	Nl	0	0	0	Nl	Nl	Nl	Full	Nl
R. tib ant	Nl	0	0	0	Nl	Nl	Nl	Full	Nl
R. gastroc med	Nl	0	0	0	Nl	Nl	Nl	Full	Nl

		SA			Amplitude (MUs)	Duration (MUs)	PolyP (MUs)	Activation	Recruitment Pattern
	IA	Fib	Fasc	Other					
R. L4 para-spinals	Nl	1+	0	0	Nl	Nl	Nl	Full	Nl
R. L5 para-spinals	Nl	1+	0	0	Nl	Nl	Nl	Full	Nl
R. thoracic PSP mid	Nl	0	0	0	Nl	Nl	Nl	Full	Nl
L. thoracic PSP mid	Nl	0	0	0	Nl	Nl	Nl	Full	Nl
L. C6 para-spinal	Nl	3+	0	0	Small	Brief	Nl	Full	Early
L. C7 para-spinal	Nl	3+	0	0	Small	Brief	Nl	Full	Early
L. C8 para-spinal	Nl	3+	0	0	Small	Brief	Nl	Full	Early
L. sternoclei-domast	Nl	0	0	0	Nl	Nl	Nl	Full	Nl
R. C6 Para-spinal	Nl	3+	0	0	Small	Brief	Nl	Full	Early
R. C7 Para-spinal	Nl	3+	0	0	Small	Brief	Nl	Full	Early
R. C8 Para-spinal	Nl	3+	0	0	Small	Brief	Nl	Full	Early

Question: What is your limited differential diagnosis?

Answer: Myasthenia gravis, amyotrophic lateral sclerosis, inflammatory myopathies, nemaline myopathy, and isolated cervical extensor myopathy.

Discussion: A brief differential diagnosis of neck extensor weakness should include myasthenia gravis, amyotrophic lateral sclerosis (ALS), inflammatory myopathies, nemaline myopathy, and isolated cervical extensor myopathy. An ideal electrodiagnostic study should be directed toward establishing a muscle or neurogenic basis for the weakness and determining the distribution of abnormalities. This patient had normal serum CK and negative acetylcholine receptor antibody studies, arguing against (although not excluding) inflammatory myopathies and myasthenia gravis. Ideally, repetitive stimulation of a proximal muscle should have been performed for myasthenia gravis, although the expected yield is low.

The abnormalities are that of fibrillation potentials, myopathic motor unit morphology, and early recruitment in cervical paraspinal muscles. The mild degree of fibrillation potentials in unilateral lumbosacral paraspinal muscles is of uncertain significance. Note that sternocleidomastoid, a neck flexor, was normal, and note also the lack of other abnormalities (myopathic or neurogenic) in extensive sampling of other limbs. This patient was diagnosed with an isolated cervical extensor myopathy, a condition of uncertain cause and classification. Atrophy of paraspinal muscles may be visible on CT or MRI in some patients. This myopathy may in fact be an axial muscular dystrophy and may overlap with other axial weakness of the trunk and low back, impairing standing up straight as well.

Clinical Pearl

A "dropped head" syndrome is seen in ALS, myasthenia gravis, inflammatory myopathies, nemaline myopathy, isolated cervical extensor myopathy, and an axial myopathy with a broader distribution, including a bent spine.

REFERENCES

1. Katz, J.S., Wolfe, G.I., Burns, D.K. *et al.*, Isolated neck extensor myopathy: a common cause of dropped head syndrome, *Neurology* 1996; 46:917–921.
2. Lomen-Hoerth, C., Simmons, M.L., Dearmond, S.J. *et al.*, Adult-onset nemaline myopathy: another cause of dropped head, *Muscle Nerve* 1999; 22:1146–1150.
3. Mahjneh, I., Marconi, G., Paetau, A., Saarinen, A., Salmi, T., Somer, H., Axial myopathy: an unrecognized entity, *J. Neurol.* 2002; 249:730–734.
4. Oerlemans, W.G., de Visser, M., Dropped head syndrome and bent spine syndrome: two separate clinical entities or different manifestations of axial myopathy?, *J. Neurol. Neurosurg. Psychiatry* 1998; 65:258–259.
5. Serratrice, G., Pouget, J., Pellissier, J.F., Bent spine syndrome, *J. Neurol. Neurosurg. Psychiatry* 1996; 60:51–54.
6. Suarez, G.A., Kelly, J.J., The dropped head syndrome, *Neurology* 1992; 42:1625–1627.
7. Swash, M., Dropped-head and bent-spine syndromes: axial myopathies?, *Lancet* 1998; 352:758.
8. Umapathi, T., Chaudhry, V., Cornblath, D., Drachman, D., Griffin, J., Kuncl, R., Head drop and camptocormia, *J. Neurol. Neurosurg. Psychiatry* 2002; 73:1–7.

SECTION VI.   EMG-GUIDED BOTULINUM TOXIN THERAPY OF FOCAL DYSTONIAS

The availability of botulinum toxin therapy (BTX) since the early 1990s has changed the treatment of many patients with focal dystonias. The efficacy of BTX has been established through controlled trials in patients with blepharospasm and cervical dystonia.[2] It was approved by the Food and Drug Administration (FDA) for use in blepharospasm in 1989 and for cervical dystonia in 2000. It appears to be effective for limb dystonias, although no clinical trial has established this. Its mechanism of action for neuromuscular junction blockade is via uptake into the presynaptic nerve terminal and cleavage by the toxin of one of three SNARE proteins required for vesicle docking, fusion, and exocytosis of acetylcholine. Botulinum toxin A (BoTox) cleaves the synaptosomal-associated protein SNAP-25, while botulinum toxin B (Myobloc) cleaves the protein synaptobrevin. The mechanism of relief of dystonia is less clear and presumably relates to changes in basal ganglia and cortical motor and sensory integration resulting from the induced weakness.

Electromyography (EMG) has two potential roles as an adjunct for botulinum toxin therapy: to *identify* which muscles should be injected by detection of abnormally firing motor units and to *find* muscles already targeted for injection. At least one study has suggested that for cervical dystonia, EMG studies were superior to clinical prediction alone for identifying which muscles should be targeted.[13] In limb dystonias, it has been shown that needle localization is more accurate in finding the targeted muscle than placement without EMG guidance (Table 1).[8] At least to date, this has not been shown to translate into a better result for the patient; as the toxin may diffuse to neighboring muscles after injection, it certainly is possible that EMG guidance does not add benefit. In general, though, the value of needle EMG for correct localization remains uncertain, and one view, dependent on the location and type of dystonia, is shown in Table 2.

Table 1.   Accuracy of Needle Placement into Intended Muscles

Intended Muscle Placement	Site of Actual Needle Placement (No. of Patients)
FCR (n = 3)	FCR (2), FDS II (1)
FCU (n = 4)	FCU (2), FDP II (1), not in muscle (1)
FPB (n = 1)	APB (1)
FPL (n = 3)	FDS II (2), not in muscle (1)
PT (n = 3)	PT (1), FDS III (1), FCR (1)
FDS II (n = 5)	FDS (1), FCR (3), not in muscle (1)
FDS IV (n = 1)	FPL (1)
FDP II (n = 4)	FDP II (2), FDP III (1), FCR (1)
FDP III (n = 3)	FDP III (2), Not in muscle (1)
FDP IV (n = 2)	FDP IV (1), FCU (1)
EIP (n = 5)	EIP (2), EDC II (2), not in muscle (1)
EDC II (n = 3)	EDC II (1), ECR (2)
ECU (n = 1)	EDC II (1)

Source: Molloy, F.M. *et al.*, *Neurology*, 58, 805–807, 2002.

Table 2.   Need for EMG Guidance in the Treatment of Various Dystonias

Focal dystonia	Usually	Sometimes	Not Usually
Facial dystonias			
Blepharospasm			X
Oromandibular	X		
Complex		X	
Cervical dystonia		X	
Limb dystonias			
Arm	X		
Leg		X	
Segmental myoclonus	X		

The approach is straightforward. Muscles that appear to be contracting inappropriately and producing the abnormal posture are targeted for injection with BTX. These muscles are usually determined by clinical inspection, and then needle EMG is used to localize the muscle, either by the presence of abundant involuntary motor unit action potentials or more commonly by asking the patient to selectively contract the muscle. Weakness and apparent clinical benefit generally are observed within days to a week and last from 2 to 6 months (typically 3 months). Injections may be repeated as long as benefit is apparent, which may be indefinite. Often, fibrillation potentials are seen with subsequent EMG-guided injections, and atrophy of the muscle becomes clinically apparent.

REFERENCES

1. Byrnes, M.L., Thickbroom, G.W., Wilson, S.A., Sacco, P., Shipman, J.M., Stell, R., Mastaglia, F.L., The corticomotor representation of upper limb muscles in writer's cramp and changes following botulinum toxin injection, *Brain* 1998; 121:977–988.
2. Ceballos-Baumann, A.O., Evidence-based medicine in botulinum toxin therapy for cervical dystonia, *J. Neurol.* 2001; 248(suppl. 1):14–20.
3. Ceballos-Baumann, A.O., Sheean, G., Passingham, R.E., Marsden, C.D., Brooks, D.J., Botulinum toxin does not reverse the cortical dysfunction associated with writer's cramp: a PET study, *Brain* 1997; 120:571–582.
4. Cole, R., Hallett, M., Cohen, L.G., Double-blind trial of botulinum toxin for treatment of focal hand dystonia, *Mov. Disord.* 1995; 10:466–471.
5. Comella, C., Buchman, A.S., Tanner, C.M., Brown-Toms, N.C., Goetz, C.G., Botulinum toxin injection for spasmodic torticollis: increased magnitude of benefit with electromyographic assistance, *Neurology* 1992; 42:878–882.
6. Farmer, S.F., Sheean, G.L., Mayston, M.J., Rothwell, J.C., Marsden, C.D., Conway, B.A., Halliday, D.M., Rosenberg, J.R., Stephens, J.A., Abnormal motor unit synchronization of antagonist muscles underlies pathological co-contraction in upper limb dystonia, *Brain* 1998; 121:801–814.
7. Guyer, B.M., Some unresolved issues with botulinum toxin, *J. Neurol.* 2001; 248(suppl. 1): I/11–I/13.
8. Molloy, F.M., Shill, H.A., Kaelin-Lang, A., Karp, B.I., Accuracy of muscle localization without EMG: implications for treatment of limb dystonia, *Neurology* 2002; 58:805–807.
9. Murase, N., Kaji, R., Shimazu, H., Katayama-Hirota, M., Ikeda, A., Kohara, N., Kimura, J., Shibasaki, H., Rothwell, J.C., Abnormal premovement gating of somatosensory input in writer's cramp, *Brain* 2000; 123:1813–1829.
10. Oga, T., Honda, M., Toma, K., Murase, N., Okada, T., Hanakawa, T., Sawamoto, N., Nagamine, T., Konishi, J., Fukuyama, H., Kaji, R., Shibasaki, H., Abnormal cortical mechanisms of voluntary muscle relaxation in patients with writer's cramp: an fMRI study, *Brain* 2002; 125:895–903.
11. Ross, M., Charness, M.E., Sudarsky, L., Logigian, E.L., Treatment of occupational cramp with botulinum toxin: diffusion of toxin to adjacent noninjected muscles, *Muscle Nerve* 1997; 20: 593–598.
12. Speelman, J.D., Brans, J.W.M., Cervical dystonia and botulinum treatment: is electromyographic guidance necessary?, *Mov. Disord.* 1995; 10:802.
13. Van Gerpen, J.A., Matsumoto, J.Y., Ahlskog, J.E., Maraganore, D.M., McManis, P.G., Utility of an EMG mapping study in treating cervical dystonia, *Muscle Nerve* 2000; 23:1752–1756.
14. Yoshimura, D.M., Aminoff, M.J., Olney, R.K., Botulinum toxin therapy for limb dystonias, *Neurology* 1992; 42:627–630.

PATIENT 62

**A 39-year-old woman with 3 to 4 years of progressive difficulty
using her right hand**

The patient has had progressive difficulty using her right hand for writing, but she has no difficulty using it for buttoning, typing, or using utensils.

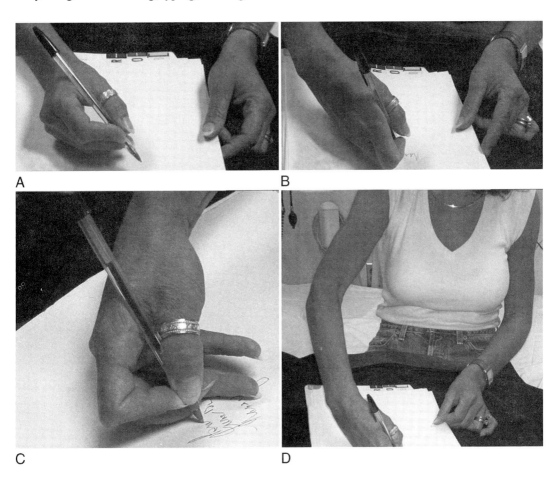

A   B

C   D

Question: Some patients with writer's cramp learn to write with the other hand. Do you think this strategy would work well for this woman over the long-term?

Answer: No. Left hand dystonia is visible in figure D.

Discussion: Note the normal posture of the hand holding the pen before writing (A) and the rapid development of dystonia when starting to write. Images (B) and (C) suggest hyperextension at the second metacarpophalangeal (MCP) joint and excessive flexion at the second proximal interphalangeal (PIP) joint. There is probably excessive flexion at the third PIP joint, as is evident in (C), in comparison to the posture of the third digit in (A). The tip of the thumb also slips off the pen in figure (B). Excessive flexion of the wrist is present in (B) and (D), and abduction of the arm at the shoulder is excessive in (D).

The predominant aspects of this dystonia are the flexion at the wrist and fingers as noted above. The hyperextension of the second MCP joint is likely compensation for the excessive flexion at the PIP joint forcing the finger to hyperextend in order to hold onto the pen. The patient reported subjectively that this seemed to be the case. The muscles and doses targeted for her treatment were as follows:

- Flexor carpi ulnaris (FCU)–30 U
- Flexor digitorum superficialis (FDS) digit 2–20 U
- Flexor digitorum superficialis (FDS) digit 3–20 U

Treatment repeated 5 times over a 1-year period seemed to be producing significant weakness but no benefit in her dystonia. Changes in her regimen including injections of FDP fourth and fifth digits and FCR also produced significant weakness but no benefit in her dystonia, so botulinum toxin treatment was abandoned. Note the dystonia present in her *left* hand that is evident in (B) and (D), where she has difficulty holding onto the paper properly. Accordingly, she would seem to be at high risk of developing writer's cramp in her left hand should she learn to write with it.

Clinical Pearls

1. Botulinum toxin is not always effective in the treatment of focal dystonias.
2. Look for subtle signs of dystonia in the other hand when observing patients with writer's cramp.

REFERENCES
1. Sheehy, M.P., Marsden, C.D., Writer's cramp: a focal dystonia, *Brain* 1982; 105:461–480.
   (Also see reference list for the introduction to this section.)

PATIENT 63

A 47-year-old man with progressive difficulty in writing for 5 years

The patient reported that he had difficulty keeping his second and third digits against the pen because of involuntary extension, and he attempted to compensate by tightening his grip with his thumb (see figure).

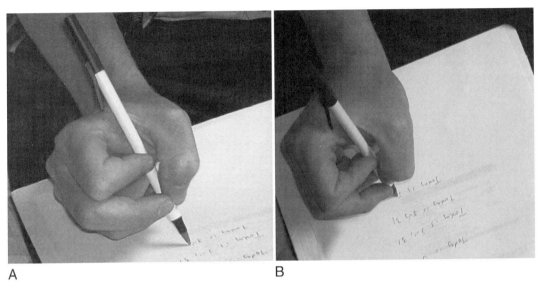

A   B

Question: What muscles and dosage would you use based on the views shown in the figure?

Answer: Extensor indicis proprius, 2.5 U; extensor digitorum communis, 5 U; flexor carpi radialis, 15 U

Discussion: This patient responded well to dosing as follows:
- Extensor indicis proprius (EIP)–2.5 U
- Extensor digitorum communis (EDC)–5 U
- Flexor carpi radialis (FCR)–15 U

The radial deviation of the wrist is difficult to appreciate in this picture. The EIP and EDC are responsible for extension principally at the MCP joints; an additional muscle that might be of value in this case is the second lumbrical (to third digit), which acts to extend the third finger at the PIP joint. This is probably the most evident aspect of his dystonia, and future injections will target this muscle as well. This patient had a good response lasting 3 months to subsequent injections.

Clinical Pearl

A wide range of individual dose responsiveness occurs with botulinum toxin treatment; some patients respond to very small doses, and others require larger doses.

REFERENCES

1. Byrnes, M.L., Thickbroom, G.W., Wilson, S.A., Sacco, P., Shipman, J.M., Stell, R., Mastaglia, F.L., The corticomotor representation of upper limb muscles in writer's cramp and changes following botulinum toxin injection, *Brain* 1998; 121:977–988.
2. Ceballos-Baumann, A.O., Evidence-based medicine in botulinum toxin therapy for cervical dystonia, *J. Neurol.* 2001; 248(suppl. 1):14–20.
3. Ceballos-Baumann, A.O., Sheean, G., Passingham, R.E., Marsden, C.D., Brooks, D.J., Botulinum toxin does not reverse the cortical dysfunction associated with writer's cramp: a PET study, *Brain* 1997; 120:571–582.
4. Cole, R., Hallett, M., Cohen, L.G., Double-blind trial of botulinum toxin for treatment of focal hand dystonia, *Mov. Disord.* 1995; 10:466–471.
5. Comella, C., Buchman, A.S., Tanner, C.M., Brown-Toms, N.C., Goetz, C.G., Botulinum toxin injection for spasmodic torticollis: increased magnitude of benefit with electromyographic assistance, *Neurology* 1992; 42:878–882.
6. Farmer, S.F., Sheean, G.L., Mayston, M.J., Rothwell, J.C., Marsden, C.D., Conway, B.A., Halliday, D.M., Rosenberg, J.R., Stephens, J.A., Abnormal motor unit synchronization of antagonist muscles underlies pathological co-contraction in upper limb dystonia, *Brain* 1998; 121:801–814.
7. Guyer, B.M., Some unresolved issues with botulinum toxin, *J. Neurol.* 2001; 248(suppl. 1): I/11–I/13.
8. Molloy, F.M., Shill, H.A., Kaelin-Lang, A., Karp, B.I., Accuracy of muscle localization without EMG: implications for treatment of limb dystonia, *Neurology* 2002; 58:805–807.
9. Murase, N., Kaji, R., Shimazu, H., Katayama-Hirota, M., Ikeda, A., Kohara, N., Kimura, J., Shibasaki, H., Rothwell, J.C., Abnormal premovement gating of somatosensory input in writer's cramp, *Brain* 2000; 123:1813–1829.
10. Oga, T., Honda, M., Toma, K., Murase, N., Okada, T., Hanakawa, T., Sawamoto, N., Nagamine, T., Konishi, J., Fukuyama, H., Kaji, R., Shibasaki, H., Abnormal cortical mechanisms of voluntary muscle relaxation in patients with writer's cramp: an fMRI study, *Brain* 2002; 125:895–903.
11. Ross, M., Charness, M.E., Sudarsky, L., Logigian, E.L., Treatment of occupational cramp with botulinum toxin: diffusion of toxin to adjacent noninjected muscles, *Muscle Nerve* 1997; 20: 593–598.
12. Speelman, J.D., Brans, J.W.M., Cervical dystonia and botulinum treatment: is electromyographic guidance necessary?, *Mov. Disord.* 1995; 10:802.
13. Van Gerpen, J.A., Matsumoto, J.Y., Ahlskog, J.E., Maraganore, D.M., McManis, P.G., Utility of an EMG mapping study in treating cervical dystonia, *Muscle Nerve* 2000; 23:1752–1756.
14. Yoshimura, D.M., Aminoff, M.J., Olney, R.K., Botulinum toxin therapy for limb dystonias, *Neurology* 1992; 42:627–630.

PATIENT 64

A 45-year-old woman with several years of difficulty with her right hand limited to writing

This patient initially held the pen normally (figure 1A), but then rapidly developed the dystonia evident in the subsequent figures.

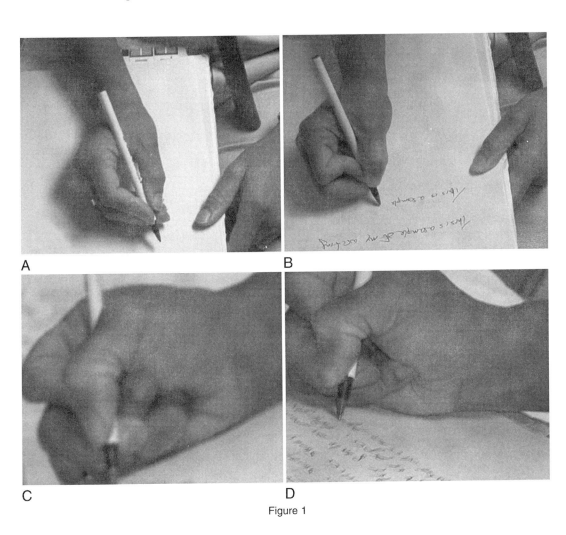

A

B

C

D

Figure 1

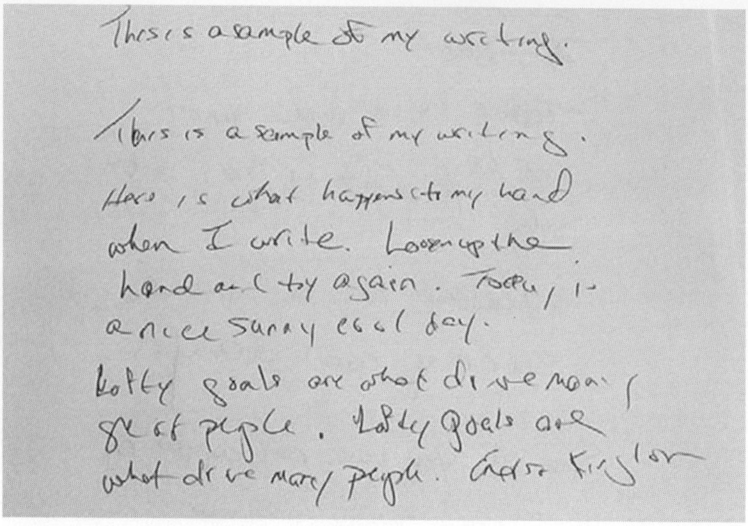

Figure 2

Question: What muscles and what doses would you use for treatment?

Answer: Supinator 20 U; Flexor digitorum superficialis, second digit 10 U; Flexor digitorum superficialis, third digit 10 U; Flexor digitorum superficialis, fourth digit 15 U; Flexor digitorum superficialis, fifth digit 5 U

Discussion: This case shares some similarities to case 62. The patient's hand appears normal while holding the pen prior to writing (see part (A) in figure). In (B) there is excessive flexion at the second PIP joint (FDS digit 2) and the thumb interphalangeal joint (flexor pollicis longus, FPL). In (C) and (D), note the excessive flexion of the other digits as well; digit 5 is digging into the palm of her hand in (C). It is difficult to appreciate from the picture, but there is also abnormal supination of the forearm and extension of the wrist (the latter best seen in (B)). Her treatment regimen was as follows and produced satisfactory results with a frequency of every 6 months:

- Supinator–20 U
- Flexor digitorum superficialis, second digit–10 U
- Flexor digitorum superficialis, third digit–10 U
- Flexor digitorum superficialis, fourth digit–15 U
- Flexor digitorum superficialis, fifth digit–5 U

Alterations to this regimen that might be considered in the future would include injection of FPL and larger doses to the FDS second digit (say, 15 to 20 U) than to the fourth digit (say, a decrease to 10 U). As apparent, treatment regimen selection is often empirically derived from trial and error after initial estimates based on the pattern of dystonia.

Clinical Pearl

Treatment regimens with botulinum toxin are empirically derived after initial estimates and trial.

REFERENCES

See reference list for the introduction to this section.

PATIENT 65

A 40-year-old physician with progressive difficulty writing for 3 years

The patient has had no difficulty with typing or writing on a blackboard.

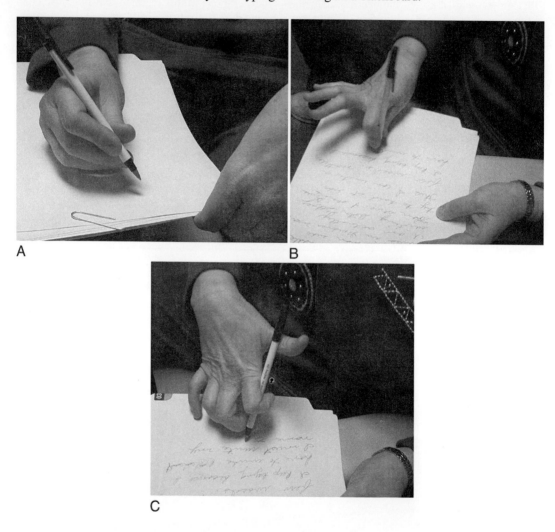

A

B

C

Question: What muscles would you target for treatment?

Answer: Finger extensors

Discussion: The figure demonstrates the normal posture of the hand holding the pen before writing (A). Within 10 seconds of writing, the patient develops involuntary extension of the third to fifth digits and can barely hold the pen (B). Soon thereafter, the second digit extends as well, and the pen drops out of the hand. To compensate, the patient typically holds the pen as shown in (C), maintaining a modest ability to write. Injection as follows resulted in moderate benefit to the patient:

- Extensor digitorum communis (EDC)—30 U
- Extensor digitorum, fourth finger—20 U
- Extensor digitorum, fifth finger—10 U

Clinical Pearl

The focal dystonia can be very dramatic, as in this case. It is worthwhile to follow such patients using photographs to assess response.

REFERENCES

1. Byrnes, M.L., Thickbroom, G.W., Wilson, S.A., Sacco, P., Shipman, J.M., Stell, R., Mastaglia, F.L., The corticomotor representation of upper limb muscles in writer's cramp and changes following botulinum toxin injection, *Brain* 1998; 121:977–988.
2. Ceballos-Baumann, A.O., Evidence-based medicine in botulinum toxin therapy for cervical dystonia, *J. Neurol.* 2001; 248(suppl. 1):14–20.
3. Ceballos-Baumann, A.O., Sheean, G., Passingham, R.E., Marsden, C.D., Brooks, D.J., Botulinum toxin does not reverse the cortical dysfunction associated with writer's cramp: a PET study, *Brain* 1997; 120:571–582.
4. Cole, R., Hallett, M., Cohen, L.G., Double-blind trial of botulinum toxin for treatment of focal hand dystonia, *Mov. Disord.* 1995; 10:466–471.
5. Comella, C., Buchman, A.S., Tanner, C.M., Brown-Toms, N.C., Goetz, C.G., Botulinum toxin injection for spasmodic torticollis: increased magnitude of benefit with electromyographic assistance, *Neurology* 1992; 42:878–882.
6. Farmer, S.F., Sheean, G.L., Mayston, M.J., Rothwell, J.C., Marsden, C.D., Conway, B.A., Halliday, D.M., Rosenberg, J.R., Stephens, J.A., Abnormal motor unit synchronization of antagonist muscles underlies pathological co-contraction in upper limb dystonia, *Brain* 1998; 121:801–814.
7. Guyer, B.M., Some unresolved issues with botulinum toxin, *J. Neurol.* 2001; 248(suppl. 1): I/11–I/13.
8. Molloy, F.M., Shill, H.A., Kaelin-Lang, A., Karp, B.I., Accuracy of muscle localization without EMG: implications for treatment of limb dystonia, *Neurology* 2002; 58:805–807.
9. Murase, N., Kaji, R., Shimazu, H., Katayama-Hirota, M., Ikeda, A., Kohara, N., Kimura, J., Shibasaki, H., Rothwell, J.C., Abnormal premovement gating of somatosensory input in writer's cramp, *Brain* 2000; 123:1813–1829.
10. Oga, T., Honda, M., Toma, K., Murase, N., Okada, T., Hanakawa, T., Sawamoto, N., Nagamine, T., Konishi, J., Fukuyama, H., Kaji, R., Shibasaki, H., Abnormal cortical mechanisms of voluntary muscle relaxation in patients with writer's cramp: an fMRI study, *Brain* 2002; 125:895–903.
11. Ross, M., Charness, M.E., Sudarsky, L., Logigian, E.L., Treatment of occupational cramp with botulinum toxin: diffusion of toxin to adjacent noninjected muscles, *Muscle Nerve* 1997; 20: 593–598.
12. Speelman, J.D., Brans, J.W.M., Cervical dystonia and botulinum treatment: is electromyographic guidance necessary?, *Mov. Disord.* 1995; 10:802.
13. Van Gerpen, J.A., Matsumoto, J.Y., Ahlskog, J.E., Maraganore, D.M., McManis, P.G., Utility of an EMG mapping study in treating cervical dystonia, *Muscle Nerve* 2000; 23:1752–1756.
14. Yoshimura, D.M., Aminoff, M.J., Olney, R.K., Botulinum toxin therapy for limb dystonias, *Neurology* 1992; 42:627–630.

INDEX

Q

Quadriceps, 72

R

Radial nerve, 208
Radial neuropathy
  proximal, 34–37
  wrist drop caused by, 36
Radiation-induced focal neuropathy, 82
Radiculoneuritis, 125
Radiculopathy
  cervical, 70
  L5, 74
  L2–L3, 86
  needle electromyography screening of, 66
Repetitive nerve stimulation
  history of, 175
  myasthenia gravis evaluations, 175, 181
Right arm weakness, 51–54
Right hand
  numbness, 144–147
  weakness of, 15–18
Right leg
  numbness of, 84–86, 91–93
  pain of, 87–90
  weakness of, 84–86, 91–93
Rippling muscle disease, 242–244
Root avulsion
  C6 nerve, 58
  case study of, 51–54

S

Saphenous nerve, 71
Sarcoid neuropathy, 114
Sarcoidosis, 114
Scapular winging, 37–40, 41–45
Sciatic nerve, 78
Sciatic neuropathy
  case study of, 78
  with myokymic potentials, 82
Sensory nerve action potentials
  abnormal median normal sural, 133–136,
    137–139
  carpal tunnel syndrome effects on, 1
  in cervical radiculopathy, 70
  dorsal ulnar cutaneous, 70
  focal neuropathy diagnosis by, 1
  generalized neuropathies evaluated using, 95
  root avulsion findings, 51–54
  saphenous, 71
  in spinal muscular atrophy, 198
  superficial peroneal, 1, 74
  sural, 130
Sensory neuronopathies, 172–174
Serratus anterior, 3t
Serum protein electrophoresis, 99
Single fiber electromyography
  neuromuscular junction disease evaluated using,
    175–176
  technical elements of, 176
Sjögren's syndrome, 174
Slow channel syndromes, 191
SMA. *See* Spinal muscular atrophy
SNAPs. *See* Sensory nerve action potentials

Spinal accessory nerve
  location of, 39
  trapezius weakness caused by lesions of, 39, 45
Spinal motor neuron gene, 198
Spinal muscular atrophy, 198
Sulfatide antibody-mediated neuropathy, 166
Superficial peroneal nerve, 71
Supinator
  anatomy of, 3t
  botulinum toxin therapy of, 257
Supraspinatus, 3t
Sural nerve, 71, 78
Sural sensory nerve action potentials, 130
Synaptic vesicles, 190
Syringomyelia, 46

T

Tensor fascia lata, 72
Teres minor, 3t
Thoracic outlet syndrome, neurologic, 46–50
Thoracoabdominal neuropathy, 103
Thymoma, 244
Tibial F-waves, 81
Tibial H-reflex, 90
Tibial nerve, 71
Tibialis anterior
  characteristics of, 72
  in foot drop, 75
Tibialis posterior, 72
Tingling in hands, 5–7, 8–11
Trapezius
  illustration of, 42, 45
  weakness of, 39, 45
Triceps, 3t
Tuberculoid leprosy, 118

U

Ulnar neuropathy
  description of, 1
  distal, 29
  at or near the elbow, 19–22, 23–26
  at wrist, 27–30
Ulnar–abductor digiti minimi studies
  generalized neuropathies evaluated using, 95
  neuromuscular junction disease evaluated using,
    175
  ulnar neuropathy at elbow evaluated using, 21,
    23–25
Ulnar–second lumbrical interosseous test, 14
Upper limb nerve innervation, 3t

V

Voltage-gated calcium channels, 186

W

Waldenstrom's macroglobulinemia, 100, 101t
Wallerian degeneration, 66
Weakness
  case studies of, 46–49, 68–70, 97–102, 153–155,
    156–157, 160–163, 199–205, 212–214,
    221–224, 225–228, 229–231, 239–241
  focal demyelination of motor axons as cause of, 83
  generalized, 126–130, 137–139, 168–171, 187–191,
    215–217

Other Titles in the Pearls Series®

Duke	**Anesthesia Pearls**	1-56053-495-8
Carabello & Gazes	**Cardiology Pearls, 2nd Edition**	1-56053-403-6
Sahn & Heffner	**Critical Care Pearls, 2nd Edition**	1-56053-224-6
Sahn	**Dermatology Pearls**	1-56053-315-3
Baren & Alpern	**Emergency Medicine Pearls**	1-56053-575-X
Jay	**Foot and Ankle Pearls**	1-56053-445-1
Concannon & Hurov	**Hand Pearls**	1-56053-463-X
Danso	**Hematology and Oncology Pearls**	1-56053-577-6
Jones, King & Wofford	**Hypertension Pearls**	1-56053-583-0
Cunha	**Infectious Disease Pearls**	1-56053-203-3
Heffner & Sahn	**Internal Medicine Pearls, 2nd Edition**	1-56053-404-4
Mercado & Smetana	**Medical Consultation Pearls**	1-56053-504-0
Waclawik & Sutula	**Neurology Pearls**	1-56053-261-0
Gault	**Ophthalmology Pearls**	1-56053-498-2
Heffner & Byock	**Palliative and End-of-Life Pearls**	1-56053-500-8
Inselman	**Pediatric Pulmonary Pearls**	1-56053-350-1
Lennard	**Physical Medicine & Rehabilitation Pearls**	1-56053-455-9
Kolevzon & Stewart	**Psychiatry Pearls**	1-56053-590-3
Silver & Smith	**Rheumatology Pearls**	1-56053-201-7
Berry	**Sleep Medicine Pearls, 2nd Edition**	1-56053-490-7
Eck *et al.*	**Spine Pearls**	1-56053-571-7
Osterhoudt *et al.*	**Toxicology Pearls**	1-56053-614-4
Schluger & Harkin	**Tuberculosis Pearls**	1-56053-156-8
Resnick & Schaeffer	**Urology Pearls**	1-56053-351-X